Psychiatry Pearls

Psychiatry Pearls

Alex Kolevzon, MD
Department of Psychiatry
Division of Child and Adolescent Psychiatry
Mount Sinai School of Medicine
New York, New York

Daniel G. Stewart, MD
Assistant Professor
Associate Director of Residency Training
Department of Psychiatry
Mount Sinai School of Medicine
New York, New York

HANLEY & BELFUS
An Affiliate of Elsevier

BS

HANLEY & BELFUS, INC.
An Affiliate of Elsevier

The Curtis Center
Independence Square West
Philadelphia, Pennsylvania 19106

Library of Congress Control Number: 2003116475

PSYCHIATRY PEARLS ISBN 1-56053-590-3

Printed in the United States

Last digit is the print number: 9 8 7 6 5 4 3 2 1

CONTENTS

CONTRIBUTORS

Malaika E. Berkeley, MD
Department of Psychiatry, Mount Sinai School of Medicine, New York, New York

Matthew Biel, MD
Department of Psychiatry, New York University School of Medicine, New York, New York

Tara Lynn Brass, MD
Department of Psychiatry, Mount Sinai School of Medicine, New York, New York

F. Tuna Burgut, MD
Assistant Professor of Clinical Neurology, Cornell Memory Disorders Program; New York Presbyterian Hospital of Cornell University, New York, New York

Anthony J. Carino
Lincolnshire, Illinois

Eran Chemerinski, MD
Department of Psychiatry, Mount Sinai School of Medicine, New York, New York

Rajendra J. Daniel, MD
Department of Psychiatry, Jamaica Hospital Medical Center, Jamaica, New York

Arthur Fox, PhD
Private Practice, New York, New York

Rivka Galchen, MD
New York, New York

Amir Garakani, MD
Department of Psychiatry, Mount Sinai School of Medicine, New York, New York

Harold W. Goforth, MD
Department of Psychiatry, Division of Geriatric Psychiatry, Duke University Medical Center, Durham, North Carolina

Tamar Hanfling, MD
Department of Psychiatry, Mount Sinai School of Medicine, New York New York

Ellen J. Hoffman, MD
Department of Psychiatry, Mount Sinai School of Medicine, New York, New York

Afia A. Hussain, MD
Department of Psychiatry, Jamaica Hospital Medical Center, Jamaica, New York

Amanda Itzkoff, MD
Department of Psychiatry, Mount Sinai School of Medicine, New York, New York

Iliyan Ivanov, MD
Clinical Instructor, Division of Child and Adolescent Psychiatry, Mount Sinai School of Medicine, New York, New York

Jacques Jospitre, Jr., MD
Department of Psychiatry, Mount Sinai School of Medicine, New York, New York

Gary P. Katzman, MD
Department of Psychiatry, Mount Sinai School of Medicine, New York, New York

Jean Kim, MD
Department of Psychiatry, Mount Sinai School of Medicine, New York, New York

Alex Kolevzon, MD
Department of Psychiatry, Division of Child and Adolescent Psychiatry, Mount Sinai School of Medicine, New York, New York

Sander Markx
Amsterdam, The Netherlands

Maureen D. Martino, MD
Instructor, Psychiatric Emergency Services, Mount Sinai School of Medicine, New York, New York

Karin Miller, MD
Department of Psychiatry, Mood and Personality Disorders, Mount Sinai School of Medicine, New York, New York

Marina Moshkovich, MD
Department of Psychiatry, Mount Sinai School of Medicine, New York, New York

Javier A. Muniz, MD
Department of Psychiatry, Mount Sinai School of Medicine, New York, New York

Lorenzo Norris, MD
Department of Psychiatry, Mount Sinai School of Medicine, New York, New York

Sarah E. O'Neil, MD
Department of Psychiatry, Massachusetts General Hospital, Boston, Massachusetts; McLean Hospital, Belmont, Massachusetts

Lori Pellegrino, MD
Department of Psychiatry, Mount Sinai School of Medicine, New York, New York

Jennifer Petras, MD
Departments of Pediatrics, Psychiatry, and Child Psychiatry, Mount Sinai School of Medicine, New York, New York

Dennis M. Popeo, MD
Department of Psychiatry, Mount Sinai School of Medicine, New York, New York

Shakil Shafqatur Rahman, MD
Departments of Pediatrics, Psychiatry, and Child Psychiatry, Mount Sinai School of Medicine, New York, New York

Michael A. Rapp, MD, PhD
Department of Psychiatry, Mount Sinai School of Medicine, New York, New York

Matthew Rottnek, MFA
Mount Sinai School of Medicine, New York, New York

Patrick Runnels, MD
Department of Psychiatry, Mount Sinai School of Medicine, New York, New York

Diane J. Sacks, MD
Director, Residency Training, Department of Psychiatry, Jamaica Hospital Medical Center, Jamaica, New York

Corbett Schimming, MD
Department of Psychiatry, Mount Sinai School of Medicine, New York, New York

Alan Schlechter, BA
Mount Sinai School of Medicine, New York, New York

Nadine Schwartz, MD
Private Practice, Philadelphia, Pennsylvania

Asher B. Simon, MD
Department of Psychiatry, Mount Sinai School of Medicine, New York, New York

Laurence J. Sprung, MD
Department of Psychiatry, Mount Sinai School of Medicine, New York, New York

Daniel G. Stewart, MD
Assistant Professor, Associate Director of Residency Training, Department of Psychiatry, Mount Sinai School of Medicine, New York, New York

Julie Stewart, PsyD
New York, New York

Thomas Stewart, BA
New York, New York

Zvi S. Weisstuch, MD
Clinical Instructor of Psychiatry and Pediatrics, Mount Sinai School of Medicine; Attending Psychiatrist, Inpatient Child and Adolescent Unit, Mount Sinai Medical Center, New York, New York

Rebecca L. West
Upstate Medical University, Syracuse, New York

Michelle Widlitz, MD
Attending Psychiatrist/Addiction Fellow, Bellevue Hospital, New York, New York

PREFACE

Psychiatry Pearls is a collection of cases designed to educate medical students, residents, and other trainees in the diagnosis and treatment of psychiatric disorders. Like other entries in the Pearl Series®, it can also help experienced practitioners hone their clinical skills and develop a deeper understanding of these illnesses. Each case begins with a brief description of relevant details from the history of present illness that vividly illustrate the patient's presentation. Past psychiatric and medical histories as well as pertinent findings from other laboratory or diagnostic examinations are also included to create a comprehensive depiction of the patient. Cases are designed to be challenging for the reader and to require the consideration of mulitple differential diagnoses, which always include underlying medical conditions that present with psychiatric symptoms.

Following the case presentation, the reader is asked to offer a diagnosis, and a detailed discussion reviews the crucial aspects of the given disorder, including options for treatment. In addition, the discussion also incorporates more current information gathered from a thorough literature review. The final part of each case is a "Pearls" section that makes 3–4 cutting edge points about important clinical considerations or comments about new directions of research, such as genetics, neuroimaging, or clinicial trials. Each case is also accompanied by a reference section designed for the reader interested in pursuing the topic further.

We extend our sincere appreciation to all of our contributors and hope that our readers will profit from all their hard work and experience.

Alex Kolevzon, MD
Daniel G. Stewart, MD

Eran Chemerinski, MD

PATIENT 1

A 38-year-old woman with fear of contamination

History of Present Illness: A 38-year old woman is referred to the psychiatric clinic by her dermatologist, who is currently treating her for an irritant contact dermatitis of both hands that resulted from repeated use of an alkaline soap. The patient has been using this soap for the past 2 weeks, thinking that its "stronger" formula would help decrease the number of times needed to wash her hands (currently about 25 times daily). She describes a recent worsening fear of germs that prevents her from leaving the house because she is afraid of touching objects outside her home. She complains of not being able to socialize with friends in public places or travel on public transportation. The patient is unable to suppress this fear, but her related anxiety is relieved at home because she is constantly cleaning the house. She was recently also forced to quit her job because of difficulty concentrating on tasks while at work, and persistent lateness. The patient endorses symptoms of depressed mood and feelings of guilt related to her inability to control the fears of contamination despite recognizing them as unreasonable.

Psychiatric History: All developmental stages were reached without difficulty. She recalls being anxious as early as childhood. During adolescence she spent long hours in her room arranging objects that she had collected from the street in an intricate fashion. She remembers that her father was also an avid collector. He had a large collection of books and would become extremely angry when people disrupted his method of organizing them. She also recalls that, despite a religious upbringing, she was always fearful of inadvertently cursing at family members. Grooming rituals such as hand washing and brushing her teeth were first experienced in college. These rituals were so time-consuming that her roommates asked her to move out because of her excessive bathroom use. She states that her mood has been "sad" most of her life and her social life very limited. She also describes episodes of alcohol abuse related to efforts to decrease the feelings of anxiety that accompany her symptoms.

Mental Status Examination: The patient is a thin woman who looks her stated age. She is neatly dressed and carries an oversized handbag that, when opened, reveals numerous packs of paper tissue that are used at all times during the interview to avoid touching objects with her bare hands. She is pleasant and has a cooperative attitude. Her eye contact is intermittent; she lowers her gaze with shame when describing some of her symptoms. Her behavior is mildly restless with constant wringing of her hands. Her voice is soft, but her speech has normal rate, spontaneity, and prosody. Her dysphoric affect appropriately reflects her mood, described as "extremely depressed and anxious." She becomes tearful when stating that her "strange" behavior has socially ostracized her. Her thought process is mostly linear, cohesive, and goal-oriented but at times appears circumstantial due to over-inclusiveness of minor details. Her thought content is plagued with multiple concerns, the most prominent of which is dying from an infectious disease due to microorganisms on objects previously touched by strangers. This concern does not reach delusional proportions because the patient is able to recognize its implausibility. She also reports being distressed by an urge to insult people whom she loves. She expresses feelings of guilt because she is "unable to control my own mind and suppress this ridiculous urge". She denies any suicidal or homicidal ideation as well as perceptual disorders such as hallucinations or illusions. She is alert and globally oriented and has intact cognitive abilities despite complaints of short-term memory deficit. Her insight and judgment are intact because she is able to assess realistically the nature of her disorder and need for treatment.

Diagnostic Testing: Complete blood count, chemistry, liver and thyroid function tests: all within normal ranges. Urine toxicology test: negative.

Questions: What are the possible diagnoses? How might this patient be treated?

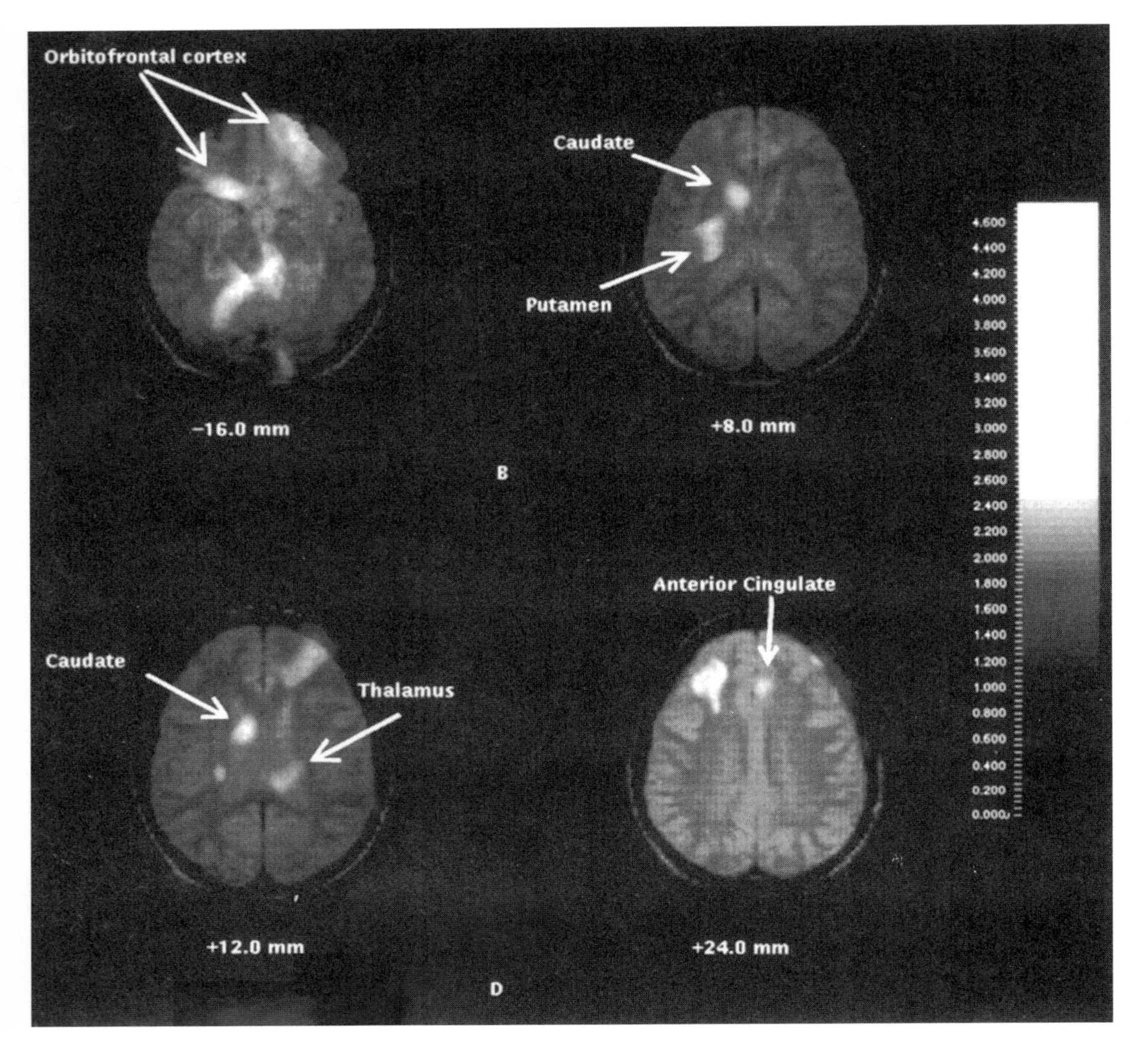

Positron emission tomographic subtraction images of provocative stimuli compared with innocuous stimuli, superimposed over magnetic resonance images for the purpose of anatomic reference, in 8 patients with obsessive-compulsive disorder (OCD). Activation during increase of OCD symptoms was found in the orbitofrontal cortex (bilaterally), right caudate nucleus, left thalamus, and anterior cingulated cortex. Other areas of activation included the right putamen and left and middle frontal cortex (not labeled). (From Rauch SL, Jenike MA, Alpert NM, et al: Regional cerebral blood flow measured during symptom provocation in obsessive-compulsive disorder using oxygen 15-labeled carbon dioxide and positron emission tomography. Arch Gen Psychiatry 1994;51(Jan):62–70, with permission.)

Diagnosis: Obsessive-compulsive disorder (OCD).

Discussion: The diagnosis of OCD was based on obsessive thoughts of contamination and compulsive cleaning. The patient also exhibited associated features such as repetitive grooming rituals, intrusive thoughts, and hoarding. Other psychiatric disorders to be considered in the differential diagnosis are schizophrenia, major depression, and autism. As opposed to delusions of thought insertion seen in schizophrenia, this patient recognized that her obsessive thoughts were products of her own mind and not based in reality. In contrast to stereotypes of autistic disorder, her compulsive rituals were accompanied by distress and ongoing attempts to resist them. Ruminations of major depressive disorder may resemble obsessive thoughts; however, the course of major depression is episodic with asymptomatic periods that this patient had seemingly never experienced.

OCD is categorized in the DSM-IV-TR as an anxiety disorder. The Epidemiologic Catchment Area program, a large community-based study, showed that 2.6% of the general population met criteria for OCD at some point in their lifetime. There is equal prevalence in adult men and women. Women may report more cleaning rituals than men, but overall there are no significant differences in symptoms between genders. Although most patients have an onset of illness at around age 20 (slightly earlier in men), OCD can be diagnosed during childhood and adolescence, as in the present patient. Mood disorders, tic disorders, eating disorders, and other anxiety disorders such as social phobia, panic disorder, and specific phobias are common comorbid psychiatric diagnoses.

The precise etiology of OCD remains unknown. Hypersensitivity of postsynaptic serotonergic receptors has been hypothesized as an underlying cause. This neurochemical hypothesis gained support from the observed efficacy of serotonergic medication in the treatment of OCD symptoms. Some pharmacologic challenge studies support this hypothesis, but the results are inconsistent. Functional neuroimaging studies suggest that the orbitofrontal cortex, cingulate, striatum, temporal lobe, and amygdala play a role in OCD. Reports of significantly higher rates of family aggregation in first-degree relatives of probands with OCD provide evidence of the importance of genetic factors. In the case of the present patient, her father's behavior suggests that he might also suffer from OCD. The results of twin studies, although inconclusive, suggest that a combination of genetic and environmental factors is important for the manifestation of OCD. Candidate gene studies are currently being conducted with the goal of understanding the molecular mechanisms of OCD. Psychodynamic theories interpret obsessive-compulsive symptoms as a regression to anal-sadistic developmental stages in response to distressing unconscious aggressive and sexual impulses.

OCD is characterized by the presence of either obsessions or compulsions that cause marked distress, are time-consuming, and significantly interfere with the person's normal occupational, academic, or social functioning. Obsessions are recurrent thoughts, impulses, or images that are experienced as intrusive and of unacceptable content. Patients recognize these thoughts as products of their own mind and make frequent attempts to neutralize them with other thoughts or actions. Compulsions are repetitive and stereotyped behaviors that the person feels driven to perform to prevent distress or a dreaded event. Patients usually characterize these behaviors as senseless and recognize that they are either not connected in a realistic way with what they are designed to neutralize or are clearly excessive. Initial resistance is typically not successful in postponing the urge to carry out these acts. Most patients with OCD report multiple symptoms, and the existence of obsessions without compensatory compulsive behavior or vice versa is infrequent. The basic types of obsessions and compulsions are remarkably limited and consistent across cultures. Fear of contamination is a commonly found obsessive thought, frequently coupled with cleaning compulsions. In the above example, the excessive time that patients typically engage in cleaning activity and the avoidant behavior that result from fear of touching objects considered as dirty usually disrupt their social life and occupational responsibilities. Fear of committing aggressive acts and preoccupation with sinful sexual thoughts are generally associated with compulsion to confess. In the type of obsessive thought characterized as need for symmetry, patients experience tension when objects or events are not arranged in a precise order. Some patients, known as "checkers," have constant doubts about having performed an action correctly, (e.g., locking the door, turning off the stove) and engage in repetitive checking behavior to prevent future hazardous situations.

At present, the data supporting psychoanalytic treatment as an effective strategy for OCD symptoms are insufficient. Cognitive behavioral and neurobiological treatments are the most frequently used approaches. Integrating the long-lasting benefits of cognitive behavioral therapy and the relatively rapid symptom relief of neurobiological therapy into a single treatment regimen may control for the shortcomings of either approach alone and result in superior outcomes. Randomized controlled studies have shown that selective serotonin reuptake inhibitors (SSRIs) are effective in the treatment of OCD. Because of their equal efficacy and more favorable side-effect profile, SSRIs have replaced clomipramine as the first-line therapy. Although optimal doses and duration have not yet been established, it is recommended that pharmacotherapy be maintained for at least 1 year. The present patient had a meaningful clinical response with paroxetine, which was increased to a daily dose of 40 mg. Her compulsive grooming behavior and obsessive thoughts diminished over the treatment course. This, along with a significant improvement in mood, permitted her to gradually engage in social activities and return to work in a part-time job outside her home. After 1 year of treatment the patient expressed a desire to continue taking the medication despite some adverse effects, such as occasional headaches and daytime sleepiness.

Unfortunately, up to 40–60% of patients do not respond to initial treatment and are thus at risk for serious social disability. In such patients, strategies such as augmentation with serotonergic agents are recommended. Open-label studies have shown that using buspirone, a 5-HT_{1A} agonist, to augment fluoxetine may be an effective strategy in resistant patients. Other neurotransmitter systems have also been involved in the pathophysiology of OCD. For example, gabapentin, a gamma aminobutyric acid (GABA) analog, was also shown to effectively augment fluoxetine. Also, dopamine antagonists such as haloperidol have been shown to be useful in combination with fluvoxamine in a subtype of patients with OCD who also have comorbid tic-related disorders. Neurosurgical techniques, such as stereotactic anterior cingulotomy and anterior capsulotomy, are used only as a last resort in selected patients with intractable symptoms. Newer treatments, such as rapid transcranial magnetic stimulation, require randomized controlled studies to evaluate their efficacy.

Pearls

1. At rest, patients with OCD have increased brain activity in the basal ganglia and frontal lobe that decreases after successful treatment. It is unclear if the activation of the frontal lobe seen in functional studies of OCD reflects a primary deficit or a compensatory response to basal ganglia dysfunction mediated by corticostriatal circuits.
2. A recent positron emission tomography study reports that lower regional cerebral blood flow (rCBF) values in orbitofrontal cortex and higher rCBF values in posterior cingulate cortex PCC predict better treatment response to SSRI medication.
3. The next step in understanding the genetics of OCD is to identify a reliable susceptibility gene (or multiple genes). The heterogeneity of the clinical phenotype, small sample sizes, and the lack of standardized criteria have hampered the interpretation of genetic studies.

REFERENCES

1. Foster PS, Eisler RM: An integrative approach to the treatment of obsessive-compulsive disorder. Comprehen Psychiatry 2001;42(1):24–31.
2. Hollander E, Kaplan A, Allen A, Cartwright C: Pharmacotherapy for obsessive-compulsive disorder. Psychiatr Clin North Am 2000;23(3):643–656.
3. Lensi P, Cassano GB, Correddu G, et al: Familial-developmental history, symptomatology, comorbidity, and course with special reference to gender-related differences. Br J Psychiatry 1996;169(1):101–107.
4. Pauls DL, Alsobrook JP, Goodman W, et al: A family study of obsessive-compulsive disorder. Am J Psychiatry 1995;152(1): 76–84.
5. Rauch SL, Shin LM, Dougherty DD, et al: Predictors of fluvoxamine response in contamination-related obsessive-compulsive disorder. A PET symptom provocation study. Neuropsychopharmacology 2002;27(5):782–91.
6. Stein DJ: Obsessive-compulsive disorder. Lancet 2002;360(9330):397–405.

PATIENT 2

A 32-year-old postpartum woman exhausted and worried about her baby

History of Present Illness: A 32-year-old woman presents to the combined psychiatric and obstetrics clinic accompanied by her husband because of his concern that she might be depressed. She is now 2 weeks postpartum from a normal spontaneous vaginal delivery of a full-term female infant. Her pregnancy was complicated by a first-trimester exposure to a poorly characterized toxic chemical at work. This exposure caused an acute episode of nausea, dizziness, and weakness.

Immediately after the exposure, the patient was evaluated in a local emergency department along with several other employees. Her exam was unremarkable, and she was discharged to routine antepartum care. There were no other antepartum complications. Her husband states that she remained worried about the possible effects of the toxic exposure on her baby and uncharacteristically went through her pregnancy worried, unhappy, and frustrated about the lack of answers from her health care providers. Her baby was a 6-pound girl, smaller than her two previous births of an 8-pound boy, now 2 years old, and an 8-pound, 9-ounce boy, now 3 years old. Her newborn girl had Apgar scores of 8 at 1 minute and 9 at 5 minutes after birth and was found to be healthy on initial pediatric exam.

Since the birth, the patient complains of exhaustion, poor sleep, and listlessness. Instead of breastfeeding, as she had done for her two previous babies, she ceded feeding of the girl to her husband with formula. She states that her milk is "no good." She comments that she barely gets out of bed, has no appetite, and frequently cries without provocation. The patient also expresses guilt about having harmed the baby and fear that her baby may not be normal. She admits to thoughts that perhaps her doctors are colluding with the managers at her workplace to "cover up" the potential consequences of the toxin exposure. She worries that the doctors are not telling her the truth and that something is really wrong with her baby.

Past Psychiatric History: The patient has never before sought psychiatric care. She denies any history of depression, including during previous pregnancies or in the postpartum period. She had taken oral contraceptives in the past without incident. Her family psychiatric history is negative. She lives with her husband of 4 years in a small apartment in a large city with their 3 children. She has limited social support and financial resources.

Mental Status Examination: The patient is an obese woman with fair hygiene and a sad, exhausted look. She is somewhat guarded on exam and has poor eye contact with paucity and low volume of speech. Her affect is constricted and apathetic. Thought process is coherent. Thought content is preoccupied with themes of guilt and paranoid ideation about medical staff and her employer. She denies perceptual abnormalities. When asked about suicide, she states that her children would be better off with "another mother" but denies a plan to hurt herself. Her insight and judgment are fair because she admits to needing help, and her impulse control is intact. Mini-mental state exam score is 27/30 because of impaired delayed recall and one error on the concentration task (serial sevens).

Laboratory Examination: Complete blood count, chemistry, urine toxicology, and thyroid function tests are within normal limits.

Questions: What is the diagnosis? How can this patient be treated?

Diagnosis: Postpartum depression with psychotic features.

Discussion: 20–40% of women report emotional problems during the postpartum period. Most of these women experience the postpartum "blues," a self-limited state of sadness, dysphoria, crying spells, and dependence. These symptoms are thought to be secondary to rapid alteration in endocrine levels and fluid shifts related to the stress of childbirth, and they typically peak on day 5 to 6 postpartum. There is a 10–15% prevalence of major depression with postpartum onset. Women at risk for postpartum depression are more likely to have a family history of depression or a past history of affective disorder associated with reproductive hormonal flux (e.g., previous postpartum depression, pregnancy, premenstrual dysphoric disorder). Recent evidence suggests that affective illness manifested during the postpartum period is hard to distinguish from affective illness at other times. The DSM-IV-TR does not distinguish between postpartum and non-postpartum presentation of mood disorders except with a modifier for "postpartum onset," which specifies that symptoms must begin within the first 4 weeks of the postpartum period. It has been demonstrated that women who have planned pregnancies in a secure environment, who enjoy supportive relationships with their partner, and who have manageable levels of life stress are less likely to experience postpartum depression. Occasionally, as in this case, the depression may be so severe that psychotic features are present.

Suicide or infanticide risks must also be carefully assessed, and hospitalization is sometime necessary. It is critical to involve the patient's partner for corroborative information, as often a depressed mother is unable to evaluate herself; she does not reliably volunteer her symptoms and tends to be focused on her baby rather than herself. In addition, there is a societal stigma against depression during what is seen by many as a "joyful time." Primary care providers sometimes "normalize" a patient's symptoms and tend to see these complaints as "extended baby blues." Postpartum depression is not a benign illness, however. It tends to be recurrent, and 40% of women who have a first depressive episode in the postpartum period will also develop a nonpuerperal depression. The risk of recurrence with subsequent pregnancy is 20%. A growing body of evidence suggests that maternal psychiatric illness is related to suboptimal mother/infant attachment, which has negative consequences for infant temperament and behavioral and cognitive development. Other sequelae of maternal affective illness are income loss, family disruption, and possible placement outside the house (e.g., foster care) that may further impair child development.

The diagnosis of postpartum depression involves a standard clinical interview and detailed corroborative information from the family. An endocrine assessment is useful to rule out thyroid dysfunction and partial or total Sheehan's syndrome. The Edinburgh Postnatal Depression Scale (EDPS) is a simple and quick screening tool that can be used as adjunct to the clinical interview. The differential diagnosis includes postpartum obsessive-compulsive disorder (OCD), postpartum psychosis, and postpartum "baby blues."

Postpartum OCD is an anxiety syndrome characterized by rapid escalation of obsessions to harm the newborn, heightened general anxiety, and disruption of the mother/infant relationship. Symptoms of OCD are limited to intrusive obsessional thoughts without evidence of accompanying compulsions. Depressive symptoms are typically not present in postpartum OCD. In postpartum psychosis, hallucinations and delusions are prominent, and there is a strong potential risk of harm to the infant. In postpartum OCD, on the other hand, patients avoid contact with their infants for fear of hurting them. They do not act on potentially harmful thoughts, and these thoughts are considered ego-alien. Postpartum "baby blues," as already mentioned, is a transient state of heightened emotional reactivity and lability that peaks 5 to 6 days postpartum.

The treatment of postpartum depression involves a combined pharmacologic and psychosocial approach. Initial pharmacotherapy is with selective serotonin reuptake inhibitors (SSRIs), titrated to effect. The dosages and duration of treatment are the same as for nonpuerperal affective disorder. Because anxiety is prominent initially, the use of benzodiazepines may also be useful. If psychotic features are present, antipsychotic medication is added. For women who are nursing, it is important to remember that there are no controlled studies of the safety of psychotropic medication in lactating women. Case reports and small case series for each of the different psychotropic medications serve as the basis of suggested treatment guidelines in the management of psychiatric illness in lactating patients. If medication is indicated, the mother needs to be provided with available information about its effects on the newborn so that informed choices can be made. The infant's pediatrician should also be involved in monitoring the infant if psychotropic medications are used during breastfeeding. Hospitalization is indicated for any suicidal or homicidal ideation. Supportive psychotherapy, interpersonal psychotherapy, and cognitive behavioral therapy have been used successfully. Psychoeducation, doula services, and visiting nurse services are useful adjuncts. After stabilization, referral to self-help groups such as Depression after Delivery and other mother/infant support groups is warranted.

The present case illustrates a more severe form of postpartum depression. Although the patient had no psychiatric history, her antepartum course contained stressors that would put her at risk for the postpartum emotional disturbances: (1) her environmental toxic exposure and resultant fear and confusion about long-term consequences; (2) toddlers at home and a husband who worked long hours and was unable to help her adequately; (3) lack of other family and social support; and (4) inadequate financial resources.

Sertraline was started on the first outpatient visit. One week later the patient's mood had not improved, and in fact she appeared even more paranoid and withdrawn. Risperidone was added. Attempts at culturally sensitive counseling for the patient's husband about postpartum adjustment were initiated. Evaluation 1 week later noted no significant change. The husband was then forced to stop working and had to care for the three children and his wife full-time. At this point hospitalization was considered, but instead a visiting nurse service began twice-weekly home-based services and daily home health services. Two weeks later there was significant improvement in energy, mood, and interests. The patient remained in the outpatient psychiatric department with plans to continue antidepressant medication treatment for 1 year. Risperidone was tapered and then discontinued after 4 months postpartum, with no recurrence of paranoid ideation. The patient was counseled on risks of recurrences in future pregnancies.

Pearls

1. Many physicians have a tendency not to treat postpartum depression effectively. It should be considered as a serious condition with significant morbidity and long-lasting negative consequences for mother and infant. The dosage and duration of medication treatment should be the same as for nonpuerperal illness.
2. Initial evaluations should always rule out endocrine abnormalities, with particular attention to potential thyroid dysfunction.
3. The risk and benefit analysis of using psychotropic medication for nursing mothers should include the documented benefits of breastfeeding and the potential adverse impact of untreated maternal illness on infant attachment and development.

REFERENCES

1. Burt VK, Suri R, Altshuler L, et al: The use of psychotropic medications during breast feeding. Am J Psychiatry 2001;158(7):1001–1009.
2. Cohen LS, Altshuler LL: Pharmacologic management of psychiatric illness during pregnancy and the postpartum period. In Dunner DL, Rosenbaum JF (eds): Psychiatric Clinics of North America Annual of Drug Therapy. Philadelphia, W.B. Saunders, 1997, pp 21–61.
3. Cox JL, Holden JM, Sagovsky R: Detection of postnatal depression: Development of the 10 item Edinburgh Postnatal Depression Scale. Br J Psychiatry 1987;150:782–786.
4. Gold L: Postpartum disorders in primary care: Diagnosis and treatment. Primary Care 2002;29(1):27–41.

PATIENT 3

A 13-year-old boy with aggressive behavior

History of Present Illness: A 13-year-old boy is brought to the emergency department (ED) from school after getting involved in a physical altercation with another student. The school report indicates that the patient grabbed the other student by the jacket during recess with no apparent provocation. The patient repeatedly stated that "the gang" would beat him up and also attempted to fight with security, accusing the guard of "being one of them." In the ED, the patient seems anxious and restless, guarded, and provocative. He is unable to provide a coherent recollection of the event, changing topics without related content, and asking every few minutes if his mother has come to the hospital. The patient becomes easily angered with rapid shifts to tears and needs significant verbal reassurance to calm down.

The patient's mother reports that the he is being seen in an outpatient clinic by a psychiatrist and is relatively adherent with monthly visits. His medication has been recently increased due to more impulsive behavior. He currently takes amphetamine/dextroamphetamine, 20 mg after breakfast at home and another 20 mg after lunch in school. The mother claims that the medication has helped him significantly with his academic work. However, as of 2 weeks ago, she has noticed that the patient has become more fidgety and "hyper," especially after the beginning of the new school year when the patient was transferred to a new class. The mother reports that she has been giving him 2 and even 3 pills in the morning because she thought that it would help him stay focused.

Past Psychiatric History: Gross motor and bowel control developmental milestones were reached at the appropriate ages. At the age of 3 years the patient had "a mild language delay" for which he received early intervention. At the age of 5 years the patient started to exhibit impulsive behaviors such as getting out of his seat in class, walking around the classroom, and constantly talking to other students. He had difficulty finishing school assignments on time. At home the patient needed to be constantly reminded and supervised with daily routines. The patient was hospitalized once at 10 years of age for hyperactive behavior, refusing to go to sleep, staying up late at night, and leaving the house without permission after his parents were asleep. He has attended a special education class since the third grade because of his disruptive behavior and poor academic performance. The patient denies alcohol or substance abuse. The parents describe a vague family psychiatric history of "mood swings" in a first cousin and paternal uncle.

Mental Status Examination: The patient looks anxious and fidgety. His speech is fast and pressured, and he jumps from topic to topic with few or no logical connections in his reasoning. Affect is labile, mostly angry and guarded. The patient states that the teachers and the students at school pick on him because "I'm different." He claims that they know he is stronger and smarter than anyone else and "all they want is to bring me down." His attention shifts quickly from one examiner to another, and he intrusively engages in conversations with other patients and staff members. When questioned about any unusual experiences, such as hearing or seeing things that other people cannot see or hear, he becomes guarded and evasive, avoids answering the question, and starts to cry when the psychiatrist inquires further. He denies suicidal or homicidal ideation.

Question: What diagnosis accounts for this clinical presentation?

Diagnosis: Comorbid attention-deficit/hyperactivity disorder (ADHD) and bipolar disorder.

Discussion: The patient's presentation is consistent with an acute onset of manic symptoms such as psychomotor agitation, irritability, grandiosity, paranoid thinking, and distractibility. The patient also presents with a history of hyperactive behavior before the age of 7 years, which supports a diagnosis of ADHD. This case is diagnostically complicated by the possibility of stimulant-induced mania. It has been documented that the first episode of bipolar disorder in children can be triggered by pharmacologic agents, particularly steroids, antidepressants, and stimulants. Stimulant toxicity, for example, can present with irritability, restlessness, paranoid delusions, and auditory and visual hallucinations.

It is possible that the current clinical presentation is related to the escalating dose of stimulant (amphetamine/dextroamphetamine) used to treat the symptoms of ADHD. This patient needed admission to the inpatient psychiatric unit for safety and observation as well as careful discontinuation of the stimulant treatment. Further evaluation, including baseline liver function tests, is required to determine the necessity of initiating treatment with a mood stabilizer.

A manic episode is defined by DSM-IV-TR as a distinct period of at least 1 week with abnormally and persistently elevated, expansiv, or irritable mood. An increasing body of research suggests the existence of early-onset childhood bipolar disorder. Twin, family, and adoption studies show that the lifelong prevalence of bipolar disorder is about 1% in the general population, and increases to between 5% and 10% in first-degree relatives. Like schizophrenia, bipolar disorder appears to be a multigenetic condition, and its expression seems significantly influenced by environmental factors. The population of pediatric bipolar illness may be small, but current research points to the early misdiagnosis of ADHD and suggests that attention deficit and hyperactivity may serve as harbingers of the developing mania. Available data strongly suggest that prepubertal childhood bipolar disorder is a nonepisodic, chronic, rapidly cycling, mixed manic state. Clinically, symptoms of mania may be discounted as severe ADHD or ignored in the context of aggressive conduct. This atypical presentation may lead clinicians to neglect the mood component.

Significant debate exists as to whether early-onset bipolar disorder is mistakenly attributed to ADHD or conduct disorder (CD) or whether ADHD and CD are frequently misdiagnosed as mania. This confusion may be the result of features common to attention deficit, disruptive disorders, and bipolar illness, and it is often quite difficult to differentiate among them reliably. Some researches emphasize the decreased need for sleep and the increased pleasure-seeking behavior as more specific for a manic episode.

Comorbid bipolar disorder and ADHD are also a widely debated topic in the child and adolescent literature, with rates of comorbidity ranging from 22% to 90% of cases. Since ADHD estimates range up to 10% of the school population, it is of extreme importance that clinicians be able to differentiate reliably between the two conditions. Although a number of ADHD and mania rating scales have been developed, their specificity remains low. No specific diagnostic instruments are available for the evaluation of early-onset manic symptoms, although the Young Mania Rating Scale may be helpful, especially in the adolescent population. The high rate of comorbid disorders in children and adolescents with bipolar disorder contributes to the severe dysfunction frequently observed. It has also been speculated that children with bipolar disorder and ADHD may have a distinct familial subtype of bipolar disorder. Stimulant-exposed adolescents with bipolar disorder may have a more severe course of illness not fully explained by ADHD comorbidity.

This pattern of comorbidity in children with bipolar disorder is unique by adult standards, especially in its overlap with ADHD, aggression, and conduct disorder. Recognition of the multiplicity of disorders should guide therapeutic options, and ADHD, oppositional behavior, aggression, and conduct disorder that was previously considered refractory to treatment may respond to mood stabilizers. An initial differential diagnosis for suspected mania should also include hyperthyroidism, substance- or medication-induced mania, postictal state, or childhood-onset schizophrenia.

Mood stabilizers are the main treatment for bipolar disorder in adults. The preparations that have been studied in pediatric populations include lithium carbonate, divalproic acid, carbamazepine, and gabapentin. No practice parameter algorithms are available for pharmacologic treatment of children with bipolar disorder. Chart review studies have found that mood stabilizers were frequently used in children with manic-like symptoms, and their use was associated with significant improvement, whereas use of antidepressant, antipsychotic, and stimulant medications was not. A number of studies have examined the safety of stimulant treatment in children with ADHD/bipolar comorbidity, but the results are mixed and inconclusive. Some studies suggest that stimulant treatment has no negative effect on the clinical course of the affective illness, whereas other studies have demonstrated adverse outcomes and significantly negative impact.

Pearls

1. It has been suggested that refractory cases of ADHD should be conceptualized as either an atypical presentation of early-onset bipolar disorder or as a comorbid ADHD and bipolar disorder condition.
2. Despite the increased risk of mood destabilization in general, selective serotonergic antidepressants have not been shown to interfere with the antimanic effects of mood stabilizers in children and adolescents.
3. Lithium is the best studied mood stabilizer in the pediatric population and has a relatively safe side-effect profile. The off-label use of anticonvulsants as mood stabilizers has increased in recent years, although the majority of data regarding safety in children have been obtained from their use in pediatric neurology. Future randomized studies will examine the mood-stabilizing properties of newer anticonvulsants and atypical neuroleptics in pediatric bipolar disorder.

REFERENCES

1. Biederman J, Mick E, Bostic JQ, et al: The naturalistic course of pharmacologic treatment of children with manic-like symptoms: A systematic chart review. J Clin Psychiatry 1998;59(11): 628–637.
2. Kim EY, Miklowitz DJ: Childhood mania, attention deficit hyperactivity disorder and conduct disorder: A critical review of diagnostic dilemmas. Bipolar Disord 2002;4(4):215–220.
3. Taylor L, Faraonte SV, Tsuang MT: Family, twin and adoption studies in bipolar disease. Curr Psychiatr Rep 2002;4(2):130–3.
4. Wozniak J, Biederman J, Richardson JA: Diagnostic and therapeutic dilemmas in the management of pediatric-onset bipolar disorder. J Clin Psychiatry 2001;62(Suppl 14):10–15.

PATIENT 4

A 61-year-old woman with hyperthermia and urinary incontinence

History of Present Illness: A 61-year-old woman with bipolar I disorder, currently hospitalized for mania, is noticed by nursing staff to have an elevated temperature of 38.4°C. Her vital signs are otherwise stable, and she is without complaints. Two hours later, the patient is noticed to be incontinent of urine and is thrashing around in her bed. Her vital signs are retaken, and the results are as follows: blood pressure, 140/80 mmHg; pulse, 100 beats/min; respiratory rate, 24 breaths/min; and temperature, 38.8°C. There are acute mental status changes, and although she remains alert, she is not oriented to time or place. When the resident attempts to take a history, she is only able to say that she "feels hot."

The patient was admitted to the psychiatric unit 5 days ago for manic behavior at home. She was brought in by her family because she told them she had "special powers" and was getting messages from God. She was sleeping only 2 to 3 hours each night and would spend most of the day reading the Bible. She also had a markedly decreased appetite with increased goal-directed activity (e.g., cleaning, writing, cooking). The family suspects that she was not taking her lithium. The patient has been hospitalized for approximately 5 days and is currently receiving lithium carbonate, 300 mg in the morning and 600 mg in the evening. In the past 2 days, the patient has received haloperidol, 5 mg intramuscularly 3 times, for agitated behavior and because she appeared to be responding to internal stimuli.

Past Psychiatric and Medical History: The patient was diagnosed with bipolar I disorder when she was 24 years old. She has had 10 hospitalizations, mainly in the context of nonadherence with medication. The patient responds well to lithium carbonate, and when she agrees to take it, she is without affective symptoms. She has never required standing neuroleptics. The patient has a medical history of essential hypertension, which is well-controlled by diet.

Mental Status Examination: The patient is an elderly woman who appears her stated age. Her eye contact is poor, and she is unable to cooperate with the interview. She is restless and shifting around on the bed, which is wet with urine. Her speech is barely audible, and she remains mute throughout most of the interview. The interviewer is unable to assess her mood, but she appears uncomfortable and irritable. She denies suicidal or homicidal ideation. She denies any auditory or visual hallucinations. She is alert but keeps her eyes closed. She is oriented to self but not to time or place. Her memory, concentration, and attention are impaired. Insight and judgment are limited.

Physical Examination: Blood pressure, 140/80 mmHg; pulse, 100 beats/min; respiratory rate, 24 breaths/min; temperature, 38.8°C. Head: normocepahlic, atraumatic, positive nuchal rigidity; pupils are 3 mm, equal, round, and reactive to light and accommodation. She is unable to cooperate with examination of her extraocular movements or the remaining cranial nerves. There is no evidence of lymphadenopathy. Lungs: clear to auscultation bilaterally. Cardiac exam: fast rate and regular rhythm; first and second heart sounds are audible, no extra heart sounds noted, and no sign of murmurs, gallop, or rub. Abdomen: soft, nontender, with positive bowel sounds. Skin/extremities: warm to the touch, no lesions or evidence of cyanosis, edema, or clubbing. Neurologic exam: patient shows significant rigidity on flexion in all four extremities and is otherwise unable to ambulate or cooperate with neurologic exam.

Laboratory Examination: WBC = 18,000, neutrophils = 60%, lymphocytes = 30%, no bands. Chemistry profile is normal. CPK = 30,000, CK-MB = 0, troponin = 0. Urinalysis: no WBC, no RBC, negative for nitrites and leukocyte esterase.

Diagnostic Examination: CT scan of the brain: no masses or hemorrhage. CSF: no evidence of infection. Blood cultures: negative.

Questions: What is the diagnosis? How should this patient be treated?

Diagnosis: Neuroleptic malignant syndrome (NMS).

Discussion: NMS is a rare but dangerous syndrome associated with antipsychotic medication. Its hallmark features are hyperthermia, rigidity, autonomic instability, and altered mental status. Other features include akinesia, dystonia, mutism, sialorrhea, incontinence, diaphoresis, pallor, and flushing.

The exact pathophysiology is unknown, but the most accepted theory is that the central and peripheral manifestations of NMS are the consequences of dopamine blockade. In addition, it is hypothesized that the severe hyperthermia is a result of hypothalamic derangement secondary to dopamine insufficiency. Presumably, the heat generated by the contracted, rigid musculature and the central derangement of temperature control combine to cause hyperthermia.

The differential diagnosis of NMS is extensive, and it is of utmost importance to remember that NMS is a diagnosis of exclusion. Initially with this patient, we needed to rule out any infectious cause of possible delirium. Urine, CSF, and blood samples were taken to check for urosepsis and meningitis. A full neurologic exam was done because neurologic phenomena such as akinetic mutism, locked-in syndrome, encephalitis, and meningitis can appear like NMS. Inhalational anesthetics can also cause a malignant hyperthermia that can appear to be NMS, but what distinguishes the two is that the hyperthermia secondary to anesthetics occurs within minutes after administration. Also, "ecstasy" (MDMA or 3,4 methylenedioxy-methamphetamine) or cocaine can cause a syndrome that may appear to be like NMS, but it can be distinguished by history or toxicology screening. Thyrotoxicosis, tetany, and acute porphyria are also in the differential and need to be ruled out. Heatstroke (which is more common in patients on neuroleptics due to medication-related impairments of heat regulation) is also in the differential, and can be distinguished from NMS by the absence of rigidity and diaphoresis. Serotonin syndrome also has a similar appearance to NMS but with prominent gastrointestinal symptoms (nausea and vomiting) and less tremor and rigidity. Finally, lethal catatonia is often indistinguishable from NMS. Most authors agree that catatonia is a final common pathway for many central nervous system disorders, and clinicians must rely on the history to distinguish between NMS and lethal catatonia.

The diagnosis of NMS is most easily made when it is seen early in the course of treatment or when the neuroleptic dose has just been rapidly increased. The majority of cases occur within the first 2 weeks of treatment. Other risk factors include agitation, dehydration, and parental administration of neuroleptics. It remains unclear whether agitation and the use of restraints are risk factors in and of themselves or whether their presence simply triggers aggressive medicating and in turn leads to NMS. HIV infection, compromised central nervous system functioning, and mental retardation have been cited as additional risk factors.

The successful management of NMS relies on early and aggressive supportive interventions. When it is suspected, a complete medical and neurologic work-up is necessary, including a complete blood count and a full chemistry profile with creatine phosphokinase (CPK) and liver enzymes. A lumbar puncture should be performed to rule out meningitis. As seen in this case, patients with NMS frequently have leukocytosis without a left shift. Elevated CPK is also frequently seen, and in severe cases it may reach 100,000 IU/L. This CPK elevation is thought to result from the muscular rigidity and elevation in body temperature seen in NMS, but injury, struggling against restraints, and repeated intramuscular injections can also cause increased CPK levels. The CPK should be serially monitored to track the syndrome's severity and course. Liver function abnormalities and electrolyte imbalances may also be seen in NMS.

In this patient the diagnosis was made mainly by the history of recent exposure to neuroleptic medication, namely the three intramuscular injections of haloperidol. In addition, physical exam revealed elevated temperature, altered mental status, rigidity, and urinary incontinence. Sepsis, meningitis, and urinary tract infection were all ruled out. The presence of elevated CPK also helped to confirm the diagnosis of NMS.

Once the diagnosis is made, the patient should be transferred as soon as possible to an intensive care unit. Antipsychotic medications should be discontinued. Patients taking anticholinergic medication should also be carefully assessed, and a slow taper is generally recommended. Intravenous fluids should be started immediately to compensate for oral restriction and to prevent volume loss from sweating. Fluids are also needed to prevent acute renal failure, because rhabdomyolysis associated with prolonged muscle contraction can cause myoglobinuria. Mechanical cooling with blankets, fans, and bathing should be started as soon as significant hyperthermia begins. If dystonia and rigidity are severe enough to limit respiratory efforts, intubation and subsequent ventilatory support may be necessary. Physical therapy interventions to decrease the associated risks of thromboembolism include frequent repositioning, range-of-motion exercises, antiembolic stockings, and kinetic nursing beds.

There is a lack of controlled studies to support the use of pharmacologic interventions in NMS. However, there is substantial anecdotal support for the use of dopaminergic agents (e.g., bromocriptine), dantrolene sodium, and benzodiazepines. Bromocriptine has been reported to decrease the duration of NMS episodes and to decrease mortality by 50%. However, it can only be administered orally (or by nasogastric tube) and has been associated with a worsening of psychosis. Dantrolene sodium is one of the hallmark medications for the treatment of malignant hyperthermia. Its mechanism of action is a blockade of intracellular calcium efflux; it thereby interferes with excitation contraction coupling. Dantrolene takes effect within minutes and reduces heat production and contraction. It can be given orally or intravenously and is given in doses from 1 to 10 mg/kg/day. Liver function needs to monitored closely with dantrolene, because it can produce hepatic toxicity. Benzodiazepines have been associated with clinical improvement in catatonia; they can also be given orally or intravenously.

The present patient was transferred within 1 hour to the medical intensive care unit (MICU), where she was placed on high-dose intravenous fluids via triple-lumen catheter. Her cardiac and respiratory functions were continuously monitored, and she did not require intubation. Intravenous benzodiazepines were used for agitation, and dantrolene was started on her second day in the MICU. CBC, chemistry profile, CPK, renal function, and liver function were monitored daily. The CPK slowly trended downward, and the patient was transferred to medicine after 7 days in the MICU.

Pearls

1. Some authors have suggested that hyponatremia can predispose to NMS. In addition, anecdotal reports show a correlation between very low levels of serum calcium and iron and more severe episodes of NMS.
2. Data about the role of anticholinergic agents in NMS are conflicting. Some reports have found these agents to be helpful and note that cholinergic rebound from abrupt discontinuation may contribute to the severity of the syndrome. However, anticholinergic agents are also known to interfere with the body's sweating mechanism and may contribute to hyperthermia, leading some clinicians to avoid their use in suspected cases of NMS.
3. Case reports have cited HIV infection as a risk factor for NMS. Some authors have observed that HIV infection of the central nervous system may increase a patient's susceptibility to extrapyramidal symptoms. This increased sensitivity may be a direct effect of HIV on the basal ganglia.
4. Electroconvulsive therapy (ECT) is seen by most authors as a second-line treatment in NMS, sometimes used after pharmacologic interventions fail. The presumed mechanism of action of ECT is the increased release of dopamine.

REFERENCES

1. Addonizio G, Susman VL, Roth SD: Neuroleptic malignant syndrome: Review and analysis of 115 cases. Biol Psychiatry 1987;22(8):1004–1020.
2. Deuschl G, Oepen G, Hermle L, Kindt H: Neuroleptic malignant syndrome: Observations on altered consciousness. Pharmacopsychiatry 1987;20(4):168–170.
3. Susman VL: Clinical management of neuroleptic malignant syndrome. Psychiatr Q 2001;72(4):325–336.

PATIENT 5

A 26-year-old man status post suicide attempt

History of Present Illness: A 26-year-old man is transferred from the medical emergency department (ED) to the psychiatric ED after receiving sutures to multiple lacerations on both wrists. The patient was initially brought to the ED by a friend who found him in the bathtub, bleeding from his wrists. When the patient is asked to move into an exam room to be interviewed, the examiner notes that he first unties and reties his shoes 3 times. When the interview finally begins, the patient reports that in recent months he has become disturbed "by his life and the way things are going." He describes feeling "ugly" and "worthless" and is "tired of dealing with everything." When asked about his suicide attempt, he states, "The past few days have been really bad.... it's all coming apart now," and begins to cry uncontrollably.

When the patient regains composure, he reports that he is a writer who has recently signed a deal to publish his novel. He was scheduled to be photographed for the book jacket cover earlier today and feels "overwhelmed" by the idea of being photographed and having the photo publicly released. When asked why he felt overwhelmed, he points to the skin around his mouth, where multiple small lesions in various stages of healing are appreciated. The patient describes an ongoing concern about the thickness of his mustache, despite being clean-shaven. He reports shaving 3 to 4 times every day and then using tweezers between shaves to prevent more growth. He endorses feeling this way for the past year, "ever since I got my nose fixed." The patient also admits to repeatedly checking for hair growth in the mirror and feeling that people in the street are constantly looking at his mustache. The patient notes that he lives alone, works from home, and has few friends. He rarely leaves the house because he does not want "to be around people." He also appears anxious to end the interview and interrupts the examiner to ask if he can go to the bathroom. When asked why, he seems embarrassed but admits to wanting to check his skin and wash his hands.

Past Psychiatric History: The patient denies any previous contact with a psychiatrist. He has never been hospitalized or taken psychiatric medication. He was referred once for depressive symptoms but never followed up.

Past Medical History: The patient admits seeing a dermatologist for "skin problems" and has a history of two rhinoplasties in the past 5 years.

Mental Status Examination: The patient is a good-looking man who appears his stated age. He is disheveled in appearance but clean-shaven. He has limited eye contact, and his speech is slow and quiet. The patient keeps his hand over his mouth throughout the interview and moves it only slightly to speak. When his hand is moved, the lesions around his lips can be seen, and some appear infected. He reports that his mood is "really bad," and his affect is constricted to the dysphoric range. He cries openly and at times uncontrollably. His thought process is linear and goal-directed. He describes feeling as though people on the street are looking at him and talking about his skin but denies other disturbance in thought content. He denies homicidal ideation but still endorses suicidal ideation. When asked about a plan, he replies, "Well, something better than cutting my wrists." He denies auditory and visual hallucinations. He is alert and oriented, with good attention and intact memory and concentration. His insight and judgment appear poor.

Questions: What is the primary diagnosis? How might the patient best be treated?

Diagnosis: Body dysmorphic disorder.

Discussion: The patient suffers from body dysmorphic disorder (BDD), also known as dysmorphophobia. It is categorized in the DSM-IV-TR as a somatoform disorder in which an individual has an excessive preoccupation with an imagined defect in appearance. This preoccupation causes significant distress and impairment in important areas of the patient's life and is not better accounted for by any other psychiatric problem. BDD is relatively common, estimated to affect approximately 2% of the population.

Any body part can be the focus of concern in BDD, but the perception of facial flaws is the most common. The perceived defect may be insignificant or even imagined. Although it is common for people to be unhappy with aspects of their bodies, the feelings of a patient who suffers from BDD extend significantly beyond unhappiness. The patient compulsively examines, attempts to hide, or changes the defect. He or she also performs repetitive behaviors such as mirror-checking, grooming, visits to doctors, and skin-picking. These behaviors and thoughts interfere with the patient's life. School and work performance also suffers, and patients may avoid relationships and social interaction but are unsatisfied with the results.

In this patient, symptoms of obsessive-compulsive disorder (OCD) became apparent initially because of the behavioral ritual that he performed prior to entering the interview room. Later, it seemed clear that body dysmorphic disorder was the primary diagnosis because of the patient's severe and persistent preoccupation with the thickness of his facial hair. He also endorsed repetitive checking and grooming compulsions. In addition, he experienced ideas of reference in which he thought other people were looking at or talking about his skin, and this experience prevents him from leaving the house. The extent of his distress is made clear by the suicide attempt that led to his initial presentation. In fact, studies have revealed that approximately 30% of patients with BDD attempt suicide. In addition, comorbid OCD and major depression are common findings in BDD. In one sample, it was noted that 12% of patients with BDD met criteria for OCD, and 37% had a history of OCD.

The treatment for BDD includes pharmacology and cognitive-behavioral therapy (CBT). In a recent study, fluoxetine was shown to be superior to placebo in alleviating the symptoms of BDD according to patient and clinician symptom-rating scales. Fluoxetine was considered effective in treating the patient's preoccupation with a bodily defect as well as the associated compulsions. Furthermore, it was noted that patients whose preoccupation was considered delusional also responded to fluoxetine. Other antidepressant medications, such as fluvoxamine and clomipramine, have also been shown to treat symptoms of BDD effectively.

Cognitive-behavioral therapy is used to treat patients with BDD by helping them to identify errors in thinking and then retraining their patterns of thinking. Patients must learn to be less "negative" and more realistic about perceived flaws. They must also learn that the perceived "flaw" will not be noticed by other people in the same manner. For instance, in the case outlined above, this young writer will eventually recognize when he enters a pattern of negative thoughts about his skin and will then be able to utilize specific strategies to modify or change those negative thoughts. He will also be encouraged to critically examine the likelihood of other people focusing on his perceived skin defect. Therapy is focused on encouraging the patient to understand his "flaw" as insignificant and to realize that others will not judge him, reject him, or be disgusted by his appearance.

The recent literature reviewing CBT interventions for the treatment of BDD has been favorable. An intervention of six highly structured sessions in which patients were taught muscle relaxation and imagery and then progressively desensitized to their "flawed" body parts showed significant symptom improvement that was maintained at a 7-week follow-up. Other studies that included CBT in individual sessions with maintenance therapy (biweekly booster sessions of therapy) and group CBT have also demonstrated significant efficacy in alleviating symptoms compared with placebo treatments.

This patient was hospitalized because of the severity of his suicide attempt and the potential for self-harm. He was started on a selective serotonin reuptake inhibitor to treat the BDD as well as the comorbid symptoms of OCD and major depression. After 10 days, the patient described improved mood and denied suicidal ideation. He was discharged to the care of an outpatient psychiatrist with the recommendation to continue pharmacotherapy and to consider initiating cognitive behavioral treatment.

Pearls

1. Many people are first diagnosed with BDD only after multiple visits to plastic surgeons or dermatologists.
2. The perceived flaw in BDD may migrate to different body parts; in this case, it appears to have gone from his nose to his skin.
3. Despite a relative paucity of research into genetics and neuroanatomy in BDD, the similarities to symptoms of obsessive-compulsive disorder may provide opportunities for future research.

REFERENCES

1. Allen A, Hollander E: Body dysmorphic disorder. Psychiatr Clin North Am 2000;23(3):617–628.
2. Looper KJ, Kirmayer LJ: Behavioral medicine approaches to somatoform disorders. J Consult Clin Psychiatry 2002;70(3):810–827.
3. Phillips KA, Albertini RS, Rasmussen SA: A randomized placebo controlled trial of fluoxetine in body dysmorphic disorder. Arch Gen Psychiatry 2002;59:381–388.
4. Phillips KA, McElroy SL, Keck PE Jr, et al:. A comparison of delusional and nondelusional body dysmorphic disorder in 10 cases. Psychopharmacol Bull 1994;30(179):179–186.

PATIENT 6

A 5-year-old boy with temper tantrums

History of Present Illness: A 5-year-old boy is brought to a psychiatrist's office for evaluation. His mother requested the evaluation due to deterioration in the child's behavior over the past 2 months. The mother states that the patient has become increasingly disobedient and ignoring directions from adults and has exhibited aggressive behavior toward younger siblings. He frequently plays roughly with his 1-year-old sister and fights with his older brother, recently scratching him on the face. The patient is described as becoming easily upset and angry. He may yell and scream, spit, kick, bite, or destroy furniture. The patient has also had occasional episodes of enuresis when his demands are not met. He has been observed torturing the family cat and used to set traps for birds to "kill them." Also of note is the fact that the patient's father was recently incarcerated. Although the patient used to see his father on rare occasions, he has not heard from him since his incarceration.

Past Psychiatric History: The patient was born at full term after a normal pregnancy. Gross motor milestones were achieved on time. At the age of 2 years the patient was babbling and used appropriately only 8 to 10 words. Speech and language evaluation at that time found more than a 50% delay in both receptive and expressive language. He continued to exhibit expressive and receptive language deficits at the age of 4 years, but treatment had decreased delay to less than 20%. He now attends a special school where he receives speech and language therapy. Since the age of 2 years, the patient has shown oppositional, defiant, and aggressive behavior toward adult authority. In school, he has initiated physical fights with other students on many occasions, attacking them with pencils or scissors that he brought from home. The patient's parents were not married and lived separately. The patient's biological father has a history of substance abuse and has been incarcerated for about 3 months. The mother is a single parent with three other young children, and the family is on public support.

Mental Status Examination: The patient looks younger than his age and is minimally related with poor eye contact. He refuses to engage and occasionally indicates "yes" or "no" answers with head movements only. His affect is angry, and mood is irritable. The patient clings to his mother and has frequent tantrums in the psychiatrist's office. He seems highly guarded and attempts to hide under the desk. He is able to calm down with verbal reassurance and, when feeling more comfortable, he starts to wander around the office, ignoring his mother's instructions to stop opening drawers and playing with the phone. He volitionally interrupts and sabotages the interview. His mother denies any self-injurious behavior or suicidal statements by the patient. There is no history of disorganized or bizarre behaviors, according to the mother. She states that "he does things he knows will drive you crazy." The patient has never reported any perceptual disturbances. Reports from school have indicated that the patient is able to engage and stay focused in activities of interest.

Diagnostic Testing: Auditory testing showed normal hearing with full range bilaterally, and neuropsychological testing indicates a normal IQ.

Questions: What is the diagnosis? What is the best treatment for this patient?

Diagnosis: Conduct disorder.

Discussion: Conduct disorder is described by the DSM-IV-TR as a repetitive and persistent pattern of behavior that violates the basic rights of others or defies major age-appropriate societal norms and rules. Aggression toward people and animals, destruction of property, deceitfulness, and theft are also included in the diagnostic criteria. This patient's presentation strongly suggests the possibility of childhood-onset conduct disorder based on the history of aggression, cruelty to animals, extreme oppositional behavior, and destruction of property. The family history of probable antisocial traits also increases the likelihood of the diagnosis, because antisocial personality disorder occurs with increased frequency in family members of children with conduct disorder. The management of this case depends on the parent's ability to control the child and on the estimated risk for potential harm to self and others. Combined behavioral and psychopharmacologic approaches may be initiated in an outpatient setting if the clinician and parent are reassured that there is no immediate safety risk.

Conduct disorder is highly prevalent and appears to occur more frequently among males. It is more likely to be seen in large families with low socioeconomic status, and familial aggregation is common. Parental substance abuse, low socioeconomic status, and oppositional behavior are key predictive factors in the progression to conduct disorder. Oppositional defiant disorder may be a precursor to conduct disorder, and a significant number of patients later develop antisocial personality disorder. In fact, one of the diagnostic criteria for antisocial personality disorder is the presence of conduct disorder before the age of 15 years. Conduct disorder is generally considered to have a relatively poor prognosis and is most probably a chronic condition that requires ongoing treatment and monitoring. ADHD has also been implicated in cases of early-onset but not late-onset conduct disorder. Genetic research has suggested an association with the DRD4 gene in children with attention-deficit hyperactivity disorder (ADHD) and concurrent conduct disorder; genetic research also suggests that this comorbidity is unlikely to be due to environmental influences independent of ADHD.

There are indications that the severity of conduct problems at a young age is associated with an increased risk of dropping out of school and unemployment by age 18 years. A substantial component of these associations may be explained by confounding factors that affect early conduct problems and opportunity later in life, such as intelligence, attention problems, and socioeconomic disadvantage. Research suggests that linkage between early conduct problems and educational underachievement and unemployment (after adjustment for confounders) is mediated by a series of adolescent behavioral processes that include patterns of peer affiliations, substance use, truancy, and problems with school authority. Increasing severity of childhood conduct problems also contributes to the risk of developing borderline and antisocial personality disorders.

Extensive comorbidity of conduct disorder with other disorders, such as depression and substance abuse, has been documented and has significant adverse effects on prognosis. Clinically significant subtypes also exist according to the age of onset (e.g., childhood-onset and adolescent-onset types), overt or covert conduct problems, and levels of restraint exhibited under stress. Conduct disorder may exist in a large portion of young patients with bipolar disorder, and in such cases the clinical presentation becomes confusing and possibly accounts for some of the documented failure to detect bipolar disorder. Conduct disorder in bipolar youths appears to be associated with a somewhat worse clinical course, and its presence may identify a subtype of very early-onset bipolar disorder.

The review of available data about the use of medication for conduct disorder in young people reveals that investigated compounds belong mainly to three classes of psychotropic drugs: mood stabilizers, neuroleptics, and stimulants (six, five, and six controlled studies, respectively). Lithium is the most documented treatment (three-fourths of trials report positive results). Lithium has been shown to be effective in treating severe aggression in children and adolescents with conduct disorder. When prescribed judiciously with careful monitoring, it can be an important part of a comprehensive treatment program. Conventional neuroleptics have also been commonly prescribed (3 of 3 studies reported positive results), and atypical neuroleptics appear promising (2 of 2 studies reported positive results). Methylphenidate improves some symptoms of conduct disorder, even in the absence of ADHD (6 of 6 studies reported positive results). Additional compounds such as carbamazepine and propranolol have also been studied and may yield some benefit. There is only a paucity of trials with antidepressants, and the evidence for their therapeutic role in pharmacotherapy of conduct disorder is still limited. Treatment should be individualized to each patient's specific condition. To be effective, treatment must address multiple foci and should continue for an extended period. Early treatment and prevention seem to improve outcomes.

Evidence suggests that family and parenting interventions also have beneficial effects on reducing criminal activity and time spent in institutions. Two forms of behavior therapy are currently seen as the most effective: parent management training and training in problem-solving skills. Parent management training assists parents in learning appropriate ways to reward positive behaviors and to prevent disruptive behaviors. Parent management training is the treatment of choice for younger children, whereas for older children it should be supplemented with training in problem-solving skills. Parent management training is one of the best-researched therapy techniques for conduct disorder, endorsed as an "empirically supported treatment" by the American Psychological Association (APA). Training in problem-solving skills is a behavior therapy that helps children learn to prioritize, to refrain from impulsive behaviors, and to consider alternative behaviors. It has led to therapeutic change in clinical samples and is characterized as a "probably efficacious treatment" by the APA. To optimize treatment efficacy, other complex prevention programs have also been developed in recent years. Results to date are mixed, but two large ongoing studies, the FAST and the LIFT studies, report positive preliminary results.

The FAST study is a conduct-problem prevention trial using a combination of social skills and anger-control training, academic tutoring, parent training, and home visiting over the course of several years. The LIFT study (Linking the Interests of Families and Teachers) uses a 10-week intervention that consists of parent training, a classroom-based social skills program, a playground behavioral program, and systematic communication between teachers and parents. The LIFT study was designed for elementary school children and their families living in at-risk neighborhoods with high rates of juvenile delinquency. In the future, conduct disorder and related problems in children and adolescents should receive higher priority for research funding and psychotherapeutic services.

Pearls

1. Patients with childhood-onset type of conduct disorder are more likely to be physically aggressive and to have disturbed peer relationships than those with adolescent-onset type. They are also more likely to have persistent conduct problems and to develop antisocial personality disorder.
2. Data from longitudinal studies indicate that children with speech and language delays are at higher risk for developing psychiatric disorders. It has also been suggested that some psychiatric disorders may indirectly be a result of speech and language impairment and that there is a probable correlation between certain types of speech and language problems and the type of psychiatric difficulty.
3. The treatment for children with conduct disorder should be multimodal and include behavioral and psychopharmacologic therapies. Limitations of both treatments include poor adherence and the fact that many youth may improve but still remain outside the range of age-appropriate functioning. There is currently no FDA-approved medication for conduct disorder.

REFERENCES

1. Brezinka V: Behavior therapy in children with aggressive dyssocial disorders. Zeitschrift fur Kinder- und Jugendpsychiatrie Psychotherapie 2002;30(1):41–50.
2. Gerardin P, Cohen D, Mazet P, Flament M: Drug treatment of conduct disorder in young people. Eur Neuropsychopharmacol 2002;12(5):361–370.
3. Steiner H, Dunne JE: Practice parameters for the assessment and treatment of children and adolescents with conduct disorder. American Academy of Child and Adolescent Psychiatry. J Am Acad Child Adolesc Psychiatry 1997;36(10 Suppl):122–139.

PATIENT 7

A 49-year-old man with generalized muscle weakness and paranoid ideation

History of Present Illness: A 49-year-old-man is brought to the emergency department by emergency medical services (EMS) with complaints of progressive weakness in his upper and lower extremities bilaterally. The symptoms began approximately 1 day prior to the current presentation, and the patient reports being in good health previously. The weakness began in both legs and arms simultaneously and became progressively more debilitating over the following 15 hours, until the patient eventually called EMS. To explain why he had become virtually paralyzed, the patient reported being poisoned by the police department. He described recently filing a lawsuit against the police for discrimination, and he now believed that they were taking revenge. He also noticed that a lock on the door of his apartment was broken a few weeks before and that since then his food has tasted different. The patient denied any mood, sleep, or appetite disturbance and also denied any history of hallucinations or other psychiatric symptoms.

During the initial evaluation, the patient became loud and verbally abusive to staff, accusing them of refusing to examine his arms and legs. A psychiatry consult was called, and the patient received haloperidol, lorazepam, and benztropine intramuscularly for agitation. The patient fell asleep and awoke several hours later complaining of worsening generalized muscle weakness and fatigue, consistent with the initial presentation. He also described difficulty breathing. On further questioning, the patient admitted to having an upper respiratory infection 1 week prior to presentation.

Past Psychiatric History: The patient denied any past psychiatric history. He has never had any contact with a psychiatrist, has never been hospitalized, and has never received any psychiatric treatment. He also denied any history of suicidality, violence, or substance abuse.

Past Medical History: The patient denies any past medical illness, has no chronic medical problems or allergies, and takes no medications on a regular basis. He reported having a brief episode of the "flu" recently.

Social History: The patient was born in Cuba and immigrated to the United States at 6 years of age. He graduated from high school and then attended college for 2 years without receiving a degree. He is divorced and has an adult daughter who lives in another state. When asked about the divorce, he evades questions but states that he has a lawsuit pending against his ex-wife and cannot discuss the details. The patient reports being self-employed as a freelance writer and is currently supported by public assistance. He denies any legal history or criminal activity.

Physical Examination: Vital signs were stable, and the patient was afebrile. He was in apparent distress, however, and reported shortness of breath and extreme weakness in all 4 extremities. Lung exam showed bilateral, diffuse, expiratory wheezing. Physical exam was otherwise unremarkable: his pupils were equal and reactive to light and accommodation, extraocular movements were intact, and there were no signs of trauma, lymphadenopathy, or jugular venous distention. His heart had regular rate and rhythm without evidence of a murmur; abdominal exam revealed a soft, nontender, nondistended abdomen, with positive bowels sounds, and no signs of rebound or guarding. There was no evidence of clubbing, cyanosis, or edema on exam of the extremities.

Neurologic Examination: Motor strength was 0/5 bilaterally in both upper and lower extremities. Deep tendon reflexes were also absent in all extremities. The patient was otherwise alert and oriented, with clear sensorium, intact cranial nerves, and no other focal neurologic deficits.

Laboratory Findings: Complete blood count: WBC = 16.0; Hgb = 14.4; Hct = 42.2; platelets = 383. Chemistry: Na^+ = 132; K^+ = 3.2; Cl^- = 104; CO_2 = 23; BUN = 5; creatinine = 0.5; glucose = 113. Blood oxygen saturation was 72% on pulse oximetry.

Mental Status Examination: The patient is a disheveled, unkempt, middle-aged man who is poorly related. He was calm and cooperative throughout the interview but was noted to have been "uncooperative with examination of his motor function," according to the emergency department chart. The patient's speech was of normal volume and rate. His mood was described as "OK," although his affect was dysphoric, incongruent, and inappropriate to the content of his speech. Thought process was circumstantial and overinclusive of details, and thought content was disturbed by clear paranoid delusions about the police poisoning his food. The patient denied hallucinations and suicidal or homicidal ideation. His insight and judgment were poor. The patient's concentration and memory were grossly intact, and he was alert and oriented to person, place, and time.

Questions: What is the diagnosis? What mistake was made early in the management of this case?

Diagnosis: Acute inflammatory demyelinating polyradiculoneuropathy (AIDP), also known as Guillain-Barré syndrome (GBS).

Discussion: AIDP was first described in 1916 by Guillain, Barré, and Strahl. It is now the most common cause of acute paralysis in the Western world with a yearly incidence of approximately 1.5 to 5 per 100,000. In the majority of cases, it is preceded by an acute infection, often of the respiratory tract, as in the present patient. AIDP may also be associated with vaccination, surgery, pregnancy, and malignancy. The exact pathogenesis remains unclear, but it is known that the demyelination of peripheral nerves occurs as a result of an autoimmune reaction triggered in most cases by an acute viral or bacterial infection.

AIDP is mostly a motor neuropathy. Muscle weakness usually starts in the lower extremities and progresses upward, usually within a few days after the initial onset of symptoms. Weakness may involve all extremities simultaneously. In some cases, cranial nerves and respiratory muscles may also be affected. This patient suffered from an atypical form of AIDP that involved all of his extremities at once and progressed rapidly to respiratory failure. Occasionally, other motor abnormalities can be seen, such as, fasciculations, myokymia, pseudospasticity, and ptosis. The absence of or decrease in deep tendon reflexes is a hallmark of the disease. Although not typical, sensory abnormalities may also be seen, such as, numbness, parasthesias, decreased vibratory sensation, and proprioceptive deficits. The nerves of the autonomic nervous system are often involved and may lead to cardiovascular complications. Patients may suffer from hypotension, and cardiac arrhythmias may develop, resulting in sudden death.

Laboratory abnormalities typically include cerebrospinal fluid (CSF) findings such as elevated CSF protein with normal cell count. Electromyography (EMG) is nonspecific but may show nerve conduction abnormalities with slowing, block, and temporal dispersion. The diagnosis of AIDP is primarily based on the clinical picture, but difficult cases can be supported by EMG findings and CSF changes.

The differential diagnosis includes Lyme disease, poliomyelitis, diphteria, vasculitis, and other neuropathies. This patient tested negative for Lyme disease. AIDP also needs to be differentiated from psychiatric illness, and conversion disorder is probably first on the list of differentials. Careful neurologic examination is therefore necessary. In AIDP, the neurologic exam shows absence of deep tendon reflexes and decreased muscle tone, as in this patient. In conversion disorder, the neurologic exam is normal.

The treatment for AIDP is supportive. All patients have to be closely monitored because respiratory failure and cardiovascular complications may develop at any stage of the disease. If a patient develops respiratory failure, intubation and mechanical ventilation should commence immediately. Beta blockers are appropriate for associated hypertension, but hypotension is usually transient and does not require specific treatment. Patients may need frequent suctioning of secretions from upper airways, and if swallowing is impaired, gastrostomy may be required. Fluid balance and nutrition should be provided, and the prevention of urinary tract infection, respiratory infection, decubitous ulcers, and pulmonary embolism is a priority. Plasmaphoresis and immunoglobulins are also used as immunotherapy. Eventually, physical and occupational therapies are essential to restore motor function. The course of AIDP is usually progressive over the first 1 to 2 weeks, followed by a gradual recovery, which is complete in the majority of cases.

In the current case, 100% oxygen was administered by mask immediately on discovering that the patient's oxygen saturation was only 72% on pulse oximetry. The patient was urgently transferred to the neurology intensive care unit. He was treated with plasmaphoresis with good response and received appropriate supportive care. After 10 days, he was successfully extubated. Physical therapy was begun, and the patient's motor function was restored to the point that he was ambulating by the day of his discharge.

While on the neurology service, the patient was followed by the psychiatric consultation liaison team. The diagnosis of delusional disorder was confirmed, based on the history of nonbizarre paranoid delusions that did not impair his functioning outside the context of the delusion itself. It is also interesting to note how the patient incorporated his medical condition into his delusional system, where his progressive paralysis confirmed the fact that his food was poisoned. The patient was prescribed olanzapine but refused to take it. Despite his delusions, he did not present a danger to himself or others, and he was discharged with a plan to continue psychiatric treatment as an outpatient.

The mortality in AIDP may approach 5% of cases and is usually due to cardiac arrhythmias, cardiac infarction, sepsis, pulmonary embolism, and aspiration. As was the case with this patient, the majority of patients recover without sequelae and are able to return to work within about 1 year. Unfortunately, in this case a formal neurologic examination was not done immediately. This omission led to the erroroneous assumption that the patient's primary problem was psychiatric and delayed appropriate care. He was also medicated with lorazepam, which placed him at additional risk for respiratory failure. The patient survived due to subsequent intubation and ventilation, good supportive care, and plasmaphoresis.

Pearls

1. Some forms of AIDP are atypical, with fulminant progression to paralysis and simultaneous involvement of all extremities.
2. Conversion disorder is a diagnosis of exclusion; therefore, a formal neurologic evaluation is mandatory in all patients presenting with motor impairment.
3. Benzodiazepines and barbiturates should be strictly avoided in suspected AIDP, because administration may contribute to respiratory compromise.
4. Medical conditions may be overlooked in patients with mental illness due to bias of the medical staff.

REFERENCES

1. Conway C.R., Bollini A.M., Graham B.G., Keefe R.S.E., Schiffman S.S.,McEvoy J.P. Sensory acuity and reasoning in delusional disorder. Comprehensive Psychiatry, 2002; 43(3): 175–8.
2. Ferraro– Herrera A., Kern H.B., & Nagler W. Autonomic dysfunction as the presenting feature of Guillain-Barré syndrome. Archives of Physical Medicine and Rehabilitation, 1997; 78(7): 777–79.
3. Halles J, Bredkjær C, Friis M: Guillain-Barré syndrome: Diagnostic criteria, epidemiology, clinical course and prognosis. Acta Neurol Scand 1988;78(2):118–122.
4. Parry GJ: Guillain-Barré Syndrome. New York, Thieme Medical Publishers, 1993.
5. Ropper AH, Wijdicks EFM, Truax BT: Guillain-Barré Syndrome. Philadelphia, F.A. Davis, 1991.
6. Taly AB, Gupta SK, Vasanth A, et al: Critically ill Guillain-Barré syndrome. J Assoc Physicians India 1994;42(11):871–874.

PATIENT 8

A 32-year-old man with depressed mood

History of Present Illness: A 32-year-old fashion photographer presented to an outpatient psychiatrist seeking therapy because of feelings of depression related to recent separation from his girlfriend of 4 months. He ended the relationship 1 month ago after his girlfriend, a fashion model, agreed to work for a photographer other than himself. He felt that she was becoming jealous of his fame. He described her as unwilling to make sacrifices for him and unable to appreciate the importance of his career. "She would insist that our relationship wasn't progressing because I was only concerned about myself." He complained that his ex-girlfriend became too dependent on him, requiring too much attention and time.

The patient met his girlfriend at a fashion event and described their initial relationship as "great." He felt that "she really understood the type of person that I am and how important my work is to the fashion industry as a whole." He spoke of initially being able to spend hours with her discussing his photographic vision and its influence on modern fashion. Mr. D described his girlfriend as "the best in the business when he was dating her" and expressed regret that she was not able to handle his fame but denied any responsibility for the deterioration in their relationship.

The patient describes sadness since separating from his girlfriend and reports feeling emptiness "like something is missing from my life." He has difficulty falling asleep and wakes up earlier than usual, getting only 4 to 5 hours of sleep at night. He complains of feeling tired with decreased energy during the day. Although he reports a lack of interest in most activities, he continues to exercise and attend social events. He also describes getting frustrated easily with other people and having ongoing conflicts with coworkers. He is working at his fourth job this year after abruptly quitting the previous three.

The patient also reports periods when he feels particularly powerful and sometimes fantasizes that he can do almost anything. During these periods he is slightly more productive but does not engage in excessive risk-taking or pleasure-seeking behavior. He admits to using cocaine intermittently over the past 10 years and describes increased use since the relationship ended. He denies any history of work-related or legal problems in connection to his cocaine use: "I'm not one of those junkies. I only snort cocaine to enhance my creative abilities and put me at ease."

Past Psychiatric History: The patient was in psychiatric treatment 3 years before the current presentation for depressed mood after being terminated from a job at a leading magazine. He saw a therapist and described the experience as initially productive. He appreciated the opportunity to express his feelings, but as the therapist began to challenge his defense mechanisms, he felt uncomfortable and terminated therapy after only 2 months. One year ago, he was prescribed sertraline (50 mg daily) by his primary care physician, who urged him to follow-up with a psychiatrist. He discontinued the sertraline on his own after 6 weeks because he noted minimal effect.

The patient describes himself as an ambitious, driven person who was born to succeed. He was raised in a chaotic environment with parents who argued frequently. His father abused alcohol and could be "charming one minute and then go into a rage the next." He describes feeling that his parents never expressed enough love for him and were not sufficiently nurturing. He nevertheless performed well in high school and college, majoring in photography and receiving significant recognition for his undergraduate work. He is currently an accomplished photographer, but mentors have criticized him for not accepting advice and becoming hostile at constructive criticism. He has also been accused by coworkers of being an exhibitionist who always needs to be the center of attention.

Mental Status Examination: The patient is a well-groomed man, with carefully styled hair and manicured nails. He is slim and appears physically fit. During the interview, he is initially concerned about the psychiatrist's credentials, closely examining the shingles on the wall. He appeared impressed by the doctor's education and told the examiner what he expected out of treatment and that he had "very special needs that must be met." The patient maintained good eye contact throughout the interview and was cooperative. His speech was normal in rate, rhythm, and volume but sometimes assumed a condescending tone. His mood was described as "down," and his affect was dysthymic and appropriate. When discussing his ex-girlfriend, however, he became visibly upset and angry. The patient's thought process was linear and goal-directed. He denied any disturbances of thought content, but he frequently had fantasies of punishing those who betrayed him. He denied any perceptual disturbances a well as suicidal or homicidal ideation. He was alert and oriented, with intact cognition, appearing intelligent, although with limited insight into the nature of his own behavior and how it affected others.

Question: What is the diagnosis?

Diagnosis: Narcissistic personality disorder.

Discussion: People with narcissistic personality disorder are characterized as having a grandiose sense of self and lack of empathy for others. The prevalence of narcissistic personality disorder ranges from 2% to 16% in the clinical population and is less than 1% in the general population, according to most epidemiologic studies. Children with narcissistic parents may develop an unrealistic sense of entitlement and self-worth and thereby are at higher risk of developing the disorder themselves. Most of the theoretical work on narcissistic personality disorder falls within the psychodynamic perspective, but recent research in psychobiology has given us new insight into possible causes of personality disorders.

The psychobiological model views personality as having many key components. Two of the most important are temperament and character. In general, temperament is thought to be the most heritable element of personality and to constitute the emotional core. Temperament traits can be seen in children at early ages and affect how they respond to certain environmental stimuli. Temperament traits start to stabilize by 3 to 4 years of age and are predictive of personality traits later in life. Character is determined not only by genetics but also in large part by culture, social environment, and random events unique to the individual. Character directly determines how we view ourselves and interact with the outside world. According to Cloniger, "temperament regulates what one notices, and in turn character modifies its meaning, so that the salience and significance of all experience depends on both one's temperament and character." A person's character is of paramount importance in determining whether an extreme temperament configuration will lead to a personality disorder.

The psychodynamic view of personality is descriptively similar to the psychobiological model but based mostly on the tripartite structure of the mind as described by Freud. This structure is encompassed by Freud's concepts of the id, ego, superego, and defense mechanisms. Psychodynamic literature describes character according to the concept of ego strength and defense mechanisms. Ego strength is defined by how a person consciously reacts to external and internal stimuli, whereas defense mechanisms are unconscious responses that protect the ego from anxiety generated by intrapsychic conflicts. The following points attempt to illustrate key concepts in the psychodynamic model of personality. Psychodynamic theory states that the components of personality grow and become organized over time in a way that allows for an organism to adapt. If interference occurs during development, a personality disorder may develop, or, as Kernberg describes, a "borderline organization" of personality can result. This borderline organization of personality is theorized to be a shared feature of all personality disorders, including narcissism. The idea of borderline organization helps to explain the observed overlap of symptoms in personality disorders.

In narcissistic personality disorder, this borderline organization leads to a poorly developed sense of self-esteem, and increased vulnerability to personal slights, real or perceived. In response, the person develops maladaptive behavior and uses immature defense mechanisms to guard vulnerable self-esteem. These actions are viewed as adequate and normal by the patient (ego-syntonic) and are generally focused on changing the environment, not the patient (alloplastic attitude).

In this patient, the diagnosis of narcissistic personality disorder was made based on the characteristic themes of grandiosity, need for admiration, and lack of empathy, which had been present in many aspects of the patient's life. In addition, this behavior was an enduring pattern manifested in how he related to other people and viewed external events. Although his insight is limited, his behavior has caused him significant subjective distress and clearly interfered with occupational goals (see Table 1 for more details).

Table 1. Comparing DSM-IV-TR Criteria to Examples from the Case Presentation

DSM-IV-TR Diagnostic Criteria	Examples from Case Presentation
(1) Has a grandiose sense of self-importance	Throughout the case, the patient spoke of his revolutionary vision for the fashion world, and although he was successful, it was not to the extent he claimed.
(2) Is preoccupied with fantasies of unlimited success, power, brilliance, beauty, or ideal love	We do not get a significant history of preoccupation with fantasies from this patient. This is typically very important, however, because many patients use fantasy to fulfill their narcissistic need for admiration
(3) Believes that he or she is "special" and unique, and can only be understood by, or associate with, other special or high-status people	This characteristic can be seen in how the patient initially views his ex-girlfriend as the"best in the business" and in his concern about the therapist's credentials.

(Cont'd.)

Table 1. Comparing DSM-IV-TR Criteria to Examples from the Case Presentation *(Cont'd.)*

DSM-IV-TR Diagnostic Criteria	Examples from Case Presentation
(4) Requires excessive admiration	This is evident in the many hours the patient may talk about himself and his need to be reassured of his ex-girlfriend's attention and devotion.
(5) Has a sense of self-entitlement	This is manifested in the patient's feeling that his ex-girlfriend should place his needs above her own.
(6) Is interpersonally exploitative	It was implied that the patient frequently used his girlfriend on his photo shoots to further his career without regard to hers. He did so without acknowledging her contribution and overvaluing his own work.
(7) Lacks empathy	The patient does not understand the feelings of his coworkers and does not realize that his ex-girlfriend's interests extend beyond his own.
(8) Is often envious of others or believes others are envious of him	The patient felt that his ex-girlfriend was jealous of him, although it was he who was jealous after she worked for another photographer.
(9) Shows arrogant, haughty behaviors	The patient's coworkers and mentors feel that he is an exhibitionist unable to accept criticism.

In the psychodynamic literature there are two predominant views on the clinical features of narcissistic personality disorder. Otto Kernberg describes the oblivious type of narcissistic patient, who tries to screen out the negative responses of others and impress people with accomplishments. In this way the oblivious type can protect fragile self-esteem from injury. The oblivious type serves as the model for the DSM-IV-TR criteria. Heinz Kohut, on the other hand, describes a type of narcissistic patient who tries to protect self-esteem by avoiding potentially harmful situations. Such people closely observe the actions of others in an effort to figure out how to behave. This careful monitoring of their environment helps them to avoid behaviors that may expose their weaknesses. They may be quiet and unassuming and often fulfill their narcissistic needs through fantasy. Although not emphasized in the DSM-IV-TR, it is important to note that both of these types exist; their common feature is the protection of a weak and fragile self-esteem.

It is also important to discuss the differential diagnosis, because many other personality disorders may be easily confused with narcissistic personality disorder. Antisocial, histrionic, and borderline personality disorders fall within the dramatic and emotional personality cluster and may exhibit significant symptom that overlap with narcissistic personality disorder. People with antisocial personality disorder can also be exploitative and lack empathy, although they are not as desperate for attention and typically have a history of criminal behavior. In histrionic personality disorder, patients need to be the center of attention but have less excessive pride and tend to be significantly more dramatic than people with narcissistic personality disorder. Borderline personality disorder may be distinguished by the presence of a fragmented and unstable self-image as well as unstable interpersonal relationships and affective lability. Narcissistic patients are typically more stable than borderline patients. They do not commit the same self-destructive acts, and their self-image tends to be more consistent over time. Narcissistic patients are able to tolerate changes in environment and relationships without the same fear of abandonment that is typically seen in borderline personality disorder.

Major depressive disorder, bipolar II disorder, and substance abuse may also be associated with narcissistic personality disorder. The patient described above, for example, would most likely meet diagnostic criteria for major depression and most probably abused cocaine. The distinction between hypomania and narcissistic personality disorder can be problematic. Both can show grandiosity in their presentation, but the hypomanic patient will have a history of significant mood cycling between episodes of mania or hypomania and depressive episodes or dysthymia.

The treatment of narcissistic personality is a significant clinical challenge. The course of symptoms tends to be chronic and lifelong, although traits may diminish after the age of 40. There is no consistent evidence that medication is useful in narcissistic personality disorder, but comorbid mood and anxiety states may be effectively treated. Insight-oriented and cognitive behavioral therapies have been found beneficial, but no conclusive evidence favors one approach over another. It is extremely difficult for such patients to relinquish the maladaptive coping mechanisms and defenses that they have developed because of their lack of ego strength and characteristically poor insight. Nevertheless, it is uniformly important to maintain a stable therapeutic framework; the therapist should be active and confront issues as necessary.

Pearls

1. The DSM-IV-TR describes the oblivious type of narcissistic patient, but a hypervigilant/sensitive type also exists. These two types may represent the opposite ends of a spectrum of narcissistic traits.
2. Narcissistic personality disorder may be distinguished from other personality disorders based on the presence of grandiosity intended to protect a sense of fragile self-esteem.
3. Although no one particular psychotherapeutic method offers a relative advantage, supportive psychotherapy should be avoided because of the tendency to reinforce maladaptive coping styles.

REFERENCES

1. Adler G: Psychotherapy of narcissistic personality disorder patient: Two contrasting approaches. Am J Psychiatry 1986;143: 430–436.
2. American Psychiatric Association Diagnostic and Statistical Manual of Mental Disorders, 4th ed, Text Revision. Washington, DC, American Psychiatric Association, 2000.
3. Gabbard GO: Psychodynamic Psychiatry in Clinical Practice, 3rd ed. Washington, DC, American Psychiatric Press, 2000.
4. Kernberg OF: Pathological narcissism and narcissistic personality disorder: Theoretical background and diagnostic classification. In Ronninggstam EF (ed): Disorders of Narcissism: Diagnostic Clinical and Empirical Implications. Washington, DC, American Psychiatric Press, 1998, pp 29–51.
5. Kohut H: The Restoration of the Self. New York, International Universities Press, 1977.

PATIENT 9

A 15-year-old girl with suicidal behavior

History of Present Illness: A 15-year-old girl is brought to the emergency department (ED) by her parents after taking "a handful of Tylenol pills." The mother reported that a few days earlier the patient had expressed concerns about an upcoming test at school for which she did not feel prepared. On the morning of the incident, the patient got out of bed about half an hour later then usual and complained of feeling tired because she did not sleep well during the night. The patient then went to the bathroom, and about 20 minutes later her mother found her on the bathroom floor crying and whispering, "I'm sorry, I'm sorry!" A bottle of Tylenol with about 10 pills left in it was found next to the patient. The parents called 911 and brought the patient to ED.

The patient reports feeling depressed "on and off all my life." She states that she had felt more worried and anxious lately because she was falling behind in school and experiencing problems with concentrating and completing homework assignments on time. The patient felt particularly concerned about a test that she was supposed to have on the day of the incident. She reported frequent awakenings during the night and remembered hearing voices telling her that she would fail the test. The patient claimed that in the morning she felt "not quite myself" and impulsively took a handful of pills. In the ED she reported feeling ashamed for "letting down my parents."

Past Psychiatric History: The patient has been in individual weekly therapy for sad feelings and crying spells since the second grade. No previous psychiatric hospitalizations were reported. Her pediatrician recently prescribed a selective serotonin reuptake inhibitor. She reported feeling "a little better" with the medication but noticed increased appetite and had gained about 8 pounds in the first 4 weeks after the medication was started. Due to concerns about weight gain she stopped the medication several weeks before the current presentation. The patient has expressed suicidal thoughts in the past but has never acted on them. No episodes of elevated mood were reported.

The patient is adopted, and no reliable family history about her biological parents is available. She was informed of her adoption years ago, and the issue seems to have been appropriately addressed through counseling. She attends regular education 10th grade class and is described by her parents as an average student, although working below her potential.

Past Medical History: The patient has a history of asthma during childhood but no other medical problems or allergies and takes no medications for any chronic medical condition.

Laboratory Examination: Complete blood count, chemistry, and thyroid function tests were within normal limits. Urine toxicology and urine pregnancy test were negative.

Mental Status Examination: The patient appears normally developed, moderately overweight, and fully oriented. She seems mildly somnolent but with good attention and concentration. She answers questions slowly and thoughtfully and does not speak spontaneously. Her affect is mildly constricted and appears sad. The patient describes her mood as "depressed for as long as I can remember." She also reports feeling chronically tired with heaviness in her arms and legs "like it's difficult to move them." The patient denies suicidal ideation and any intent or plan during the ED evaluation, but she did express suicidal remarks in the past, as reported by her parents. Both patient and parents deny suicide attempts in the past. The patient does not appear acutely psychotic, but when questioned she admits to hearing voices "telling me bad things about myself" that usually occur during night hours when she has difficulty falling asleep. She also admits to frequently feeling scared, as though "something bad is going to happen."

Questions: What is the diagnosis? What should be included in the differential diagnosis?

Diagnosis: Adolescent major depressive disorder.

Discussion: The essential features of major depressive disorder, as defined by the DSM-IV-TR, are the presence of 5 or more depressive symptoms for at least a 2-week period and a clinical course characterized by discrete depressive episodes without a history of manic, mixed, or hypomanic episodes.

As with other psychiatric disorders, most studies dealing with the genetics of depression have been limited to adults. However, several studies suggest that there is continuity between childhood- and adolescent-onset depression and adult depression. More direct estimates of the heritability of depressive symptoms or episodes in children and adolescents indicate that genetic contributions are greater than 50%. Twin studies have also suggested that depression in young people is heritable. Most researchers conclude that major depression in children and adolescents is familial but that the magnitude of familial risk varies according to a multitude of experimental factors.

This patient has been diagnosed with major depression based on the presence of symptoms of depressed mood, decreased concentration and energy level, impaired sleep, and suicidal thoughts and behavior. It is important to specify retrospectively the duration of the current depressive symptoms because a major depressive episode can also develop in the context of dysthymic disorder. Dysthymic disorder is typically characterized by chronically depressed mood for more days than not over the course of at least 2 years. It may be diagnosed in children when the mood is irritable or depressed and when symptoms occur for only 1 year. When major depression occurs on top of dysthymic disorder, it is known as "double depression." The results from the laboratory tests in the ED are helpful to rule out depressive disorder secondary to a medical condition, such as hypothyroidism, or a substance-induced mood disorder. A depressive episode in adolescence may also be the first presentation of bipolar disorder. The absence of any history of expansive or elated mood temporarily rules out bipolar disorder in the current patient. However, it is possible that in a 15-year-old girl with a major depressive episode, especially given the presence of psychotic symptoms, bipolar disorder may still develop. The presence of auditory hallucinations is notable in this patient, and the nature of the hallucinations should be elucidated, particularly whether their content contains any potential commands. It is therefore important to consider whether the diagnosis should also include "with psychotic features." The proper disposition from the ED setting for this patient is acute hospitalization for safety concerns.

Most adolescents recover from first depressive episodes, but different studies have demonstrated that between 30% and 70% experience one or more depression recurrences during adolescence or adulthood. Depression is more likely to recur in patients with a family history of major depression, comorbid dysthymia and anxiety, negative cognitive styles, exposure to family conflict, and abuse. Longitudinal data from studies examining adolescents with depression, 14 to 16 years of age, have shown that this population is at increased risk for adverse outcomes later in life between the ages of 16 and 21 years. Studies have also suggested that early depression is associated with an increased risk of major depression and anxiety disorders later in life. Findings from comorbidity studies demonstrate a close correlation between depressive and anxiety symptoms over time.

Results of magnetic resonance imaging (MRI) studies have shown that increased white matter hyperintensities in children with psychiatric disorders are predominantly located in the frontal lobes and are associated with bipolar, depressive, and conduct disorders. Volumetric MRI studies of mood disorders have revealed volume differences in the amygdala and basal ganglia of subjects with bipolar disorder and depression compared with controls. Volumes were increased in bipolar subjects and decreased in depressed subjects. A common finding to both major depression and bipolar disorder was a decrease in prefrontal cortical volumes. It has been suggested that underdevelopment of the prefrontal cortex leads to loss of cortical modulation of the limbic emotional network. This loss may result in unipolar depression or mood cycling, depending on the abnormalities of the subcortical structures involved. In functional MRI (fMRI) studies, decreased physiologic activity in the dorsal prefrontal cortex has also been demonstrated during major depressive episodes, specifically in areas implicated in language, selective attention, and visuospatial or mnemonic processing. In addition, these abnormalities reverse with symptom remission. Areas of "deactivation" during the depressed state may reflect neurophysiologic interactions between cognitive and emotional processing and may relate to the subtle cognitive impairments associated with major depression.

Community surveys evaluating the prevalence of emotional distress among adolescents who presented to a general practitioner's office showed that, although only 12% of patients presented with psychological complaints, about 50% of these patients had clinically significant levels of psychological distress, and 22% had suicidal ideation. Suicidal ideation is frequently associated with mood disorders. Suicide attempts occur 3 times more often in adolescent girls than in adolescent boys, but completed suicide occurs 4 to 5 times more often in adolescent boys. Adolescents with suicidal ideation typically have poor coping strategies and deficient problem-solving skills. Risk factors for suicide in adolescents include previous suicide attempts, male gender, a history of aggressive behavior, substance abuse, depression, and access to a gun. Risk factors for girls include previous suicide attempts, pregnancy, a history of running away, and a mood disorder. In the United States, the most common method of suicide among adolescents is the use of a firearm, which accounts for about two-thirds of suicide among boys and about half of suicides among girls. The second most common method of suicide among adolescent boys is hanging, and among girls it is the ingestion of toxic substances. The persistence of suicidal ideation or a family's inability to adhere to outpatient treatment requires psychiatric hospitalization to secure the patient's safety.

The overall findings of meta-analysis studies indicate that several different psychosocial interventions for childhood and adolescent depression result in clinically significant treatment gains. Treatment with pharmacologic agents such as antidepressants for depressed youths is only modestly effective. To date, research into the safety and efficacy of these medications has lagged behind clinical practice. Nevertheless, many adolescents are treated with antidepressants and mood stabilizers. Early evidence with the selective serotonin reuptake inhibitors is more encouraging than with tricyclic antidepressants (TCAs), for example, which have not been shown to be more effective than placebo in children and adolescents. Concerns about the safety and effectiveness of TCAs and the monoamine oxidase inhibitors have left disappointingly few pharmacologic treatment options for depressed children and adolescents. Recently, investigators have begun to examine the use of newer antidepressant medications in children and adolescents with major depression. Pharmacokinetic studies of sertraline, paroxetine, and nefazodone have been performed in depressed youths, and the results of these studies have provided data for rational administration strategies and also indicate that these agents may be well tolerated in children and adolescents. Further evidence that newer antidepressants are well tolerated by depressed youths has also been obtained in both open-label and double-blind studies. However, high rates of placebo response in depressed children and adolescents make such studies difficult to interpret.

Pearls

1. Recent MRI studies show significant differences in prefrontal cortical volumes in patients with familial and nonfamilial childhood onset of depression. Subjects with familial depression had smaller left prefrontal cortical volumes, and subjects with nonfamilial depression had increased left prefrontal cortical volumes compared with controls. These findings may suggest that cortical volume differences are a result of degenerative processes in familial depression and maturational irregularities in nonfamilial depression.
2. All of the new classes of antidepressant medications exhibit similar clinical efficacy; typically their side-effect profiles govern psychiatrists' decision making when treating adolescents.
3. Depressed youths who present with psychotic symptoms, psychomotor retardation, medication-induced mania or hypomania, or a family history of bipolar disorder are at increased risk for developing bipolar disorder.

REFERENCES

1. Drevets WC: Functional anatomical abnormalities in limbic and prefrontal cortical structures in major depression. Progr Brain Res 2000;126:413–431.
2. Findling RL, Reed MD, Blumer JL: Pharmacological treatment of depression in children and adolescents. Pediatr Drugs 1999;1(3):161–182.
3. Michael KD, Crowley SL: How effective are treatments for child and adolescent depression? A meta-analytic review. Clin Psychol Rev 2002;22(2):247–269.
4. Todd RD, Botteron KN: Family, genetic, and imaging studies of early-onset depression. Child Adolesc Psychiatr Clin North Am 2001;10(2):375–390.
5. Wagner KD, Amborsine PJ: Childhood depression: Pharmacological therapy/treatment (pharmacotherapy of childhood depression). J Clin Child Psychol 2001;30(1):88–97.

PATIENT 10

A 24-year-old man with paranoid thinking

History of Present Illness: A 24-year-old man, accompanied by his mother, is brought to the emergency department by emergency medical services because he has been "acting strangely" at home. When the psychiatrist goes to interview the patient, he is sitting quietly on the floor in the corner of the room. He is reluctant to speak with the psychiatrist but eventually agrees to be interviewed. He states immediately that he has done nothing wrong. With prompting, he begins to describe that he has been unable to leave his home for the past 2 weeks because he is frightened for his safety. "The computer store," he begins, "down the street from my house has been keeping records on me." When asked what kind of records, he replies, "records about everything." He notes that about 4 weeks ago, when he walked by the computer store, one of the employees nodded to him on the street. He was confused about how the employee recognized him, since they had never met before. The patient made a point of walking back to his house through an alternate route to avoid seeing the man again. Later that night, when he logged onto his own computer to check his e-mail, he noticed that the first site he visited contained an advertisement for the same computer store. He was shocked, he reported, as to how they had gotten into his computer to place the advertisement. He began to research the company on the internet and was impressed by how clever they were. No matter where he looked, he found no evidence that they were hacking into people's computers. He signed up for their site, hoping to gain access to more information, but after he signed up, he noticed that every time he logged on to their site, the page opened by greeting him with his own name!

He describes feeling as though "something else was going on." He reports thinking that the employees of the store were watching him, and he began to avoid the computer store altogether. Soon after, he noticed other people on the street looking at him. Even on buses and subways, he found that he was recognized everywhere. "How could they disseminate information on me so fast?" he asked. "It's almost unbelievable." Several days before the current presentation, the patient described seeing a man in a dark suit standing across the street, watching him. Suddenly he understood what was going on: "They think I know too much." When asked what he knows and why "they" would be interested, he became furious with the interviewer and began to yell, "like I would tell you, for all I know, you're one of them too!" Despite numerous attempts to elicit more information, the patient fell silent and refused to answer further questions, replying, "Go to hell, I'm onto you now," to each question.

Corroborative information from the mother indicated that his behavior had gradually begun to change over the past 8 months since he lost his job as a clerk at a local store. He began to spend all his time at home on the computer or watching television. "He would just sit there, staring at the screen, like in a trance. He wouldn't even respond if I called his name half the time." His mother had thought that he was depressed about losing his job, but when she asked him what actually happened at his job, he would only say, "Those bastards, they should all rot in hell." When the patient's mother eventually went to ask the owner of the local store what had happened, the owner told her that he was as confused as she, because one day the patient just stopped coming to work. The owner had not seen the patient for about a week, until he appeared suddenly to say that they were going to be sorry for what they did to him.

The mother reports that her son has always been a "good kid," and she is now frightened by what is happening to him. Recently she has had extreme difficulty understanding what he is talking about most of the time and has noticed that he gets angry with only the slightest provocation. He has been screaming at his mother and grandmother when asked even simple questions. He also stopped eating, was not sleeping well, and was no longer bathing or cleaning his room. For the past 3 days, the patient had locked himself in his room and would not come out. Finally, his mother became so concerned that she called EMS, and the patient was brought to the emergency department for evaluation.

Past Psychiatric History: The patient refused to answer questions regarding past psychiatric symptoms, treatment, or hospitalizations. He also refused to provide information about recent or past substance abuse. According to the patient's mother, he has no past psychiatric history and no known substance abuse. She describes his behavior as undergoing a significant change beginning approximately 8 months ago.

Past Medical History: Although the patient refused to cooperate with questions about past medical history or a medical review of symptoms, he has no known medical problems and takes no medication on a regular basis. The patient's physical exam was unremarkable.

Laboratory Examination: Complete blood count, chemistry, vitamin B_{12}, folate, RPR, thyroid function tests, and urine toxicology were within normal limits.

Diagnostic Testing: Computed tomography of the brain showed no evidence of mass, infarct, or bleeding.

Mental Status Examination: The man appears somewhat younger than his stated age. He is sitting in the corner of the examination room, disheveled and wearing dirty clothing. He has no abnormal involuntary movements, but during the course of the interview, he frequently looks up at the security camera on the ceiling. His speech is terse and loud but not pressured. When asked to describe his mood, he replies, "How would you feel?" He appears guarded and highly irritable, and his affect is appropriate to the content of his speech and congruent with his mood. He is perseverative on the topic of the computer store, and his thought process remains vague and evasive. He denies auditory or visual hallucinations as well as suicidal or homicidal ideation. When asked about feelings of paranoia, he states, "Oh that's great, go ahead and write me off as crazy. You'll see." He is oriented to place and time. His judgment and insight are impaired.

Questions: What is the diagnosis? What significant differential diagnoses should be considered?

Diagnosis: Schizophrenia, paranoid type.

Discussion: Psychosis has had multiple descriptions throughout the history of psychiatry, from a loss of ego boundaries to a formal thought disorder. Even within the DSM-IV-TR, there is disagreement about what constitutes psychosis in the definitions of the psychotic disorders. Psychosis is most typically defined as the presence of hallucinations or delusions, and this is how it is generally conceptualized by nonpsychiatric medical professionals. But psychiatrists tend to describe three constituents of psychosis: hallucinations, delusions, and formal thought disorder. Psychosis is then defined as the presence of any of these three constituents to the degree that grossly impairs reality testing. Of note, patients with a psychotic disorder typically have a clear sensorium, whereas other illnesses that might present with psychosis (e.g., delirium) are not categorized as "primary" psychotic disorders. Because the patient's sensorium was clear (he was awake, alert, and oriented), it was not likely that he was delirious. Furthermore, his medical work-up was negative, also supporting a primary psychotic process rather than a psychotic process secondary to a general medical condition.

Psychosis is a hallmark of schizophrenia, although it is by no means the only disorder in which psychosis appears. Numerous psychiatric disorders (see Table 1) and medical disorders (see Table 2) can present with psychosis.

Table 1. The Differential Diagnosis of Psychosis in Psychiatric Illness

Primary psychotic disorders
- Schizophrenia
- Schizophreniform disorder
- Brief psychotic disorder
- Delusional disorder
- Schizoaffective disorder

Mood disorders
- Major depression with psychotic features
- Bipolar mood disorder

Anxiety disorders
- Obsessive compulsive disorder
- Posttraumatic stress disorder

Personality disorders
- Schizotypal personality disorder
- Paranoid personality disorder
- Schizoid personality disorder
- Borderline personality disorder

Cognitive disorders
- Dementia
- Delirium

Other disorders
- Autistic disorder
- Factitious disorder
- Malingering

Table 2. The Differential Diagnosis of Psychosis in Medical iIlness

Substance-induced
- Amphetamines
- Hallucinogens
- Alcohol
- Barbiturate withdrawal
- Cocaine
- Phencyclidine
- Ketamine
- Wernicke-Korsakoff syndrome

Infectious
- AIDs
- Creutzfeld-Jakob disease
- Neurosyphilis
- Herpes encephalitis

Neurologic
- Epilepsy
- Neoplasm
- Cerebral vascular disease
- Huntington's disease
- Metachromatic leukodystrophy
- Normal pressure hydrocephalus

Metabolic/toxic
- B_{12} deficiency
- Carbon monoxide poisoning
- Heavy metal poisoning
- Homocystinuria
- Pellagra
- Wilson's disease

Others
- Systemic lupus erythematosus
- Acute intermittent porphyria
- Fabry's disease
- Fahr's disease
- Head trauma

The history remains the most important tool for directing attention toward a medical cause of psychosis. A thorough history and review of symptoms should be performed, asking specifically about medications, drug abuse, changes in appetite, fatigue, weight loss or gain, bowel habits, cold or heat intolerance, and sleep. Vital signs are used as a blunt screen for an infectious or toxic-metabolic abnormality. Altered blood pressure, heart rate, temperature, and respiratory rate can point toward specific medical causes, such as infectious, substance-induced, or toxic-metabolic. The physical examination is another good screening tool and should be performed on all patients presenting with psychosis, especially psychosis of acute onset in an emergency department. Findings on physical examination that suggest a medical cause include cherry red skin (carbon monoxide poisoning); moon facies, buffalo hump, truncal obesity with appendal wasting, and ecchymosis (steroid use); or dependent edema, dry skin, thinning hair, and goiter (hypo- or hyperthyroidism). Laboratory tests are obtained to rule out certain obvious medical causes of psychosis. Complete blood count, blood chemistries, vitamin B_{12}, folate, RPR, thyroid function tests, and urine toxicology are ordered for every patient. Other laboratory tests are done as appropriate and might include lumbar puncture, CT or MRI of the head, EEG, and heavy metal screen.

Multiple street drugs can induce a psychotic syndrome, and a detailed drug use history should be taken for every patient with psychotic symptoms, along with a thorough toxicology screen. PCP intoxication can look identical to schizophrenia, and patients who are cocaine-intoxicated can present with agitation, impaired reality testing, and hallucinations (typically tactile hallucinations of bugs crawling on the skin). Alcohol intoxication can present with auditory hallucinations, and such patients are particularly prone to acting on hallucinatory commands to harm themselves or others. Alcohol withdrawal, on the other hand, often presents with visual hallucinations.

Once medical and substance-related causes have been eliminated, the differential diagnosis of psychosis can continue along specifically psychiatric avenues. Psychotic symptoms may be present in multiple psychiatric syndromes (see Table 1), which can be divided by whether they are primarily psychotic disorders, mood disorders, anxiety disorders, personality disorders, cognitive disorders, or other disorders. Each of these disorders is discussed in detail in other cases in this text. The present discussion focuses on the differential diagnosis of psychosis with delusions as the presenting symptom. The major neuroanatomic and neurochemical findings, as well as the proposed causes of schizophrenia are discussed in case 12. For a discussion of the clinical features, subtypes, epidemiology, and treatment of schizophrenia, see case 11.

Paranoia was originally equated with any delusion, but it has come to be synonymous with delusions of persecution. Bizarre delusions are defined as fixed, false beliefs that are not only improbable but essentially impossible; they are typical of schizophrenia, paranoid type. In schizophrenia, there is often a mix of bizarre and nonbizarre delusions. Bizarreness is important diagnostically, because in delusional disorder, for example, the delusions are not bizarre. In delusional disorder, the delusions are also confined to a particular area or idea, and other areas of social and occupational functioning are not significantly impaired. In schizophrenia, on the other hand, the person's functioning is impaired in many, if not most, areas of life. The current patient not only has delusions but also has become impaired in occupational, social, and self-preservative functioning. In schizoaffective disorder, the symptoms are the same as for schizophrenia, apart from the presence of mood symptoms.

Patients with primary mood disorders can also be psychotic and may have delusions, hallucinations, or thought disorder. But psychotic features of mood disorders tend to be held within the confines of mood symptoms, and when the mood disorder has been successfully treated, the psychosis retreats. Delusions may also occur in major depression with psychotic features as well as in either the manic or depressed phases of bipolar I disorder. Delusions in mood disorders tend to be "mood-congruent;" that is, they match the mood of the patient. For example, a manic patient may have delusions of grandeur, whereas a depressed patient is more likely to have delusions that his organs are rotting inside his body. Similarly, patients with anxiety disorders who have delusions tend to have them specifically in relation to the anxiety-producing ideas or emotions. For example, a patient with posttraumatic stress disorder related to the attacks on the World Trade Center might present with the delusion that the security guards in the emergency department were working for the Taliban and were going to kill him.

Delusions in personality disorders have a somewhat different presentation. Personality disorders are defined by their persistence across time and context, whereas the axis I disorders (e.g., schizophrenia, major depression, bipolar disorder) tend to have periods of exacerbation and remission. That being said, in many of the personality disorders, delusional content is often vague and fluctuating with life stressors over time. However, in one personality disorder in particular—paranoid personality disorder—the delusional element is pronounced and persistent. A person with paranoid personality disorder has an unrelenting distrust and suspiciousness of others that spans across the person's entire interactional pattern. Such a person sees others as malevolent in general and interprets the actions of others as attempts at exploitation or harm. Similarly, the loyalty of friends is suspect, and hidden meaning is found in benign events. In the primary psychotic disorders, on the other hand, delusions tend to be more specific and often confined to a particular person or group of people.

The diagnosis of schizophrenia was based on numerous factors. First, the patient meets the criteria for active psychosis. He has positive symptoms (in this case, delusions as well as disorganized speech and behavior) and some negative symptoms (in this case, social withdrawal and avolition).

Second, consider the time course of his symptoms. He had more than 1 month of active psychotic symptoms, and, including the prodromal phase (discussed in case 11), he had significantly altered functioning for more than 6 months. He may have had some depressive symptoms initially, but it is more likely, given the progression of his illness, that these were early negative symptoms of schizophrenia. The patient was admitted to the hospital because his judgment was severely impaired by his psychosis, and he was a potential risk to himself and the community. Although at first he refused treatment, he ultimately agreed and was treated with antipsychotic medication—in this case, risperidone. Eventually he became less paranoid and developed moderate insight into the nature of his symptoms. The patient was discharged from the hospital after several weeks, and outpatient follow-up was arranged to provide psychosocial support and medication management.

Pearls

1. The social history is the key to differentiating delusional disorder from paranoid schizophrenia. The patient with delusional disorder is much less impaired in other areas apart from his or her delusion, whereas the patient with schizophrenia will have gross impairments in most areas of functioning.
2. The paranoid type of schizophrenia tends to have a relatively later onset than other types of schizophrenia. There also tends to be a somewhat better functional prognosis that may be related to the lesser prominence of negative and cognitive symptoms.
3. Syphilis used to be a fairly common cause of psychotic symptoms. Although it is rare to see such a case today, we still perform a VDRL for every patient with the first presentation of psychosis.

REFERENCES

1. Andreasen NC, Black DW: Introductory Textbook of Psychiatry, 3rd ed. Washington, DC, American Psychiatric Association, 2001.
2. American Psychiatric Association: Diagnostic and Statistical Manual of Mental Disorders, 4th ed, Text Revision. Washington, DC, American Psychiatric Association, 1994.
3. Sadock BJ, Sadock VA: Kaplan and Sadock's Comprehensive Textbook of Psychiatry, 7th ed. Philadelphia, Lippincott Williams & Wilkins, 1999.
4. Sims AC: Symptoms in the Mind, 3rd ed. Philadelphia, W.b. Saunders, 2002.

PATIENT 11

A 25-year-old woman found unresponsive

History of Present Illness: A 25-year-old woman is brought to the emergency department (ED), apparently unresponsive. She was found lying on a park bench by police, and when they could not arouse her, they called an ambulance to have her transported to the ED. Her vital signs are normal: blood pressure, 115/80 mmHg; heart rate, 76 beats/min; temperature, 98.6°F; and respiratory rate, 16 breaths/min. Physical examination reveals no signs of trauma or obvious injury. The patient is gaunt and looks malnourished. Her eyes are closed, and she does not respond to voice or sternal rub. Strangely, when the ED physician tries to move her arms, he meets strong resistance and moves her arm to a new position only with great effort. Even more to his surprise, he finds that her arm stays in the new position, even after he releases it.

Luckily, the patient had identification in her purse, which, with some prying, was taken from her on admission. The mother is contacted. The mother states that she is frightened after hearing of her daughter's condition because nothing like this has happened to her before. The mother is nevertheless relieved to know that they have found her daughter, who recently disappeared. Until about 3 months ago, the daughter lived with the mother but had not been seen since then. The patient's mother describes her as a cooperative child who never made unreasonable demands and was quiet and introspective while growing up. According to the mother, the patient finished high school and had started classes at a community college. However, she had to stop school after only one semester because of poor academic performance. She returned home and has not mentioned going back to college since. The patient spent most of her time doing clerical work in the family real estate business. She had become more withdrawn over the past year, but the mother interpreted this behavior as being "a little down" because her only friend had graduated from college and was now engaged to be married. Approximately 7 months ago, the patient's mother became more concerned because her daughter had become reclusive, missing work and often spending many days at a time in her room. She would come out only to eat a few morsels of food and then quickly retreat to the confines of her room. The mother says that at this point her daughter appeared preoccupied with whether the food she was eating had been "killed in a morally acceptable way." She expected her daughter to "snap out of it" but eventually told her that she was going to take her to see a doctor. The next morning the patient disappeared from her mother's house (3 months before the current presentation).

Past Psychiatric History: According to the mother, the patient has no history of psychiatric illness and, as far as the mother knows, never used drugs. The mother recalls a cousin with mental illness who is now in an "institution."

Past Medical History: The patient has no medical problems, takes no medication, and has no known allergies.

Laboratory Examination: Emergency lab tests reveal the following:

• White blood count	6,000
• Hemoglobin	13.3
• Sodium	141
• Potassium	4.1
• Calcium	10.3
• Magnesium	2.0
• Phosphorus	2.1
• Arterial blood gases	Within normal limits
• Pulse oximetry	Oxygen saturation of 97% on room air.

Diagnostic Testing:

- A stat CT scan of the head reveals no evidence of bleeding, mass, or infarct.
- CSF extracted via a lumbar puncture is clear.
- Preliminary CSF results from the laboratory demonstrate no obvious signs of infection; cultures and PCR are pending.

Mental Status Examination: The patient is a slightly cachectic-looking woman, lying with eyes shut on a stretcher. She does not respond to questioning or touch. She does not move spontaneously, and, when placed, her extremities hold their position. Limbs have cogwheel rigidity on flexion and extension. There is no spontaneous speech and therefore no way to evaluate mood, affect, thought process, or thought content. Orientation cannot be assessed, nor can judgment or insight.

Question: What is the most likely psychiatric diagnosis?

Diagnosis: Schizophrenia, catatonic type.

Discussion: Schizophrenia has a worldwide prevalence between 1% and 1.5%. It has an equal prevalence in men and women, although men and women tend to present at different ages and may have a different course of illness. The age of onset in men is typically between 15 and 25 years; in women, between 25 and 35 years. In general, women are thought to have a slightly better outcome than men, perhaps because men may have more prominent negative symptoms that more dramatically impair social functioning.

Schizophrenia has three main symptom complexes: positive symptoms, negative symptoms, and cognitive symptoms. The DSM-IV-TR focuses on positive and negative symptoms for making the diagnosis (see Table 1). Positive symptoms include hallucinations (sensory perceptions that do not exist in reality), delusions (fixed, false beliefs that are not amenable to contradictory evidence), bizarre behavior, and thought disorder (expressed as disorganized or illogical speech). Negative symptoms are symptoms in which behaviors that are considered normal are absent. Examples include affective flattening (decreased affective expression or responsiveness), alogia (impoverished thought), avolition (poor or absent motivation), anhedonia (decreased participation and interest in pleasurable activities), and inattention (poor social relatedness).

The cognitive symptoms of schizophrenia are the best predictors of functional outcome; they include impairments in working memory (the ability to hold information in memory to perform tasks), executive functioning (the ability to plan and execute plans), and intelligence (patients with schizophrenia have a mean drop of 10 IQ points shortly after their first psychotic episode). There is no pathognomonic finding for schizophrenia, and each of the active symptoms associated with the disorder may also be found in other disorders. Schizophrenia is, therefore, an amalgam of multiple findings: at least two positive symptoms or one positive and one negative symptom.

The time course of the disease is important for diagnosis and prognosis. Schizophrenia has a prodromal phase, in which the person presents as strange or mildly bizarre, with a withdrawal of interest in social activities and a possible preoccupation with internal ruminations or ideas. This stage can persist for months to years, and some evidence indicates that the occurrence of schizophrenia can be at least partially predicted from examining children for certain behavioral abnormalities. The second stage of schizophrenia is the active phase, in which the symptoms that are typically present for diagnosis are prominent (positive, negative, and cognitive). This phase is essentially one of remissions and exacerbations, often regardless of treatment. The third phase of schizophrenia is the residual phase, in which the positive symptoms have subsided, but the cognitive and negative symptoms remain prominent. To make the diagnosis of schizophrenia, the presentation of all three stages together must have lasted at least 6 months. If the entire course of the illness has lasted from 1 to 6 months, the most appropriate diagnosis is schizophreniform disorder; if the illness has lasted less than 1 month in total, the diagnosis is brief psychotic disorder. The fact that the current patient has been having active symptoms for more than 1 month, along with prodromal symptoms for greater than 6 months, makes schizophrenia the most likely diagnosis. The differential diagnosis of psychosis is covered in the discussion for case 10.

Table 1. Negative and Positive Symptoms of Schizophrenia

Negative Symptoms	Positive Symptoms
Affective flattening	Hallucinations
• Unchanging facial expression	• Auditory
• Decreased expressive gestures	• Somatic-tactile
• Poor eye contact	• Olfactory
• Affective nonreactivity	• Visual
• Inappropriate affect	Delusions
• Lack of vocal prosody	• Persecutory, jealous
Alogia	• Guilt
• Poverty of speech	• Grandiosity, religious
• Thought blocking	• Somatic
• Increased response latency	• Ideas of reference
Avolition	• Being controlled or mind reading
• Poor grooming and hygiene	• Thought broadcasting, insertion, or withdrawal
• Poor performance at work or school	Bizarre behavior
• Physical anergia	• Clothing, appearance
Anhedonia	• Social, sexual
• Decreased recreational interests, activities	• Aggression/agitation
• Decreased sexual interest, activity	• Stereotyped behavior
• Poor ability for intimacy, closeness	Positive formal thought disorder
• Decreased or absent relationships with friends, peers	• Derailment
Attention	• Tangentiality or circumstantiality
• Social inattentiveness	• Incoherence or clang associations
• Inattentiveness during testing	• Illogical speech

Schizophrenia also has multiple subtypes. For each subtype, the primary diagnostic criteria remain the same, and the subtypes are defined by which symptoms have particular prominence. The paranoid type is characterized by preoccupation with delusions or auditory hallucinations; importantly, flattened affect and disorganization of speech or behavior are not as prominent. The disorganized type is just the opposite: disorganized speech and behavior as well as flat or inappropriate affect are more pronounced than delusions or hallucinations. In the undifferentiated type of schizophrenia, there may be multiple symptoms consistent with several subtypes, but none are more pronounced than others. The residual type is defined by the absence or reduction of positive symptoms but a persistence of the negative symptoms.

The catatonic type of schizophrenia deserves special mention because of its complexity. Although previously common, it has now become somewhat rare in developed countries. The classic feature of catatonia is a disturbance of motor function. Patients who present with this subtype of schizophrenia can have catatonic stupor (slowed motor activity, often to a point of immobility) or be selectively mute (responding selectively or not at all to questions or commands). Interestingly, when patients present with selective mutism, they are often able to write answers to questions. The prototypic presentation is catatonic rigidity, a bizarre posturing in which patients assume strange poses that range from statuesque to grotesque; these postures are rigidly held for hours or days. These patients show catatonic negativism that is characterized by resisting movement by an examiner. If they can be moved, patients with catatonia often demonstrate waxy flexibility and maintain whatever new posture into which they are placed. This patient demonstrates both qualities: catatonic negativism and waxy flexibility. Catatonic patients can also have periods of intense movement or agitation, including repetitive, stereotyped behaviors (called stereotypies), and they can also alternate rapidly between stupor and excitement without warning. In a catatonic state, close medical supervision is necessary because patients can suffer from malnutrition, exhaustion, or hyperpyrexia. Catatonia is also not specific to schizophrenia. It can occur in any disorder in which psychosis is present, including bipolar I disorder and major depression with psychotic features. Furthermore, catatonia can present in many medical diseases that can mimic schizophrenia or cause psychosis.

Lorazepam is typically the treatment of choice for catatonic states, given as a 1- to 2-mg injection. This regimen often breaks the catatonia, but it may reappear and require repeated treatment. Alternatively, electroconvulsive therapy (ECT) is sometimes used to treat catatonia. Antipsychotics are typically avoided at first, because catatonia may initially appear similar to neuroleptic malignant syndrome (NMS) and akinesia, both of which are caused by antipsychotic medications.

However, the standard of care for the treatment of schizophrenia in general begins with the use of antipsychotic medications. All antipsychotics currently available are antagonistic at dopamine receptors in the brain. There are two main categories of antipsychotics: the typical antipsychotics and the atypical antipsychotics. All typical antipsychotic medications are considered equal in efficacy, although they differ in potency. All are antagonistic at dopamine type 2 (D2) receptors and exert their effects primarily on positive symptoms. Prototypic examples of typical antipsychotic medications are chlorpromazine (low potency) and haloperidol (high potency). The primary difference between these medications is their side-effect profiles. Low-potency antipsychotics tend to have more anticholinergic side effects (sedation, orthostatic hypotension, dry mouth), whereas high-potency antipsychotics tend to have more dopaminergic side effects (parkinsonism, extrapyramidal symptoms, tardive dyskinesia).

Newer antipsychotics also have varying degrees of dopaminergic blockade but impact other neurotransmitter systems, including serotoninergic, muscarinic, and alpha-adrenergic receptors. Readers interested in a more detailed discussion are referred to any standard textbook of psychopharmacology. For current purposes, let it suffice to say that atypical antipsychotics are generally considered equally efficacious as typical antipsychotics in targeting positive symptoms but may be more effective in targeting negative symptoms. The prototypic atypical antipsychotic is clozapine, which is also the only antipsychotic to demonstrate increased efficacy in schizophrenia. Clozapine provides a significant improvement in 30% to 60% of patients refractory to typical antipsychotic medications. This medication has a multitude of potential side effects, which include orthostatic hypotension, sedation, weight gain, sialorrhea (drooling), tachycardia, constipation, and tremor. Clozapine also carries a risk of very serious side effects, including agranulocytosis, seizures, hyperglycemia, and diabetes mellitus. Hence, it is used only when patients are refractory to other antipsychotic medications. Other atypical antipsychotics include risperidone, olanzapine, quietiapine, ziprasidone, and aripiprazole; each varies in its side-effect profile (see Table 2).

The advent of antipsychotic medications about 50 years ago revolutionized the treatment of schizophrenia. Before such medications, patients were typically institutionalized for most, if not all, of their

Table 2. Some Common Antipsychotic Medications and Their Major Side Effects

Medication	General Grouping	Some Side Effects
Chlorpromazine	Low Potency Typical Antipsychotic	*Common:* sedation, hypotension, jaundice *Serious:* seizures, agranulocytosis, aplastic anemia
Haldoperidol	High Potency Typical Antipsychotic	*Common:* EPS, akathesia, insomnia, sedation, weight change, gynecomastia, galactorrhea *Serious:* NMS, TD, ADR, seizures, jaundice, arrhythmia, hyperpyrexia, dystonia
Risperidone	Atypical Antipsychotic	*Common:* agitation, EPS, headache, constipation, dyspepsia, tachycardia, somnolence *Serious:* hypotension, TD, NMS, hyperglycemia, diabetes mellitus, seizures (rare), QT prolongation
Olanzapine	Atypical Antipsychotic	*Common:* somnolence, EPS, weight gain, asthenia, dry mouth, constipation, tremor, orthostatic hypotension *Serious:* hypotension, EPS (rare), TD, NMS, diabetes mellitus, hyperglycemia, seizures (rare), priapism (rare)
Clozapine	Atypical Antipsychotic	*Common:* drowsiness, sialorrhea, tachycardia, constipation, EPS, increased sweating, tremor, fever, weight gain *Serious:* seizures, leukopenia, agranulocytosis, NMS, TD, pulmonary embolism, hyperglycemia, diabetes mellitus, paralytic ileus, hepatitis, cardiac arrhythmia/arrest/CHF (rare)

NMS, neuroleptic malignant syndrome; TD, tardive dyskinesia; ADR, acute dystonic reaction; EPS, extrapyramidal symptoms

adult lives. Institutions were essentially cities unto themselves, with tens of thousands of patients in residence at any given time. With antipsychotic medications, the number of patients institutionalized has been dramatically reduced to a fraction of the original numbers. However, current pharmacologic treatments are far from curative or even restorative. Patients with schizophrenia remain functionally impaired to varying degrees throughout their lifetime.

Other interventions in the treatment of schizophrenia are primarily psychosocial. Individual and group psychotherapy, as well as structured, daily programs that provide vocational, social, and family education and support, have been used with varying degrees of success. These psychosocial interventions are now considered an essential component of the life-long care that most patients with schizophrenia require.

Pearls

1. When evaluating a patient who presents as unresponsive, always consider medical causes (e.g., CNS infection) and life-threatening psychiatric causes (e.g., neuroleptic malignant syndrome) first.
2. Some preliminary evidence indicates a genetic component in catatonia with linkage to chromosomes 15 and 22.
3. Electronconvulsive therapy (ECT) is considered by many to be the treatment of choice for pregnant women who present with catatonia.

REFERENCES

1. American Psychiatric Association: Diagnostic and Statistical Manual of Mental Disorders, 4th ed, Text Revision. Washington, DC, American Psychiatric Association, 1994.
2. Arana GW, Hyman SE, Rosenbaum JF: Handbook of Psychiatric Drug Therapy, 4th ed. Lippincott Williams & Wilkins, 2000.
3. Bleuler E: Dementia Praecox or The Group of Schizophrenias. Translated by Joseph Zinkin, MD. New York, International Universities Press, 1950.
4. Ferrill MJ, Kehoe WA, Jacisin JJ: ECT during pregnancy: Physiologic and pharmacologic considerations. Convul Ther 1992; 8(3):186–200.
5. Sadock BJ, Sadock VA: Kaplan and Sadock's Comprehensive Textbook of Psychiatry, 7th ed. Philadelphia, Lippincott Williams & Wilkins, 1999.
6. Stober G, Pfuhlmann B, Nurnberg G, et al: Towards the genetic basis of periodic catatonia: Pedigree sample for genome scan I and II. Eur Arch Psychiatry Clin Neurosci 2001;251(Suppl 1):125–130.
7. Stompe T, Ortwein-Swoboda G, Ritter K, et al: Are we witnessing the disappearance of catatonic schizophrenia? Comp Psychiatry 2002;43(3):167–174.

PATIENT 12

A 45-year-old woman in a shelter

As a consulting psychiatrist for a homeless shelter, you are asked to see a client who has recently arrived. The client is waiting at the door of your office and politely opens the door for you when you arrive. She states, "I have an appointment with you today," and begins to follow you into your office. When you ask her to wait a few more minutes, she replies, "Okay, sure," and remains standing directly outside your office door. When you call her into the office, she enters, smiling broadly, and sits down in the chair across from you, appearing very relaxed.

History of Present Illness: The client begins talking even before she sits down and reports the following: "I have had bad experiences with psychiatrists for the past year, so you will understand if I am not clear right away because the time that I told him of the things that he wasn't helping me with, he just kept raising my medication and it didn't help. I just kept getting worse and worse and not being able to think, and they all seem to think that the answer is just to switch medicines or to take away my kids, they are all grown now, but I didn't to raise them because they took them away, but I call them, but not anymore since they are grown. I don't even know where they are now, but I know that they are okay because they are good kids. When I was a kid I used to spend my summers in Asbury Park on the beach. Do you like the beach? It's nice, the beach, all the sand and sun. It was sunny yesterday, but today it's raining, which I don't like as much because I don't have a raincoat, but I will be getting one for Christmas, do you celebrate Christmas?"

She denies all psychiatric symptoms and states that she just needs a refill of her medication, olanzapine, which she has been taking for the past two years.

Past Psychiatric History: Corroborative information gained from the client's mother describes her as never being academically successful. She went to a special education school until the 10th grade, when she dropped out to have her first child. She has been in and out of relationships throughout her life, the longest of which lasted about 4 months. Each of her three children is from a different father, and she does not see them.

When she was 22, the client became very "depressed" after her only friend was killed in a car accident. Of note, the mother states that the person was not a close friend but someone with whom she worked at a local hardware store. At that time, the client was seen by a psychiatrist who prescribed sertraline. The mother is not sure whether the patient took the medication regularly, but about 2 weeks after starting it, she began acting "very strangely." She would sit and stare at the television, and even though the television was off, she would become highly irritated if someone stepped in front of the screen. Eventually she was hospitalized and started on "some other medications" with some improvement. Even with the medications, according to the mother, the client "has never been the same." The mother describes a course of illness that went through phases over the years. At times the patient would seem "okay," engaging in conversation and making sense for the most part. Then, all of a sudden, she would act like a different person; withdrawn; sitting around the house all day long; wearing multiple jackets in the middle of summer with gloves and a scarf; refusing to take her sunglasses off even at the kitchen table. At these times, the daughter's speech would get more and more confused, and she would have to go back to the hospital for a time. After about 5 years, the client left home, and now the client's mother hears from her only when she is hospitalized, which is about 3 times each year.

The client has a history of marijuana use that began at age 13 years but states that she has not used the drug in years because it seems to make her feel "funny in a way that it did not used to." She denies other drug use, including alcohol. She smokes one pack of cigarettes per day. The client also denies any current or past medical illness, and the internist who works at the shelter confirmed that there is no indication of medical problems, according to past records.

Mental Status Examination: The client is a middle-aged woman who appears her stated age, appropriately groomed with fairly good hygiene. She is restless throughout the interview, sitting on the edge of her chair most of the time and tapping her feet. She has no obvious abnormal involuntary movements. Her speech is mildly pressured, although she can be interrupted. When interrupted, she states, "I'm sorry," and falls immediately silent until asked another question. The rate of her speech is not fast, and the rhythm seems fairly regular. Her mood is euthymic. Although her affect is inappropriate at times and she laughs at peculiar moments, there are no signs of lability. Her thought process is moderately disorganized. Although one can follow her thought process with some difficulty, she is clearly tangential. She denies paranoid ideation, hallucinations, delusions, obsessions, ideas of reference, and other disturbances of thought content. Her judgment seems to be moderately impaired, as does her insight into the nature of her illness. She denies homicidal or suicidal thoughts or impulses.

Questions: What is the diagnosis? How is the patient's history different from a typical presentation of bipolar illness?

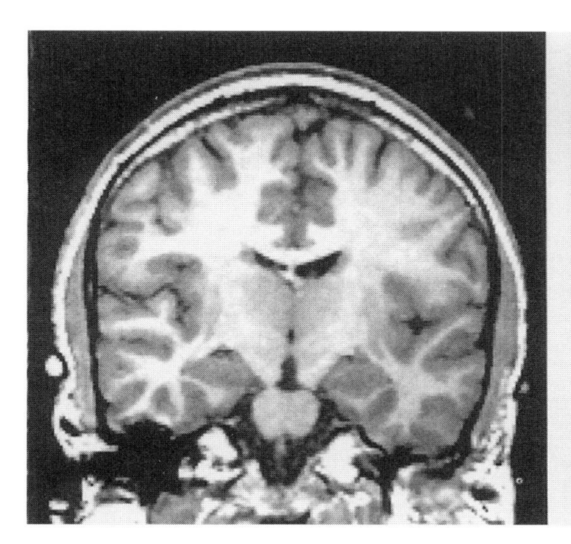

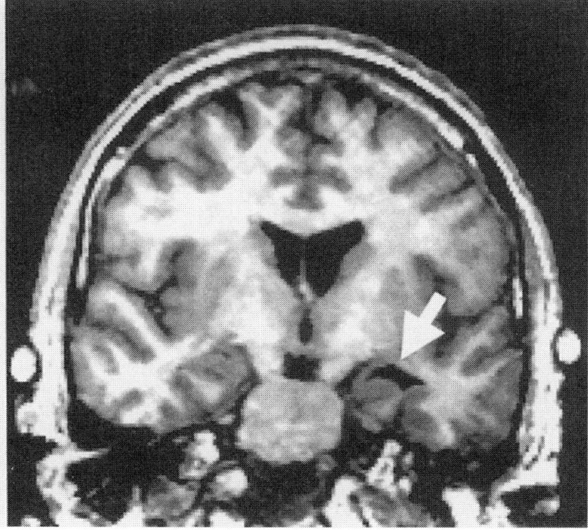

Magnetic resonance images of a normal control *(left)* and a patient with schizophrenia *(right)*. Note the increased CSF in the lateral ventricles, left Sylvian fissure, and left temporal horn *(white arrows)* in the MR image of the patient with schizophrenia. Furthermore, tissue reduction in the left superior temporal gyrus of the patient with schizophrenia can be seen in comparison with the control image. (From Shenton ME, et al: Abnormalities of the left temporal lobe and thought disorder in schizophrenia: A quantitative magnetic resonance imaging study. N Engl J Med 1992;327:604–612, with permission. Copyright 1992, Massachusetts Medical Society. All rights reserved.)

Diagnosis: Schizophrenia, disorganized type.

Discussion: The diagnosis is schizophrenia, disorganized type, but this patient presents a fairly difficult diagnostic challenge because many aspects of her case suggest either schizoaffective disorder or bipolar disorder. The diagnosis of schizophrenia requires 1 month of active symptoms (hallucinations, delusions, and/or formal thought disorder) as well as a total length of illness of 6 months, including the prodromal, active, and residual phases (see case 11). Although the pressured and disorganized quality of the patient's presentation might suggest mania, this type of presentation can also be typical of disorganized schizophrenia. Patients seem to move all over the place as they speak (tangentiality) with the inappropriate laughter and giddiness that can also accompany mania. However, clues in the current presentation and in the past psychiatric history favor a primary psychotic process over a primary mood disorder. For example, the patient's first presentation, although it seemed like depression, was unsuccessfully treated with antidepressants and developed into a psychosis. And even after treatment, the patient did not return to her premorbid state of functioning but instead remained significantly impaired. This aspect of the case raises the question of whether the client's initial presentation was actually related to the negative symptoms of schizophrenia (see case 11) rather than depression. Furthermore, patients with bipolar illness tend to function at or close to their baseline in between episodes of mania or depression. Patients with schizophrenia tend to remain impaired throughout their lives after the onset of illness, never returning to their premorbid level of functioning. Her subsequent episodes of illness did not appear to have a prominent mood component but instead focused on bizarre and inappropriate speech and behaviors. Although the diagnosis of schizoaffective disorder must be considered, there is insufficient information to suggest that the patient had a mood-related episode that meets criteria for a depressive or manic episode.

Often patients with psychotic disorders who are decompensating in the context of stopping their medication require inpatient hospitalization because the impaired ability to care for themselves puts them at significant risk in the community. However, this patient convincingly denied any suicidal or homicidal ruminations or impulses. Despite her impaired judgment and insight, the olanzapine was restarted in the outpatient setting, and the patient was monitored closely over the next few days. Soon after, she became more organized in her thinking and was clearly improving. This patient was able to avoid hospitalization and was counseled on the importance of continuing her medication.

The remainder of this discussion focuses on etiologic theories and neuropathologic findings in schizophrenia. For a review of the clinical features, subtypes, epidemiology, and treatment of schizophrenia, see case 11; for the differential diagnosis of psychosis, see case 10. Schizophrenia is most likely not one disease. This idea is entertained largely because findings about schizophrenia in neuroanatomic, neurophysiologic, genetic, and neurofunctional investigations are plagued by inconsistent results and because different patients have varying degrees of response to pharmacotherapeutic interventions. Hence, it is considered by most experts to represent a final common pathway of a multitude of diseases. However, there are some cardinal findings in schizophrenia, which are reviewed below.

Schizophrenia is currently viewed as a neurodevelopmental disease. In other words, it is believed that something occurs along the path of development of the organism to produce the illness. Whether this developmental abnormality results from a combination of genetic factors or from an environmental insult during fetal development, birth, or later remains to be discovered. But schizophrenia is now seen as likely representing the culmination of numerous factors that converge to produce the illness. This view has been known as the diathesis-stress model, which attempts to integrate biological and environmental factors in disease formation. A simplified explanation of this model suggests that vulnerability (diathesis) to a particular disease is acted upon by an environmental influence (stress) to produce disease. In this model, having the diathesis alone does not produce disease, nor does the stressor alone. It is therefore considered a "two-hit" hypothesis because both stress and diathesis are required to produce disease.

Several neuropathologic findings have recently been described in schizophrenia. An increase in ventricular volume has been shown in schizophrenia (see figure, p. 43) and may be a result of a decrease in axons, neuropil (the axonal and dendritic branches of neurons), or supporting structures (myelin and oligodendrocytes). There is no solid evidence for a global loss of axons in schizophrenia, although some neuroanatomic findings are consistent with abnormal patterns of axonal migration during development.

Reductions in the volume of various brain structures have also been noted in schizophrenia. For example, reductions in temporal lobe volume, including the hippocampus, parahippocampal gyrus, and amygdala, have been described. A decrease in the size of dorsal thalamic nuclei has also been found in schizophrenia, whereas examination of other subcortical structures has revealed no consistent findings. In schizophrenia, increases in neuronal density have been found in the prefrontal cortex—a part of the frontal lobes that is believed to be responsible for executive functioning. Various white matter-related findings have also been found in schizophrenia and are outlined below.

The discovery that antipsychotic medications are antagonistic at dopamine type 2 (D2) receptors led to the dopamine hypothesis, which has been the major theory of schizophrenia for the past 25 years. In this theory, dopaminergic overactivity or an increased sensitivity to dopamine is thought to be responsible for producing the symptoms of schizophrenia. Evidence that dopamine-releasing agents (like amphetamines) produce psychotic symptoms and findings of increased dopamine content and higher D2-receptor density in schizophrenia lend support to this theory. However, medication effects confound these results. Antipsychotic medications are efficacious primarily for positive symptoms, although some of the atypical antipsychotics have mild beneficial effects on negative symptoms as well. Unfortunately, providing relief of positive symptoms does not return the patient to a premorbid state of functioning. Such patients remain functionally impaired throughout life, suggesting that dopamine has a modulatory impact on the disease state but may be the downstream effect of some other, more far-reaching insult to the brain.

Phencyclidine and other N-methyl-D-aspartate receptor antagonists produce a schizophrenia-like psychosis. This finding has led to the idea that glutamate dysfunction is involved in schizophrenia, and accumulating evidence supports the theory that chaotic glutamate transmission may play a role in schizophrenia. Dysfunction of GABAergic circuits has also been proposed in schizophrenia, with data building for various abnormalities in GABAergic cell number, density, and function in schizophrenic brains.

White matter, specifically oligodendrocytes and myelin, have recently become the subject of investigation in schizophrenia. Ultrastructural abnormalities in oligodendrocytes and the myelin sheath have been described as well as a downregulation of myelin-related genes in the prefrontal cortex of schizophrenic patients. Furthermore, neuroanatomic investigations of white matter in schizophrenia using new MRI techniques have discovered abnormalities in both coherence and orientation of white matter in frontal and temporal lobes. These findings are exciting and may mark a new era in understanding the etiology of at least a subset of patients with schizophrenia.

Pearls

1. Patients with schizophrenia have been found to have problems with smooth visual pursuit. Although not universal, disinhibition of saccadic eye movements is frequently observed. Because eye movements are partially controlled by the frontal lobes, this finding is consistent with theories of schizophrenia that implicate the frontal lobe.
2. Patients with disorganized schizophrenia are often significantly impaired in their ability to learn information and to organize their thoughts and actions in meaningful ways. These cognitive impairments are considered poor prognostic factors.
3. In trying to differentiate schizophrenia from schizoaffective disorder, it is important to note that negative symptoms may present like depression and positive symptoms may present like mania.

REFERENCES

1. Friston KJ: Schizophrenia and the disconnection hypothesis. Acta Psychiatr Scand Suppl 1999;395:68–79.
2. Gluck MR, Thomas RG, Davis KL, Haroutunian V: Implications for altered glutamate and GABA metabolism in the dorsolateral prefrontal cortex of aged schizophrenic patients. Am J Psychiatry 2002;159(7):1165–1173.
3. Hakak Y, Walker JR, Li C, et al: Genome-wide expression analysis reveals dysregulation of myelination-related genes in chronic schizophrenia. Proc Natl Acad Sci USA 2001;Apr 10;98(8): 4746–4751.
4. Harrison PJ: The neuropathology of schizophrenia: A critical review of the data and their interpretation. Brain 1999;122:593–624.
5. Selemon LD, Goldman-Rakic PS: The reduced neuropil hypothesis: A circuit based model of schizophrenia. Biol Psychiatry 1999;145(1):17–25.

PATIENT 13

A 43-year-old woman with confusion

History of Present Illness: A 43-year-old woman walks into the medical emergency department (ED) naked and confused at 2:15 in the morning. On initial triage, vital signs are stable, but the patient appears to have an unsteady gait and tremor. The patient vomits shortly after being seen. She is oriented to person only, unaware of her location, the date, or any of the events leading up to her presentation. She cannot provide her address or any identifying information, except to mumble "depakote, lithium, Tegretol, lots," when asked what medications she is taking. She is confused at several points during the interview but never lethargic, and her thought process is disorganized. She repeatedly laughs inappropriately and does not appear concerned by the fact that she has arrived without clothing. She remains calm in the ED but does not understand why she is there or how she arrived. No prior charts are available to review the history, and the patient is unreliable due to confusion and unable to provide contact information.

It is a cold evening, with a temperature of approximately 45°F, and the patient is noted to be shivering. There are no other signs of hypothermia, and there is no evidence of bruising or physical trauma. Blood work is drawn, and a psychiatric consult is called.

Mental Status Examination: The patient is well-groomed despite being without clothes. She is wearing hospital pajamas and covering herself with a blanket around her shoulders. She sits calmly in a chair and is cooperative with the interview. Her speech is soft, mumbling, dysarthric, and almost incoherent at times. Her psychomotor behavior is affected by a tremor, but no other abnormal movement or agitation is observed. She appears euthymic and seems to understand questions related to her mood. Her affect is inappropriate at times; she smiles oddly with frequent laughing. Her thought process is disorganized; she does not answer questions directly and goes off on tangents or includes many irrelevant details in her responses. She appears internally preoccupied during the interview, frequently staring into space, although it is difficult to assess directly whether she is experiencing auditory hallucinations. There is no evidence of suicidality or homicidality based on observations in the ED. She is alert but oriented to person only; she is able to name the month but gives the wrong date and day of week. She is able to name the city but does not know that she is in a hospital and cannot identify her location.

Physical Examination: Temperature, 36.7°C; heart rate, 55 beats/min; blood pressure, 130/80 mmHg; respirations, 18 breaths/min General: She is a well-nourished, well-appearing adult in no apparent distress. HEENT: No evidence of head trauma. Pupils are equal and reactive to light, extraocular movements are intact, and the oropharynx is clear. Oral mucous membranes are dry, and there are no signs of goiter or JVD. Cardiac: Decreased rate to 55 beats/min but regular rhythm with no murmurs, gallops, or rubs. Chest: Clear to auscultation bilaterally. Abdomen: Soft, nontender, nondistended, with positive bowel sounds. Extremities: No signs of clubbing, cyanosis, or edema.

Neurologic Examination: Mild ataxia, coarse tremor, and hyperreflexia. Cranial nerves 2–12 are intact, but nystagmus is observed; strength is 4/5 upper and lower extremities; sensation is difficult to test; coordination is impaired.

Diagnostic Testing: Computed tomography (CT) of the brain: no signs of mass, bleeding, or infarct. Electrocardiography (EKG): normal sinus rhythm at 58, with T-wave flattening. Electroencephalography (EEG): diffuse slowing, no seizure foci.

Laboratory Examination: Complete blood count showed elevated white blood cells to 12.3, with no left shift. Chemistry showed mild dehydration; serum toxicology was negative. Liver, thyroid function tests, and urinalysis were within normal limits. Carbamazepine and valproic acid levels were undetectable. The serum lithium level was 2.3 mEq/ml. Alcohol level was negative.

Question: What is the most probable cause of this patient's confusion?

Diagnosis: Lithium toxicity.

Discussion: Lithium is the most commonly used acute and prophylactic treatment for bipolar I disorder. It is also used as an adjunctive treatment in resistant schizophrenia, major depressive disorder, and agitation. Serum levels are checked initially, with each dose change, and every 6 months once the patient is euthymic and stabilized. Values considered to be therapeutic are between 0.6 and 1.2 mEq/ml for maintenance therapy and between 1.0 and 1.5 mEq/ml for the treatment of acute mania. Lithium toxicity is considered a medical emergency and can result in death or permanent neuronal damage. It has become increasingly important for the general medical practitioner to become familiar with the pathogenesis of lithium toxicity, because several symptoms of early toxicity overlap with common side effects: fine tremor, gastrointestinal upset, muscle weakness, and EKG changes, such as T-wave flattening—all of which this patient demonstrated. Another common side effect is polyuria with secondary polydipsia. This side effect may develop in patients who have therapeutic levels as well as those who are overtly toxic. Polyuria with secondary polydipsia can be treated by decreasing the lithium dose, using sustained-release lithium, or adding a potassium-sparing diuretic, such as amiloride. However, with the addition of a diuretic, the lithium dose must be monitored carefully, along with potassium levels.

This patient had several of the hallmark signs of lithium toxicity. She presented with mental status changes and signs of neurotoxicity, such as impaired coordination and gait, tremors, muscle weakness, and hyperreflexia. She also had EKG changes, although T-wave flattening and bradycardia are commonly noted in patients who are not toxic. In this case, the lithium level was elevated. Alcohol intoxication also had to be considered in this clinical picture. In any patient presenting with mental status changes, the differential diagnosis includes central nervous system disorders, metabolic disorders, illicit drug or alcohol use and withdrawal, medication toxicity, overdose, primary psychiatric disorders, seizure disorders, and endocrinologic disorders such as thyrotoxicosis. In this case, a primary seizure disorder might be suspected due to the change in mental status and the fact that the patient may be taking two anticonvulsants, both of which were at undetectable serum levels. However, seizures and EEG changes can also be part of the lithium neurotoxicity syndrome. All of these factors must be considered in forming a differential, and in this case an EEG is warranted. Typical EEG manifestations include diffuse slowing, widening of the frequency spectrum, and potentiation and disorganization of background rhythm. To confound the diagnosis, however, EEG changes can also be seen in patients who do not have signs and symptoms of neurotoxicity.

Central nervous system toxicity is the hallmark of lithium intoxication. Acute lithium toxicity may appear clinically similar to encephalopathy or delirium because of symptoms of disorientation, distractibility, memory impairment, fluctuation of consciousness, sleepiness, incoherence, delusional thinking, and hallucinations. On neurologic exam, hyperreflexia, hypertonia, myoclonus, ataxia, and coarse tremor can be seen with moderate toxicity. As toxicity progresses, stupor, seizures, fasciculations, spasticity, rigidity, choreoathetosis, paresis, paralysis, and eventually coma may develop. Persistent or long-lasting neurologic sequelae have been termed syndrome of irreversible lithium-effectuated neurotoxicity (SILENT). The most common symptoms of SILENT are persistent cerebellar symptoms, but other manifestations may include persistent papilledema, optic neuritis, isolated downbeat nystagmus, peripheral neuropathy, and myopathy. A review of over 40 cases of this syndrome revealed a wide range in lithium levels from 0.25 to 7.4. In other words, patients who were toxic did not necessarily have what are considered to be "toxic" lithium levels.

Specific risk factors for developing lithium neurotoxicity at therapeutic serum levels are rapid dosing, concomitant administration of neuroleptics, preexisting EEG abnormalities, genetic susceptibility, and undetected or preexisting cerebral pathology. Women and elderly patients are considered to be at higher risk for toxicity. Any new medications or recent dose changes should be reviewed for a potential interaction and possible etiology of the toxicity. Chronic medical conditions that increase the risk of developing lithium neurotoxicity are congestive heart failure, diabetes, hypertension, and chronic renal failure. Some chronic psychiatric conditions, including depression and schizophrenia, may also increase risk. Other acute conditions that may increase the risk of developing neurotoxicity are infections, electrolyte imbalance, and hyperthermia.

Several commonly administered over-the-counter and prescription medications are known to affect lithium metabolism and result in higher serum levels. Many medications have been implicated, including nonsteroidal anti-inflammatory drugs (NSAIDs), angiotensin-converting enzyme inhibitors (ACEIs), calcium channel antagonists, diuretics, and antipsychotics. NSAIDs, such as indomethacin, have been shown to increase lithium concentrations by 30–59% in controlled studies. Aspirin, however, does not appear to affect steady-state levels. ACEIs have been shown to increase lithium serum concentrations and to increase the risk of subsequent toxicity. Nifedipine, a calcium channel antagonist, has also been shown to decrease lithium clearance. Thiazide diuretics are thought to increase lithium concentrations by increasing its reabsorption in the proximal tubule. In combination with antipsychotics, lithium treatment may worsen extrapyramidal side effects or increase the risk of their emergence. The risk of neurotoxicity may also be increased with concomitant lithium and antipsychotic treatment, although this combination has been found to be clinically useful.

Treatment depends on the severity of toxicity. Activated charcoal is not effective because it does not bind lithium ions. Initial management involves protecting the airway, checking chemistry to assess renal function, and ordering a lithium level to help assess extent of toxicity. Gastric lavage may be helpful in acute ingestion of lithium. Several studies suggest that whole bowel irrigation with polyethylene glycol to remove unabsorbed lithium from the GI tract may be helpful, especially with the sustained lithium tablet, although this technique may lead to further volume depletion. Volume resuscitation should then be the focus, using normal saline to reverse and prevent volume depletion. Patient must be monitored for hypernatremia during volume repletion, especially those with diabetes insipidus, which is a common side effect of chronic lithium treatment. The focus then shifts to removing the lithium from the body.

Hemodialysis is the treatment of choice for severe toxicity in any patient with coma, convulsions, respiratory failure, deteriorating mental status, or renal failure, regardless of the lithium level. Dialysis is rarely indicated with serum lithium levels lower than 2.5 mEq/ml; however, guidelines have not been firmly established. There is some debate about the preferred extracorporeal treatment modality for severe intoxication. High-volume continuous venovenous and arteriovenous hemofiltration may be preferable to intermittent hemodialysis, especially if the patient is hemodynamically unstable. Although continuous hemodialysis may remove lithium more slowly, intermittent hemodialysis bares the risk of a "rebound" concentration—a subsequent increase in lithium level after hemodialysis is completed. Despite evidence of moderate toxicity, the above patient remained hemodynamically stable, had normal renal function, and responded to volume repletion. Lithium levels and neurologic status were monitored in a medical setting until levels trended down to less than 1.0 mEq/ml and the patient's sensorium was clearing. It was determined that the patient had not attempted an overdose because the symptoms had developed over several days and were thought to be due most probably to recent medication changes.

Pearls

1. Lithium toxicity is not measured by serum level alone; patients may be lithium-toxic even within the therapeutic range of serum levels.
2. Lithium levels must be checked for 3 to 4 days, even after dialysis. This point is especially important to remember in dealing with a patient taking sustained-release lithium.
3. The most common change on EKG is T-wave flattening or inversion, which may be seen in up to 30% of patients and is generally reversible after cessation of therapy. However, lithium is contraindicated in patients with sick sinus syndrome, and, in rare cases, ventricular arrhythmias and congestive heart failure have been associated with lithium therapy.
4. On laboratory examination, lithium is widely known to cause a benign leukocytosis, and neutrophil and eosinophil counts may be elevated without affecting function.
5. TSH should be checked every 6 months, because up to 5% of patients will develop hypothyroidism.

REFERENCES

1. Adityanjee: The syndrome of irreversible lithium-effectuated neurotoxicity (SILENT). Pharmacopsychiatry 1989;22:81–83.
2. Finley PR, Warner MD, Peabody CA: Clinical relevance of drug interactions with lithium. Clin Pharmacokin 1995;29(3):172–191.
3. Groleau G: Lithium toxicity. Emerg Med Clin North Am 1994;12(2):511–531.
4. Kaplan HI, Sadock BJ: Lithium. In Kaplan and Sadock's Synopsis of Psychiatry, 8th ed. Philadelphia, Lippincott Williams & Wilkins, 1998.
5. Kores B, Lader MH: Irreversible lithium neurotoxicity: An overview. Clin Neuropharmacol 1997;20(4):283–299.
6. Okusa MD, Crystal LJT: Clinical manifestations and management of acute lithium intoxication. Am J Med 1994;97(4):383–389.
7. Timmer RT, Sands JM: Lithium intoxication. J Am Soc Nephrol 1999;10:666–674.
8. Van Bommel EF, Kalmeijer MD, Ponssen HH: Treatment of life threatening lithium toxicity with high-volume continuous venovenous hemofiltration. Am J Nephrol 2000;20(5):408–411.

PATIENT 14

A 52-year-old man with command auditory hallucinations

History of Present Illness: A 52-year-old man walks into the psychiatric emergency department with the chief complaint of "hearing voices telling me to kill myself and others." The patient reports a long history of hearing voices but states that this episode began a few hours ago. In response to the clinician's questions, he describes hearing two male and three female voices that seem to come from "outside my head." He states that he hears the voices "all the time" and that they do not "come and go." He denies any coping mechanisms to help reduce the intensity of the voices. He states that, although the voices tell him to "kill others," they do not specify whom he should kill. When asked what other things the voices are telling him, he adds, "They're telling me to leave my shelter." He also reports feeling "depressed" and states, "If you let me go, I'll kill myself or somebody else." The patient also volunteers that he sees "a refrigerator door opening and closing" and "little animals running around." He endorses all symptoms of depression, including decreased sleep, decreased appetite, poor concentration, hopelessness, feelings of worthlessness, and guilt. He was discharged from the psychiatric inpatient unit 3 days ago; at that time, he was without any psychotic or depressive symptoms. The patient reports that after discharge he returned to his homeless shelter and bought $200 of crack cocaine, which he used over the past 2 days. He also drank two 40-oz beers each day since his discharge.

Past Psychiatric History: The patient has a history of multiple psychiatric hospitalizations, and a review of old charts shows a prior diagnosis of major depressive disorder, recurrent, with psychotic features. He frequently is not adherent with outpatient appointments, and this problem has reportedly led to a return of depressive and psychotic symptoms in the past. He has an intermittent history of crack cocaine and alcohol abuse. He reports past heroin abuse and is currently maintained on methadone as an outpatient. He denies current heroin abuse, although he admits to being administratively discharged from several methadone maintenance programs when urine toxicology screens returned positive for heroin. He denies any history of violence but says that he has been incarcerated for drug possession and selling methadone. He has a remote history of three suicide attempts, all of which occurred under the influence of substances. Once he also took "a few pills" after an argument with his mother when "she was getting on my case." He denies being hospitalized after any of his suicide attempts.

Laboratory Examination: Urine toxicology screen: positive for methadone and cocaine. Blood alcohol level: 0.800

Mental Status Examination: The patient is a fairly well-kempt man who arrives with a packed duffel bag. He appears his stated age and has intense eye contact. He is initially cooperative, but as the psychiatrist becomes more inquisitive about his specific symptoms, he becomes agitated, stating, "Why are you asking me so many questions?" He appears restless and at times agitated during the interview, but when not obviously observed, he is seen calmly reading the sports section of the newspaper. His speech is loud but with normal rate and articulation. He describes his mood as "depressed," and his affect is tearful during the interview. He does not appear to be responding to internal stimuli. Thought process is logical and goal-directed, without any looseness of associations or flight of ideas. There is no evidence of circumstantiality or tangentiality. He endorses suicidal ideation but lacks a specific plan. He endorses homicidal ideation but lacks a specific victim, stating, "I'll kill anybody who gives me a hard time." He is alert and oriented, and concentration, recall, and retention are not impaired. The patient has limited insight into his substance abuse or his need for continued psychiatric outpatient care. His judgment is fair in that he is seeking medical care for his psychotic symptoms, and he reported to the ED when he began to feel that he "might lose it".

Question: Which diagnosis most likely accounts for this patient's presentation?

Diagnosis: Malingering.

Discussion: Malingering is listed in the DSM-IV-TR as a condition not attributable to a mental disorder. Rather, it is the intentional production of false or grossly exaggerated physical or psychological symptoms, motivated by external incentives. According to Philip Resnick, an expert in the field, "there is no other syndrome that is so easy to define but so difficult to diagnose."

The incidence of malingering is unknown, but it is relatively common. It is found most frequently in settings with large male populations, such as the military and prisons, although it can also occur in women. Malingering usually stems from one of the following goals: to avoid punishment (pretending to be insane at the time of a crime), to avoid combat (or conscription into the military), to gain monetary compensation (social security disability), or to gain admission to a psychiatric hospital to avoid arrest or for free room and board (also known as "three hots and a cot").

In the list of differential diagnoses, one should first consider factitious disorder, which is characterized by physical or psychological symptoms that are intentionally produced or feigned to assume the sick role. The motive in factitious disorder is primarily unconscious (i.e., the patient has a need to be taken care of by others), whereas the motive in malingering is an external incentive, such as shelter or escape from the police. However, many authors consider them overlapping syndromes because financial gain or avoidance of specific obligations may also be a potential motive in factitious disorder and psychological gain may play a role in malingering. Other differential diagnoses include hypochondriasis (i.e., preoccupation with the fear of having or contracting a serious disease), somatization disorder (i.e., multiple somatic complaints that cannot be explained by physical and laboratory examinations), and conversion disorder (i.e., motor impairment or neurologic symptoms that are unintentionally formed and unconsciously motivated).

Malingering is commonly seen with substance abuse, as in the patient described above. This patient would also meet criteria for polysubstance dependence (alcohol, opiates, and cocaine). With the diagnosis of malingering, it is often appropriate to consider personality disorders. Lying is one of the defining characteristics of antisocial personality disorder, and patients with histrionic personality disorder may use deception (or dramatic exaggeration) to enhance their approval with others. Exaggeration and lying are often also used by patients with borderline personality disorder to idealize and devalue others, and narcissistic patients may be prone to exaggeration to protect fragile self-esteem.

To make a diagnosis of malingering, one should look for symptom inconsistency. There may be inconsistency in the observed symptoms themselves. For example, this patient was quite distressed and agitated while talking to the examiner but appeared relaxed when he thought he was not being observed. There are also frequently inconsistencies between what the malingerer reports and how genuine symptoms typically manifest themselves. For example, the patient in this case states that he hears voices "all the time," while most patients with true hallucinosis report that voices are not continuous but intermittent. Also, most patients with chronic auditory hallucinations have coping mechanisms to help diminish the intensity of the voices (e.g., listening to music), whereas malingerers do not. Malingerers sometimes report that their auditory hallucinations contain stilted language and far-fetched commands, such as the patient in this case describing voices that tell him to "kill myself and others" and "to leave my shelter." In contrast, most patients with genuine psychotic illness report auditory hallucinations that comment on their actions or say that two voices are talking to each other. One should note that visual hallucinations are reported more frequently by malingerers than by genuinely psychotic individuals. Dramatic or bizarre visual hallucinations should raise suspicions of malingering.

The physician should also be aware of the absence pf psychotic signs on mental status exam. This patient's thought process was goal-directed and without any formal thought disorder. Malingerers are rarely able to feign disorganized speech, such as tangentiality, circumstantiality, neologisms, or word salad. Although some malingerers may successfully feign psychosis on specific tests, psychological testing should be obtained in suspected malingerers. Specifically, the Minnesota Multiphasic Personality Inventory (MMPI-2) and the Structured Interview of Reported Symptoms (SIRS) are the most useful psychological tests to ascertain psychosis.

In the management of a suspected malingerer, all efforts should be made to avoid becoming angry (a common response to malingerers) because it will disrupt the rapport and lead the patient to become more guarded, thereby confounding the clinician's ability to make a reliable diagnosis. After completing the examination, the physician may decide to confront a potential malingerer with his or her suspicions. The suspected malingerer should be given every opportunity to "save face." However, if the patient does not confess to malingering and if the physician is unable to confirm the diagnosis, difficult cases of suspected malingering in the ED may require inpatient hospitalization for diagnostic purposes. Careful and intensive treatment of malingered symptoms usually reveals the relevant and underlying issue. Interestingly, hospitalized psychiatric patients with genuine illness are quite astute in detecting a malingerer among them; they have been known to tell malingerers to stop acting.

This patient was admitted to an extended observational unit in the ED for 24 hours. His vital signs were monitored every 4 hours to ensure that he was not in alcohol withdrawal. He slept soundly at night and ate breakfast, lunch, and dinner, often complaining that the portions were too small. He also complained that staff were not helping him because his requests for benzodiazepines were repeatedly denied. The following day, he requested to speak with the psychiatrist, stating that "I'm just going to go if you're not going to admit me." The patient then admitted that he was not hearing voices and did not want to kill himself or anybody else, adding, "I was just saying that because I thought you would have to admit me."

Pearls

1. In the interview of suspected malingerers, the clinician should ask open-ended questions that are carefully phrased to avoid giving clues about the nature of true psychotic symptoms. Patients who report suspicious symptoms should be questioned about them in great detail.
2. In malingered depression, patients tend not to exhibit the associated physical signs, such as psychomotor retardation, constipation, and slowed speech. Truly depressed patients also frequently experience a diurnal variation in mood symptoms, in which mood is worse in the morning. In general, malingers tend to be unaware of the subtler aspects of symptomatology.
3. Malingerers are typically more willing to call attention to their symptoms than other patients. They can also attempt to intimidate the clinician and may accuse staff of thinking that they are faking. In patients with genuine pathology, such accusations are extremely rare.
4. Ganser's syndrome is a controversial condition associated with malingering that occurs in prison inmates. It is characterized by giving approximate and incorrect answers to simple questions (e.g., 2 plus 2 equals 5). It is classified in the DSM-IV-TR as a dissociative disorder but may be a type of malingering because patients are typically trying to escape punishment or avoid responsibility for their actions.

REFERENCES

1. American Psychiatric Association: Diagnostic and Statistical Manual, 4th ed., Text Revision. Washington, DC, American Psychiatric Association, 1994.
2. Kaplan H, Sadock B: Synopsis of Psychiatry, 8th ed. Baltimore, Williams and Williams, 1998.
3. Resnick PJ: The detection of malingered psychosis. Psychiatr Clin North Am 1999;22:159–172.
4. Rosenhan D: On being sane in insane places. Science 1973;172:250–258.
5. Wiley SD: Deception and detection in psychiatric diagnosis. Psychiatr Clin North Am 1998;21:869–893.

PATIENT 15

A 46-year-old woman with ataxia and facial tics

History of Present Illness: The patient is a 46-year-old woman being transferred from internal medicine after stabilization from an overdose of lithium carbonate. She reports losing her job 6 months ago and soon after began to experience symptoms of depressed mood, insomnia, and hopelessness that eventually led to the current suicide attempt. She also describes increasing isolation because she is unable to enjoy social activities. On admission to the psychiatric ward, however, the patient's chief complaints are multiple facial tics and difficulty with walking due to lower extremity tremors. The symptoms began 6 months ago, and she describes a history of multiple car accidents as a result of "paralysis" and also complains of feeling embarrassed in public because of facial tics. She denies current depressive symptoms and states that she is anxious to return home despite her continuing motor symptoms. Two days prior to her planned discharge, the patient reported having a seizure. Evening nursing staff noted tonic clonic contractions of her extremities without loss of consciousness, bowel or bladder incontinence, or postictal confusion. A thorough neurologic evaluation, including electroencephalography (EEG) and magnetic resonance imaging (MRI), was negative. The patient has no significant past medical history.

Past Psychiatric History: The patient had one previous major depressive episode 20 year before the current admission after a divorce from her first husband. She has a remote history of opioid dependence (oxycodone) but has been clean for 2 years and regularly attends Narcotics Anonymous. She denies any other past psychiatric illness. She describes multiple potentially lethal suicide attempts over the past 6 months, including drinking ammonia, and complains that her husband never took her symptoms seriously. She was not able to tolerate several antidepressant trials and reports no effect with her current regimen of citalopram with lithium augmentation.

Laboratory Findings: Lithium level < 0.2. Complete blood count: normal. Chemistry: normal. Liver function tests: normal. Thyroid function tests: normal. Urine toxicology: negative. MRI with gadolinium: normal. EEG: normal.

Mental Status Examination: The patient is a well-groomed woman dressed in tight-fitting clothing with bright colors. She wears excessive make-up and appears younger than her stated age. The patient's behavior is restless with obvious facial tics that vary in severity and frequency, although she appears calm and cooperative. Her tics seem to transiently improve while she is concentrating on speaking. Her speech has normal rate, rhythm, and volume. Her mood is described as "good," although her affect is superficially euthymic, labile, and inappropriate at times when she smiles while discussing suicide attempts. Her thought process is circumstantial but logical, and she denies any thought content or perceptual disturbance. No active suicidal or homicidal ideation is elicited at this time. Her judgment and insight are impaired because she does not understand the seriousness of her suicide attempt or the psychological component of her motor symptoms.

Questions: What is the diagnosis? How are the patient's neurologic and psychiatric symptoms related?

Diagnosis: Conversion disorder with comorbid major depression

Discussion: Conversion disorder is characterized by motor and sensory symptoms that appear neurologic in origin but are actually related to psychological factors. Prevalence rates vary, but it is clearly more common in females. Depression, anxiety, and schizophrenia are common comorbid conditions and increase the risk for suicide. The cause of conversion disorder is unclear, but several theories exist. Psychoanalytic theory dictates that conversion symptoms are a physical manifestation of unconscious conflict and allow the patient to express the need for help while still shielding the conscious from painful emotions. Secondary gain may also play a potential role because physical symptoms are more likely than psychiatric symptoms to warrant exemption from responsibilities. Biological factors are also considered relevant, and recent neuroimaging studies have revealed changes in cerebral metabolism in conversion disorder.

The diagnosis requires at least one symptom affecting voluntary motor or sensory function, a psychologically stressful precursor, and symptoms that must not be feigned or intentionally produced. Common motor symptoms include paralysis, gait disturbance, tremors, and tics. Blindness, paresthesias, and anesthesia are the most common sensory symptoms. Pseudoseizures are frequently associated with conversion disorder, as noted in the patient's history of present illness. Pseudoseizures in general are more likely to occur in patients with an underlying seizure disorder, although such was not the case in this example. Pseudoseizures may be difficult to distinguish from true seizures, even to an experienced clinician, except that they lack EEG changes or postictal increases in prolactin concentrations. Another characteristic feature of conversion disorder is an entity known as la belle indifference; although not a reliable diagnostic measure, it describes the patient's frequent lack of concern about presumably serious deficits. This lack of concern was evident in this patient, who was anxious to be discharged home despite her symptoms. A history of substance abuse and cluster B personality disorders are also more common in patients with conversion disorder. This patient had histrionic personality traits and also admitted to a history of oxycodone dependence.

The primary task in diagnosing conversion disorder is to rule out underlying organic pathology. In fact, a significant percentage of patients diagnosed with conversion disorder are eventually discovered to have neurologic or nonpsychiatric disorders that may have explained the conversion symptoms. Hypnosis, amobarbital, and benzodiazepines are sometimes used as diagnostic interventions, and the resolution of symptoms under their influence confirms the presence of conversion disorder. Many neurologic disorders, brain tumors, and diseases of the basal ganglia can also cause conversion symptoms. Conversion disorder should be viewed as a diagnosis of exclusion, appropriate only after thorough medical and neurologic evaluations do reveal no other pathology. Other somatoform disorders, such as hypochondriasis and somatization disorder, are also important to consider. However, somatization disorder includes symptoms that affect several other body systems and presents as a more chronic illness. In hypochondriasis, the patient does not have actual deficits but is instead concerned about the presence of illness. Malingering and factitious disorder are also important differential diagnoses but present as consciously feigned or exaggerated symptoms (see appropriate cases).

The diagnosis in this patient was based on clear evidence of neurologic symptoms without an underlying organic cause. She was experiencing significant conflict in her marriage at the time, in addition to suffering from a major depressive episode that was so severe that it led to a suicide attempt with an overdose of lithium. These issues were thought to meet the criteria of a psychologically stressful precursor to the conversion symptoms. In addition, these symptoms were not likely to have been intentionally produced. It is unlikely that the patient purposefully became involved in multiple car accidents in the context of feigned paralysis. Finally, the presence of histrionic personality traits, pseudoseizures, a history of substance dependence, and the absence of any explanatory neurologic condition as corroborative evidence made conversion disorder the most likely diagnosis.

Conversion disorder is typically transient, with spontaneous symptom resolution. A minority of patients experience additional episodes in the context of psychosocial stressors. Most symptoms last less than 1 month, and the longer the symptom duration, the worse the prognosis. This patient actually had a history of many years of similar symptoms characterized by a relapsing and remitting course with exacerbations that occurred in the context of major depressive episodes. Her symptoms improved moderately with an increase in citalopram and successful treatment of her depression on the inpatient unit. Treatment options are limited, although insight-oriented psychotherapy, behavioral therapy to reduce stress, and benzodiazepines may be effective. Reassurance through routine physical and neurologic examinations may also benefit the patient. In this patient, brief psychotherapy helped her develop insight into the psychological nature of her neurologic symptoms and seemed to offer emotional relief and a reduction in the frequency of symptoms. On discharge, the patient was continued on antidepressant treatment and referred for individual, weekly psychotherapy with a psychiatrist who intended to continue an insight-oriented approach.

Pearls

1. A recent single photon emission computerized tomography (SPECT) study in patients with conversion-related sensorimotor deficits revealed a consistent decrease of regional cerebral blood flow in the thalamus and basal ganglia contralateral to the deficit.
2. Another neuroimaging study found right hemisphere structural lesions or physiologic dysfunction in patients with nonepileptic seizures (i.e., pseudoseizures) associated with conversion disorder.
3. Conversion symptoms may occur because susceptible individuals have underlying cerebral pathology that affects circuits controlling emotional processing and sensorimotor function.

REFERENCES

1. Benbadis SR, Hauser WA: An estimate of the prevalence of psychogenic non-epileptic seizures. Seizure 2000;9:280–281.
2. Devinsky O, Mesad S, Alper K: Nondominant hemisphere lesions and conversion nonepileptic seizures. J Neuropsychiatry Clin Neurosci 2001;13:367–373.
3. Halligan PW, Bass C, Wade DT: New approaches to conversion hysteria. Br Med J 2000;320:1488–1489.
4. Vuilleumier P, Chicherio FA, Schwartz S, Slosman D, Landis T. Functional neuroanatomical correlates of hysterical sensorimotor loss. Brain, 2001;124:1077–1090.
5. Yazici KM, Kostakoglu L: Cerebral blood flow changes in patients with conversion disorder. Psychiatry Res 1998;83:163–168.

PATIENT 16

A 26-year-old woman with fear and anxiety

History of Present Illness: A 26-year-old woman presents to an outpatient psychiatrist's office for an initial consultation. Over the past few months she has become progressively fearful and distressed, with depressed mood and frequent feelings of anxiety. She reports that whenever she is around people, she has trouble making eye contact and starts to feel sick with fluttering in her stomach, sweaty palms, racing heartbeat, and a dazed feeling. These feelings occur mostly around strangers but sometimes even around friends and family. She describes being withdrawn and depressed lately as a result, avoiding going out with friends and recently even quitting her part-time job as a clerk because she cannot tolerate interacting with coworkers. She also complains of sleeping poorly and has been tearful and upset because of the distress that she feels. She says that the anxiety occurs mainly around people—not in other contexts; but despite her awareness of these symptoms and their triggers, she feels that she cannot control their onset. She describes her appetite and energy level as "okay" and denies any suicidal ideation or psychotic symptoms. She occasionally uses alcohol at parties, up to two drinks at a time when she does go out, but denies using it otherwise and denies other drug use.

Past Psychiatric History: The patient briefly saw a therapist during her sophomore year in college for symptoms of depression and tried sertraline prescribed by her primary care physician. She stopped taking the medication after a few months because she felt better. She denies ever being hospitalized in a psychiatric unit but reports that her mother was once hospitalized because of anxiety and depression. Her maternal grandfather also has a history of alcohol abuse.

Past Medical History: The patient denies any current medical problems and does not take any medications except for a multivitamin.

Mental Status Examination: The patient is a well-related, mildly anxious, well-groomed woman with poor eye contact. She is restless and tearful at times throughout the interview. Speech is regular in rate and rhythm, with an anxious tone. Mood is both anxious and depressed. Her affect is mood-congruent, appropriate, and constricted to the anxious range. Thought process is logical, goal-directed, and coherent. No suicidal or homicidal thoughts, auditory or visual hallucinations, or delusions are endorsed. She also denies any obsessions or compulsions. Insight and judgment appear fair to good. The patient is aware of her symptoms but feels that she cannot consciously stop them.

Diagnostic Testing: She recently had a routine physical exam at her internist's office and reports that all blood work, including thyroid function tests, was within normal limits.

Questions: What is the diagnosis? How might this patient be treated?

Diagnosis: Social phobia.

Discussion: Social phobia, also known as social anxiety disorder, is characterized, according to the DSM-IV-TR, by excessive anxiety when the affected person is exposed to certain social or performance situations. Specifically, these situations involve an intense fear of potential judgment and humiliation in front of other people. The anxiety does not necessarily come in the form of panic attacks but typically results in physiologic symptoms, such as blushing, sweating, dry mouth, stomachaches, headaches, trembling, and palpitations. These symptoms may also serve to reinforce the person's fears of being perceived by others as awkward or nervous. The anxiety is consciously recognized as excessive and undesirable and can lead to marked avoidance of the triggering situations and social contacts. Some classic triggers include public speaking, use of public bathrooms, meeting strangers at parties, or any kind of performance-related event (e.g., piano recital).

People who suffer from social phobia tend to become isolated and also may have occupational impairment, leading to a higher risk of depression and substance abuse. Approximately one-third of patients with social phobia meet criteria for major depression, and substances such as alcohol are frequently abused because of their potential to alleviate symptoms of anxiety in social situations. Social phobia can be generalized, or it may occur in the context of specific trigger situations, such as performance. The generalized subtype has been shown to cause a greater degree of impairment and typically has an earlier age of onset. Patients with social phobia also may have higher rates of sexual dysfunction compared with the general population.

Social phobia may be the most common anxiety disorder, and anxiety during public speaking is probably the most prevalent symptom. The lifetime prevalence ranges from 2% to 13%, depending on whether commonly related phobias such as fear of using the bathroom are included. The peak age of onset is during the teenage years, although the onset varies on average from 5 to 35 years of age. Social phobia is often comorbid with other diagnoses (in 70% to 80% of cases), most frequently specific phobia or agoraphobia. This level of comorbidity is worrisome because it increases the risk of suicidality. And, despite the marked impairment and distress that social phobia causes, only about 5% of sufferers seek psychiatric help.

Social phobia is likely a multidetermined illness, with genetics, personality traits, and environmental factors playing a role. The disorder may result from a genetic predisposition to heightened sensitivity to perceived rejection by others. It is also three times more likely to occur in first-degree relatives compared with the general population. Although more conclusive twin studies need to be done, initial studies reflect a higher concordance rate in monozygotic compared with dizygotic twins. Studies also have noted that patients with social phobia tend to have lower levels of dopaminergic binding compared with normal controls, and this trait may be linked to less assertive behavior. Patients with social phobia also may have a more hypersensitive sympathetic axis, leading to increases in the release of norepinephrine and epinephrine during stressful situations. Premorbid risk factors for social phobia include childhood traits associated with behavioral inhibition in unknown situations (e.g., shyness) and environmental factors such as parents who tend to be more overprotective and rejecting, exposure to domestic violence, death in the family, early parent-child separation, and other childhood traumas.

Psychoanalytic theories of social phobia indicate its relation to anxiety hysteria, a term referring to anxiety as a manifestation of an unresolved childhood conflict. Even when the person with social phobia has grown into adulthood, conscious or unconscious reminders of this unresolved conflict can trigger the same feelings of anxiety. Cognitive-behavioral theories, on the other hand, regard social phobia as resulting from automatic negative cognitions regarding social interactions (e.g. "I'm no good compared to everyone, I look like the idiot here"). Over time this chronic pattern of negative generalizations becomes a self-reinforcing phenomenon that leads to social inhibition. The symptoms of anxiety become conditioned to recur during social interactions and thereby reinforce the cycle of self-humiliation and loss of control.

Social phobia is classified as one of the anxiety disorders, and the most common differential diagnoses include panic disorder with agoraphobia, avoidant personality disorder, major depressive disorder, and schizoid personality disorder. In this patient, panic disorder symptoms are evident, but they are largely present within the confines of social situations, as is more characteristic of social phobia. If the symptoms occurred at random or in nonsocial situations, and if the patient had stayed inside as a result of fear of random recurrence of symptoms, panic disorder with agoraphobia may have been the appropriate diagnosis. The symptoms of social phobia often overlap with those of avoidant personality disorder, and the main difference between the two is that social phobia refers to a constellation of physiologic symptoms as opposed to the underlying personality traits that can be associated with these symptoms. Some studies have reported that the majority of people with social phobia also have an avoidant personality disorder. In this patient, more questions about self-perception, interpersonal relationships, and coping style would need to be asked to consider possible personality traits.

This patient also mentions feeling depressed, and although an increased risk of major depression is associated with social phobia, she denies most symptoms of depression with the exception of sleep disturbance and depressed mood. It is nevertheless important to continue to monitor her for the development of additional depressive symptoms. Patients with social phobia also should be carefully screened for substance abuse, especially alcohol. This patient mentions mild use of alcohol socially, but the degree of use does not appear to affect her level of functioning and is probably not a causative factor in the present symptomatology. Rather, this patient appears to use alcohol to self-medicate in order to reduce her feelings of anxiety in social situations. Medical conditions such as cardiac arrhythmias or thyroid gland dysfunctions should also be ruled out because of their potential to cause or exacerbate symptoms of anxiety.

Psychotherapy and pharmacotherapy are both indicated in the treatment of social phobia to address the physiologic symptoms and the psychological triggers or underlying basis for the symptoms. Some controlled studies have shown that a combined approach of psychotherapy and psychopharmacology is probably more effective than either alone, but this disorder is nevertheless considered highly treatable.

Psychopharmacologic interventions for both acute and maintenance therapy include antidepressants such as the selective serotonin reuptake inhibitors (SSRIs), monoamine oxidase inhibitors (MAOIs), and venlafaxine. Of interest, tricyclic antidepressants (TCAs) have been shown to be less effective in social phobia than in generalized anxiety or panic disorder, although the reason remains unclear. Other medications that may be used include benzodiazepines, buspirone, and beta blockers such as propranolol. Also of potential benefit as second-line treatments are gabapentin, pregabalin, and clonidine; more randomized, controlled trials are needed to confirm their efficacy. One recent study with paroxetine indicates that treatment for at least two months increases the likelihood of reducing symptoms of social phobia. Some studies have also shown that higher doses of SSRIs or venlafaxine are needed for remission of symptoms of social phobia compared with major depression, panic disorder, or generalized anxiety disorder. Psychotherapeutic approaches include cognitive-behavioral therapy to retrain irrational cognitions and desensitize fear-provoking situations and psychoanalytic psychotherapy to address the unconscious conflicts that lead to the anxiety.

Pearls

1. The treatment of social phobia with SSRIs may require higher doses at a longer duration than typically needed for major depressive disorder, panic disorder, or generalized anxiety disorder.
2. Different studies have shown cognitive-behavioral therapy to be more effective than placebo for the treatment of social phobia, with treatment effects comparable to those of SSRI and benzodiazepine therapy and somewhat less effective than MAOIs.
3. Some studies have postulated that the generalized and nongeneralized forms of social phobia are two separate illnesses with separate etiologies. The generalized form has been associated with alterations of dopamine and serotonin transmission and the nongeneralized form with adrenergic abnormalities.
4. One recent study using functional magnetic resonance imaging noted heightened activity in patients with social phobia in the amygdala and hippocampal regions in response to angry and fearful faces compared with normal controls.

REFERENCES

1. Gwosdow A, and Psychiatric Times staff: Maximizing outcomes in social anxiety disorder. Advances in Psychiatric Medicine: Supplement to Psychiatric Times, January, 2003.
2. Kaplan HI, Sadock BJ (eds): Synopsis of Psychiatry, 8th ed. Baltimore, Williams & Wilkins, 1998, pp 603–609.
3. Lepine J: The epidemiology of anxiety disorders: Prevalence and societal costs. J Clin Psychiatry 2002;63(Suppl 4):4–8.
4. Massion AO, Dyck IR, Shea MT, et al: Personality disorders and time to remission in generalized anxiety disorder, social phobia, and panic disorder. Arch Gen Psychiatry 2002;59:434–440.
5. Stein DJ, Stein MB, Pitts CD, et al: Predictors of response to pharmacotherapy in social anxiety disorder: An analysis of 3 placebo-controlled paroxetine trials. J Clin Psychiatry 2002;63:152–155.
6. Stein MB, Goldin PR, Sareen J, et al: Increased amygdala activation in angry and contemptuous faces in generalized social phobia. Arch Gen Psychiatry 2002;59:1027–1034.

PATIENT 17

A 33-year-old man referred for being "weird"

History of Present Illness: A 33-year-old man presents to a shelter. He is referred to the staff psychiatrist by the intake team because they found him to be "weird." The client at first refuses to speak, insisting that he has no need for psychiatrists. When he is told that needs to speak with the doctor in order to stay at the shelter, he begrudgingly agrees.

When the man first enters the office, he does not sit down, even when invited. Instead, he goes directly to the window and stares out of it, saying nothing. When asked for his name, he replies without looking away from the window. He continues to examine the scene outside the window as well as the window frame and screen while tersely answering questions about how he arrived at the shelter, where he lived before, and other basic demographic information. He reveals quite reluctantly that he had been living on the streets for the past 8 years and would not have come to the shelter except for the fact that "it is just too cold … out there." Suddenly he sits down but continues to stare out the window. When asked what outside the window has his attention, he says, "Nothing," and quickly turns away and begins to stare at the floor. When asked about current psychiatric symptoms, he vehemently denies the presence or history of hallucinations, paranoia, racing thoughts, changes in mood, risk-taking behavior, and suicidal or homicidal thoughts.

Past Psychiatric History: Eventually, with gentle encouragement, the client begins to tell a vague and incomplete history of his life. He reports that he has lived most of his life alone. His parents are described as "crazy. My mother was always in the hospital, and I think she took a medicine called thorazine." He also reveals that he ran away from his foster home at age 16, because he "didn't get along" with his foster parents. Eventually he got a job as a security guard in a factory and volunteered to work the night shift. He set up a cot in a closet of the factory and slept there, never needing to find his own apartment. He notes that this arrangement also prevented him from having to "deal with people," whom he reportedly finds "stupid."

He denies ever having a sexual relationship of any kind, stating that "women are a waste of time." When asked what he likes to do, he replies that he is "homeless. What should I be doing?" He denies having any friends, saying, "I told you that people are stupid. Why would I have stupid friends?" When the psychiatrist comments that he must be quite a survivor to have made a life for himself under such difficult and lonely circumstances, the client retorts that he would rather be alone than have to spend time talking to someone as stupid as a psychiatrist.

The client denies any past psychiatric symptoms and claims that he has never been hospitalized. He also denies any history of substance abuse or sexual or physical abuse. He has no significant medical problems and takes no medications on a regular basis.

Mental Status Examination: The client appears his stated age. He is fairly well related, despite his apparent disinterest and indifference to the interviewer. Eye contact is poor. No psychomotor agitation or retardation is observed, nor does he demonstrate any abnormal involuntary movements. His speech is terse and nonspontaneous for the most part, although there are moments when he speaks in more than monosyllables, demonstrating that the rhythm, rate, and volume of his speech are normal. He describes his mood as "fine," although he appears irritated. His affect is constricted in the irritable range but is congruent with his mood and appropriate. In the realm of thought process, he is vague but with clear, coherent, and logical answers to all questions. Thought content is unremarkable, as he denies suicidal or homicidal rumination, obsessions, and delusions of any kind. Insight is limited, and his judgment is grossly intact (he came in from the cold) but not sophisticated. He is oriented to time, place, and person.

Diagnostic Testing: The client refuses any further work-up and states that he is unwilling to meet with the psychiatrist again because he has no interest in "wasting my time."

Question: What is the most likely diagnosis?

Diagnosis: Schizoid personality disorder.

Discussion: Schizoid personality disorder is defined primarily by a detachment from interpersonal or social interactions as well as a restricted ability to express emotion in interpersonal contexts. These limitations in functioning are demonstrated through (1) lack of close relationships (including family life), (2) predilection for solitary activities, (3) disinterest in sexual relationships, (4) general anhedonia, (5) lack of close friendships, (6) indifference to praise or criticism, and (7) emotional flattening that often appears as coldness and detachment. Four or more of these indications are required for the diagnosis. Schizoid personality disorder is coded on axis II and, like all personality disorders, reflects a stable pattern of interaction that generally begins by early adulthood and persists in multiple contexts. This client demonstrates each of these symptoms. Psychiatrists do not typically make a diagnosis of a personality disorder in one meeting with the patient, choosing instead to meet multiple times to rule out any axis I disorder and to explore the social history in greater detail. However, because patients with schizoid personality disorder typically do not seek or accept evaluation or treatment, the diagnosis is often tentatively made after one interview.

The differential diagnosis of schizoid personality disorder includes schizophrenia, schizotypal personality disorder, paranoid personality disorder, avoidant personality disorder, other psychotic disorders or mood disorders with psychotic features, pervasive development disorders, and substance abuse. Patients with schizoid personality disorder are often misdiagnosed as schizophrenic; however, there are important distinctions between the two diagnoses. Patients with schizoid personality disorder lack psychotic symptoms and a formal thought disorder and typically have a more successful work history. Despite these distinguishing features, schizophrenia and schizoid personality disorder overlap on multiple domains, most notably social withdrawal and emotional flattening, making the distinction between the two at times difficult. Schizotypal personality disorder, on the other hand, is differentiated from schizoid personality disorder by a different set of criteria. Schizotypal patients tend to demonstrate more of the odd-relatedness and perceptual abnormalities of schizophrenia than patients with schizoid personality disorder. Patients with paranoid personality disorder are more likely to have paranoia rather than indifference as a central theme in their avoidance of social interactions, and paranoid patients tend to be more engaged with people, although quite distrustful. Avoidant personality disorder is an important differential diagnosis to consider because of significant overlap in the realm of social isolation. The patient with avoidant personality disorder, however, has a desperate wish to participate in social activities, a feature obviously lacking in schizoid personality disorder.

This patient has significant symptoms of social isolation and emotional constriction but does not demonstrate psychotic symptoms, making the diagnosis of schizophrenia unlikely. He is also not oddly related, as we would expect in schizotypal personality disorder. Although the nature of his social behavior is somewhat guarded, it does not have the distinctly victimized and paranoid quality of paranoid personality disorder. One also does not get the impression that this patient is desperately looking for contact with others, as would be the case in avoidant personality disorder. He denies any history of substance abuse, and there is no obvious reason to suspect a pervasive developmental disorder based on the current history.

Schizoid personality disorder is considerea a "schizophrenia spectrum disorder" because of overlap of some symptoms and because schizoid personality is sometimes found in patients who progress to schizophrenia, at least in retrospect. The appropriateness of schizoid personality disorder as an intermediate point in the development of schizophrenia has been suggested, and although 30% of schizophrenic patients examined retrospectively were found to have premorbid schizoid personality disorder, this point remains contentious and controversial. Clearly, given that not all patients with schizoid personality disorder progress to schizophrenia, it is likely that, if the two disorders are related, they exist on a continuum of severity in relation to each other. The prevalence of schizoid personality disorder in the general population has previously been estimated at up to 1.4%, although a recent study found a prevalence of approximately of 1.7% in a community sample. Siblings of patients with schizophrenia tend to have a higher prevalence, up to 3.4% in one study, but this finding has not been consistently replicated. Given the symptoms of social withdrawal and disinterest in patients with schizoid personality disorder, the diagnosis may lend itself to an underrepresentation selection bias in studies examining its prevalence.

Little is known about schizoid personality disorder because patients rarely present for treatment and even more rarely consent to involvement in research. The accumulation of data about schizoid personality disorder tends to come from studies that examine the spectrum disorders in siblings of patients with schizophrenia. Therefore, findings about schizoid personality disorder may well be subject to significant selection bias. Patients with schizoid personality disorder who do not have siblings with schizophrenia are not well represented in research, and the patients with schizoid personality disorder who are studied may represent a particularly severe form of the disorder if the possibility of genetic loading is considered. That being said, patients with schizoid personality disorder have a significant degree of overlap with schizophrenic patients. Schizoid personality disorder occurs more frequently in among siblings of people with schizophrenia than in the general population. However, the incidence of schizoid personality disorder within families of people with schizophrenia is not different from the incidence in families with members suffering from affective psychoses. This finding suggests that schizoid personality disorder in siblings may correlate better with psychosis in general than with schizophrenia per se. Patients with schizoid personality disorder also have been found to have a preponderance of negative schizophrenia-like symptoms, antisocial traits, and disorganization. Some have even suggested that schizoid personality disorder be considered a risk factor for schizophrenia with predominantly negative symptoms. Schizoid patients also have poorer performance on verbal fluency tests, more like schizophrenic siblings than normal controls.

Although investigators have been reluctant to conclude that the overlap of schizoid personality disorder symptoms and schizophrenia are related to a similar etiology, one could make the argument for similar processes at work on some level. Dopaminergic dysregulation, chaotic glutamate and GABA states, and deficiencies in myelin and oligodendrocyte structure and function have been proposed as etiologic bases for schizophrenia, and it is possible that one or all of these abnormalities are present as well in schizoid personality disorder to some degree. However, no large-scale investigations into these possibilities have been published to date. Similarly, no large-scale neuroimaging investigations have been made into schizoid personality disorder. These areas await exploration.

Pharmacologic therapy for schizoid personality disorder has not been formally investigated. In the rare instances when patients present for treatment, clinicians tend to use low-dose antipsychotic medications. The atypical antipsychotics, which may have a positive effect on the negative symptoms of schizophrenia, may be a more reasonable choice than typical antipsychotics, which have the potential to worsen negative symptoms. Uncontrolled studies suggest that psychodynamically oriented psychotherapy may have some efficacy in the treatment of schizoid personality disorder. Similarly, psychoeducation has been proposed as a possible treatment strategy in patients who consent to treatment. This patient refused treatment. He was unwilling to meet with the psychiatrist again and within a few days, when the weather warmed, he left the shelter, stating that the preferred the solitude of the park.

Pearls

1. There have been only two genetic linkage studies in schizoid personality disorder. One study demonstrated an association between the dopamine D2 receptor Taq A1 allele and schizoid/avoidant traits. The other study suggested a link between the 480-bp VNTR 10/10 allele of the dopamine transporter DAT1 gene and schoizoid/avoidant traits.
2. Studies that examine schizoid personality disorder may be confounded by underrepresentation of subjects, given the social isolation and indifference of people with the diagnosis.
3. The relative risk of schizoid personality disorder has been examined in a group of people exposed to maternal famine during intrauterine life. Exposed people showed a twofold increase in the occurrence of schizoid personality disorder.

REFERENCES

1. Chang CJ, Chen WJ, Liu SK, et al: Morbidity risk of psychiatric disorders among the first-degree relatives of schizophrenia patients in Taiwan. Schizophr Bull 2002;28(3):379–393.
2. Cuesta MJ, Gil P, Artamendi M, et al: Premorbid personality and psychopathological dimensions in first-episode psychosis. Schizophr Res 2002;58:273–280.
3. Cuesta MJ, Peralta V, Zarzuela A: Are personality traits associated with cognitive disturbance in psychosis? Schizophr Res 2001;51:109–117.
4. Gilvarry CM, Russell A, Hemsley D, Murray RM: Neuropsychological performance and spectrum personality traits in the relatives of patients with schizophrenia and affective psychosis. Psychiatry Res 2001;101:89–100.
5. Maier W, Falkai P, Wagner M: Schizophrenia spectrum disorders: A review. In Maj M, Sartotius N (eds): Schizophrenia, 2nd ed. New York, John Wiley & Sons, pp 317–365.
6. Rodriguez Solano JJ, Gonzalez De Chavez M: Premorbid personality disorders in schizophrenia. Schizophr Res 2000;44:138–144.
7. Torgesen S, Kringlen E, Cramer V: The prevalence of personality disorders in a community sample. Arch Gen Psychiatry 2001;58;590–596.

Amir Garakani, MD
Alan Schlechter, BA

PATIENT 18

A 16-year-old girl with amnesia

History of Present Illness: A 16-year-old girl is brought to a comprehensive psychiatric emergency program (CPEP) by her parents on the advice of the high school guidance counselor. She was sent to the counselor earlier that day after one of her teacher's saw a pencil drawing on her desk depicting acts of violence and bloodshed involving teenagers. The school principal suspended her indefinitely and told her that she needed to be evaluated by a psychiatrist. The patient says that she has no memory of making the sketch. She states that she blacked out and lost all sense of time, and when she returned to consciousness, the drawing was on her desk. The patient admits that the picture looks like her distinct drawing style. The teacher can neither confirm nor deny the girl's account but states that at times she has slept during class.

The patient can recount several incidents over the past few months in which she slipped, usually without warning, into an unreal, suspended state and reportedly lost contact with the world around her. She has no idea how long the incidents lasted or what happened during the time. Her friends and family first started to notice these episodes about 6 months ago and are intimately familiar with this odd behavior. Her voice changes suddenly, and she begins speaking nonsense about unknown people and places. She assumes many eccentric characters, each with a different name. There were at first six, but now at least 12 people, including one who identifies herself as the patient. They can talk to each other and to the people around her. Two voices in particular, an 18th century matriarch and the patient's namesake, fight over how she looks, dresses, and speaks. The matriarch scolds her and tells her that she and her friends are corrupted. The episodes last for 30 seconds or several minutes, after which the patient has no memory of what occurred. Episodes occur intermittently, from daily to weekly, with no known provoking or alleviating factors. The girl's only knowledge of the incidents comes from what witnesses tell her.

Past Psychiatric History: The parents report no difficulty in the patient's birth or with speech or motor function during early childhood. She had no problems concentrating at home or in school and was, in fact, placed in accelerated classes. She played normally and got along with her sister and friends. At age 15, the patient was raped by a man who was staying at her home. Several weeks later the family physician informed the patient that she had contacted a chlamydial infection and treated her accordingly with antibiotics. She had no previous history of sexual activity. The patient stopped dating her boyfriend, whom she knew before the attack, and said that she did not want to date anyone ever again. Her family and friends noticed that she did not like to be touched and always seemed especially jumpy. Her friends are concerned that she has been engaging recently in uncharacteristic behavior: smoking cigarettes, using marijuana, wearing provocative clothing, getting body piercings, and talking constantly about religious rituals and rebirth. Once an honor student, her grades have suffered dramatically, although she will not admit this problem. Her parents also report that she is increasing verbally and physically abusive with her younger sister, seemingly for no reason. The patient admits to having brief bouts of crying every night before she sleeps, despite not feeling sad or scared about anything. She has highly vivid dreams in which she sees a landscape of unrecognizable dead bodies and blood.

Mental Status Examination: The girl is tall and thin and appears her stated age. She wears a white blouse revealing her waist and a pierced navel. Her natural brown hair has blond highlights, and she uses excessive amounts of make-up. She maintains good eye contact and answers all questions. She sits relaxed in her chair but plays with her hair and blouse in a suggestive manner. Speech is fluid with normal rate, rhythm, and volume. She says that she is "happy" now, despite what happened to her today. Her affect is inappropriate, as she smiles and shows little emotion in describing how she was raped. Her thought process is overall goal-oriented. She denies any paranoid ideation or delusions but has magical thinking, believing that she can talk to the spirits of the dead. She denies any perceptual disturbances. There is no current suicidal ideation or plan, but she admits to having occasional thoughts of cutting her wrists. The patient has never had thoughts about hurting anyone, and she is confused about her dreams about murdered people. She is awake, alert, and oriented to person, place, and time. Impulse control is poor, given her recent drug use and violent outbursts. Her insight is limited, although she admits to the presence of recent changes in her mood and behavior. Judgment is impaired because she continues to deny the impact of these changes on her friends and family.

Diagnostic Testing: EEG is unremarkable.

Question: What is the most likely diagnosis?

Diagnosis: Dissociative identity disorder (DID).

Discussion: DID is characterized by the presence of two or more distinct identities within a single person (DSM IV-TR). The identities, known as personality states or alters, recurrently take control of the person's behavior, leaving the alter personalities and, most often, the host in a state of relative amnesia. The change in name from multiple personality disorder to DID emphasizes the distinction between a patient having more than one personality and the current notion that personality dissociates into multiple identities. Five primary symptoms of DID have been accepted: identity confusion, identity alteration, amnesia, depersonalization, and derealization. DID has an estimated prevalence of 1%, but significant controversy surrounds its etiology, diagnosis, and treatment. DID has not been subjected to the same experimental rigor as many other psychiatric diseases.

The relationship between past trauma and amnesia illustrates the prevailing etiologic theory of DID. The behavioral state model, or posttraumatic stress disorder (PTSD) model, identifies the encapsulation of traumatic experiences in patients with DID as a method to allow more normal maturation in other developmental dimensions. A disorder in the development of the orbitofrontal cortex (OFC) has been targeted as a possible neurodevelopment of DID. The OFC may serve to allow experiences of the past, present, and future to consolidate into a unified sense of self. When abuse overwhelms the child's sense of the internal and external world, moments are compartmentalized to allow the child to develop in other ways. With repeated trauma these moments develop into whole periods of lost memory. As alters develop, they manifest different aspects of personality that the patient cannot resolve. Common alter states include an aggressive persona, a suicidal persona, or an eroticized persona, and most were seen in the present case. It must also be stressed that in certain cases alters can share information among themselves, as in this patient, whereas in other situations they are completely isolated. The average patient with DID has 13 to 15 identities, but at the time of diagnosis the median number is actually three. This discrepancy in the number of identities may be due to increased awareness of the clinicians witnessing the progression of the disorder from its onset.

DID is often considered a severe complex form of PTSD due to the almost universal presence of a history of repeated physical or sexual abuse. The validity of the diagnosis has been questioned because of the high comorbidity with PTSD, borderline personality disorder (BPD), and schizophrenia, which are high on the list of differential diagnoses. Common to any of these diseases is generalized irritability, anxiety, and poor impulse control with increased levels of risk-taking behavior and substance abuse, as in this patient. Although auditory hallucinations can be present in DID, they are typically of a different character from those found in schizophrenia. For example, the auditory hallucinations heard in DID come from internal identities, as in this patient, whereas hallucinations seen or heard in patients with schizophrenia are more often felt to be coming from outside sources. Other dissociative disorders (dissociative amnesia, dissociative fugue, depersonalization disorder, dissociative disorder not otherwise specified) and depression are also commonly on the differential list for DID.

The increased diagnosis of DID over the past 20 years can be attributed to heightened awareness of DID; increased reporting of child, sexual, and physical abuse; and improvement of diagnostic criteria and instruments. The Structured Clinical Interview for DSM-IV Dissociative Disorders (SCID-D) and Dissociative Disorder Interview Schedule (DDIS) assess degrees of amnesia, depersonalization, derealization, identity confusion, and identity alteration symptoms. They have strongly diagnostic and interrater reliability and are useful in delineating DID from PTSD, BPD, and schizophrenia. The Dissociative Experience Scale (DES) is a self-report measure that can serve as a screening tool and is also used to monitor the progression of treatment. Cultural factors, such as magical thinking and folklore, and substance abuse must always be ruled out. In children and adolescents with DID, presentation is similar to that of adults, but there are often helpful informants, such as teachers and relatives, who can help identify fantasy play such as imaginary friends and daydreams. The present patient was diagnosed with DID based on amnestic periods in which her voice changed suddenly and she appeared to become an 18th century matriarch. The information provided by family, friends, and her teacher was essential in verifying her diagnosis because the patient (as is typical of patients with DID) was not reliable enough to provide an accurate history.

Patients treated for DID can often find resolution of their dissociated identities; however, the treatment can take years (3–5 on average), and it is typically a significant clinical challenge. Psychotherapy is identified as the primary treatment for DID, along with hypnosis, and pharmacology may be a useful adjunctive therapy. The therapist must maintain neutrality among the alternate personalities, encouraging each one to enter into therapy and avoiding use of one alter against the other. Often, as with the present patient, voices command the patient to perform acts, comment negatively about the patient, and argue with each other. The patient may attempt to enact past experiences with the therapist playing the role of the abused or the abuser. This strategy gives the therapist the opportunity to redirect the patient and attempt to reconcile past experiences. Pharmacologic adjuncts include clonazepam, clonidine, carbamazepine, and lithium to treat comorbid symptoms; however, no agent has been shown to be specifically effective in DID. Cognitive behavioral therapy can be used effectively to limit self-destructive behavior. Inpatient treatment should be considered in cases of acute crisis or when the patient is a potential risk to self or others.

Pearls

1. The emphasis on trauma as the inducing element of DID has bolstered scientific support for this controversial diagnosis. Given the existing bias, DID may in fact be underdiagnosed by psychiatrists.
2. Despite the presence of EEG abnormalities in different identities and an association between dissociative symptoms and seizure disorders, little evidence supports changes in brain wave patterns in DID. EEG is probably not a reliable diagnostic test.
3. Eye movement desensitization and reprocessing (EMDR) involves the stimulation of subconscious memories to heighten recall and awareness of past trauma. EMDR and hypnosis are sometimes used to treat DID, although their efficacy has not been conclusively demonstrated.
4. A common autonomic manifestation of DID is the experience of tension headaches when a patient switches between alters.

REFERENCES

1. Burton N, Lane RC: The relational treatment of dissociative identity disorder. Clin Psychol Rev 2001;21(2):301–320.
2. Fine CG, Berkowitz AS: The wreathing protocol: The imbrication of hypnosis and EMDR in the treatment of dissociative identity disorder and other dissociative responses. Eye Movement Desensitization Reprocessing. Am J Clin Hypnosis 2001;43(3-4):275–290.
3. Forrest KA: Toward an etiology of dissociative identity disorder: A neurodevelopmental approach. Conscious Cogn 2001;10(3):259–293.
4. Gleaves DH, May M: An examination of the diagnostic validity of dissociative identity disorder. Clin Psychol Rev 2001;21(4):577–608.
5. Kluft RP: Dissociative identity disorder. In Michelson LK, Ray WJ (eds): Handbook of Dissociation: Theoretical, Empirical, and Clinical Perspectives. New York, Plenum Press, 1996, pp 337–366.
6. Putnam FW, Loewenstein RJ: Dissociative identity disorder. In Kaplan and Sadock's Comprehensive Textbook of Psychiatry. Phildelphia, Lippincott Williams & Wilkins, 2000, pp 1552–1564.

Amanda Itzkoff, MD

PATIENT 19

A 27-year-old woman with suicidal ideation

History of Present Illness: A 27-year-old woman is brought by her boyfriend to the psychiatric emergency department (ED), complaining of "excruciatingly painful depression" and suicidal ideation with a plan to take an overdose of venlafaxine, prescribed by her psychiatrist for depression. On the day before her presentation, the patient and her psychiatrist discussed how successful her treatment had been over the past 6 months, and the psychiatrist even suggested reducing the frequency of visits. In light of her recent treatment success, the patient describes feeling perplexed by the relatively sudden feelings of hopelessness, emptiness, and anxiety and refers to the experience as "a depressive crash." After her boyfriend left for work, these feelings deepened, and she began to have thoughts of suicide. Feeling alone and frightened, the patient attempted to phone her psychiatrist. When she was unable to reach her, she became so angry that she hurled the telephone at the wall. The patient reports feeling like her thoughts were racing and like she had stepped outside her own body. She also describes feeling empty and abandoned by both her boyfriend and her psychiatrist. Moments of panic-like anxiety reportedly alternated with periods of desperate depression because of the fact that her boyfriend would likely "break up" with her, "just like my psychiatrist did." She phoned her boyfriend at work and told him of her suicidal plans, and he immediately returned home to bring her to the ED.

The patient has been living with her boyfriend for 1 year. She is currently unemployed and takes one part-time college class; she denies any specific career plans. The boyfriend reports that he cares deeply for her but that the relationship has been "difficult." He states that the patient moved in with him only 3 months after they met, and he feels that this may be the reason for their frequent conflict. The patient reports that she has suffered from "intractable depression" for 12 years but that the regimen of venlafaxine, 150 mg/day, which was started 6 months ago, has been helpful. She admits that her mood seems to be chronically low. She refers to her current psychiatrist as a "genius" and states that she has been free of symptoms for the past 4 months.

Past Psychiatric History: The patient describes being a happy, well-adjusted, and obedient child without significant medical or psychiatric problems. At age 13 she began dating against her parents' wishes and shortly thereafter became sexually involved with multiple partners. She drank alcohol, smoked marijuana, and used intranasal cocaine with several of her sexual partners. She had many loud arguments with her parents about her disobedience. At age 15 she had her first depressive episode, which was characterized by increased appetite, weight gain, decreased interest in activities, and diminished concentration with decreased school performance. She was diagnosed with "depression" and treated with psychodynamic psychotherapy. The patient states that the psychiatrist was "cruel" and only wanted to "make my life more painful than it already was." Since that time, the patient states that her mood has been persistently sullen and downcast. At age 18 she left home for college "to get away from my parents." Her father, who was described as an alcoholic, died when the patient was 24 years old. Soon afterward she attempted suicide by "taking some pills." After the suicide attempt she remained on an inpatient psychiatric unit for 6 months. She had multiple medication trials, including paroxetine, fluvoxamine, sertraline, and citalopram but discontinued each because of reportedly intolerable side effects.

Personal History: The patient lives with her boyfriend, whom she met 15 months before the current presentation. She describes an immediate and intense bond between them and is often comforted by his stable and close-knit family structure. Soon after moving in with her boyfriend, she feared that he would leave her because of their arguments, and her depressive symptoms subsequently recurred.

Mental Status Examination: The patient is a slightly overweight woman who appears her stated age. The ends of her hair show traces of pink hair dye growing out. She has a tattoo on her right hand of a heart with a man's name written in it. She makes good eye contact. At times she clenches her fists and pounds on the table. Speech is generally within normal limits, but when she refers to her father or former psychiatrist, she speaks at a louder volume. She states that her mood is "terribly depressed."

Her affect is labile, ranging from anger and frustration to dysthymia, but generally negative. Thought form is goal-directed and without evidence of circumstantiality or tangentiality. She is slightly paranoid about being "left" at the hospital and asks the examiner not to leave her alone. She states that she is no longer suicidal because she is "comforted" by the examiner. She has never had homicidal ideation and denies auditory or visual hallucinations. Impulse control is impaired as evidenced by fits of temper. Insight and judgment are impaired; she does not appear to understand the nature of her symptoms or how they affect others.

Question: What diagnosis best explains the patient's symptoms and behavior?

Diagnosis: Borderline personality disorder (BPD).

Discussion: According to the DSM-IV, BPD is characterized by a pervasive pattern of instability of mood, impulse control, interpersonal relationships, and self-image. The disorder begins in adolescence or early adulthood, but a formal diagnosis before the age of 18 requires the presence of symptoms for at least 1 year. Personality disorders, in general, are diagnosed only on the basis of enduring, inflexible, and maladaptive patterns of behavior that cause significant distress to the person. BPD occurs in approximately 2% of the general population and approximately 20% of psychiatric inpatients. It is diagnosed 3 times as often in women and is commonly comorbid with axis I disorders, particularly mood disorders. The cause is likely to be multifactorial, with genetics and early childhood experience playing major roles. Histories of childhood trauma, neglect, and abuse are common in patients with BPD. BPD is also more common in first-degree relatives of patients diagnosed with BPD, substance abuse, and depression. There are no diagnostic tests for BPD, although studies have indicated that persons with BPD may have certain neuroendocrine abnormalities, including chronically low serotonin and abnormalities in thyrotropin-releasing hormone.

Although the present patient may meet criteria for the diagnosis of major depressive disorder, the presence of BPD accounts for the full spectrum of her symptoms and behaviors. Her history is significant for the pattern of intense interpersonal relationships, frantic attempts to avoid abandonment, multiple suicidal gestures, mood shifts in response to interpersonal events, impulsivity, and inappropriate anger that defines BPD. Other diagnoses considered in the differential include bipolar I disorder, bipolar II disorder, histrionic personality disorder, and dependent personality disorder. Patients with BPD have exceptionally labile moods, often leading to an initial diagnosis of an axis I disorder reflective of the symptoms at the time of presentation. However, mood shifts in patients with BPD tend to be in response to interpersonal events. Mood symptoms that occur independently of a comorbid mood disorder tend to shift rapidly and resolve quickly, usually within hours or days. Despite the multiplicity of affects experienced by patients with BPD, they often complain of feeling chronically depressed. In addition, many patients with BPD suffer from comorbid axis I disorders, as is likely the case with the present patient. Axis I disorders most commonly seen in patients with BPD include mood disorders, anxiety disorders, posttraumatic stress disorder, and substance use disorders. Eating disorders are particularly common in female borderline patients.

This patient's history exemplifies the chaotic lives experienced by patients with BPD. Her extreme sensitivity to perceived rejection by her psychiatrist is characteristic of the disorder as are the disproportionate effects of this perception on the patient's mood, behavior, and self-image. Her suicidal gesture may be viewed as an angry, maladaptive response to a stressor rather than as a product of depression. It may also be viewed as a frantic effort to avoid abandonment and an effort to perpetuate a dependent relationship. All of these factors are common unconscious motivators in patients with BPD. In addition, it is common for borderline patients to make unconscious attempts to sabotage their own treatment. The present patient, in wishing to overdose on a medication that has been helpful to her is both an undermining of treatment and a demonstration of hostility toward her psychiatrist.

In 1975, Kernberg conceptualized BPD in a group of patients with particular primitive defense mechanisms. Chief among the primitive defense mechanisms used by people with BPD is splitting, which causes them to idealize some people and devalue others or to oscillate between idealization and devaluation of the same person over time. They often idealize relationships with potential caregivers, leading them to make unrealistic demands and eventually causing the failure of such relationships. The present patient uses this characteristic borderline defense in devaluing a prior therapist and idealizing the current therapist. Another primitive defense mechanism described by Kernberg is projective identification, a process in which the patient induces the feeling states in others that the patient is unconsciously unwilling or unable to experience personally. Kernberg also described the contradictory concept of self that leads to identity disturbance, also known as identity diffusion, in persons with BPD. These disturbances are manifested in their lack of goals, multiple major changes in life plans, or attempts to "adopt" the identities of others. At times of extreme stress, they may also experience transient paranoid or dissociative symptoms.

The tendency to impulsivity in patients with BPD is particularly concerning, because they often make disastrous decisions. The present patient's impulsivity is evidenced by her sexual promiscuity and substance use. Other may spend exorbitantly, binge and purge, or engage in other risky behaviors without understanding their motivations. These behaviors often occur in response to psychosocial stressors or to alleviate chronic feelings of emptiness. The borderline patient's inability to control anger results in potentially physical confrontations.

Of utmost concern is the tendency to repeated suicide attempts or gestures and self-mutilating behavior. Suicide threats should not be discounted in borderline patients; it is estimated that 8% to 10% of patients with BPD commit suicide.

The American Psychiatric Association guidelines support the use of psychotherapy with symptom-targeted medications in the treatment of BPD. Effective therapy for patients with BPD is likely to be extended and should involve clear limit-setting and appropriate therapeutic boundaries. Dialectical behavior therapy, a form of cognitive-behavioral therapy, has been shown to have efficacy in reducing suicidal behaviors in suicidal or parasuicidal patients with BPD. Pyschodynamic psychotherapy, also called transference-focused psychotherapy when applied to the treatment of BPD, has been shown to be an effective treatment. Both dialectical behavior therapy and psychodynamic psychotherapy have been examined in randomized, controlled trials. Pharmacotherapy should be used as an adjunct for the diminution of symptoms as well as the treatment of comorbid disorders. Pharmacologic treatment includes selective serotonin reuptake inhibitors (SSRIs) as the main first-line agents; second-line agents include mood stabilizers, monoamine oxidase inhibitors (MAOIs), and low-dose neuroleptics.

The present patient was hospitalized on an inpatient psychiatric unit and began dialectical behavior therapy. The patient and her psychiatrist established a hierarchical plan in which they first focused on the most self-destructive aspects of the patient's behavior, including suicidal gestures and misuse of medication. The patient also participated in group therapy, which validated her suffering while encouraging reflection rather than impulsivity. The patient was continued on venlafaxine, with the agreement that she would use the medication only as prescribed, for the treatment of mood lability, rejection sensitivity, impulsivity, and inappropriate anger. Valproate was added to assist in impulse control. Although some patients require low-dose neuroleptics for the treatment of dissociative or paranoid symptoms, the present patient's perceptual symptoms resolved during the course of her inpatient therapy. After discharge, the patient continued to have twice-weekly sessions with her psychiatrist and participated in group therapy once a week. She required an additional inpatient hospitalization after her boyfriend began a new job that required him to travel often. After this discharge, the patient enrolled in school again and was able to work part-time at the school book store. With these stabilizing factors in place, the patient is maintained on venlafaxine and twice-weekly therapy.

Pearls

1. Several studies have reported that 40% to 71% of borderline patients relate a history of childhood sexual abuse compared with 19% to 46% of controls. Early-onset abuse in particular is a predictor of BPD. Parental neglect and parental substance abuse are also strong predictors of BPD.
2. Recent studies have shown low 5-HT synthesis capacity in corticostriatal pathways in the brains of patients with BPD and impulsivity. Neuroimaging studies have also reported decreased volumes of the amygdala and hippocampus in patients with BPD.
3. There is an interesting relationship between BPD and posttraumatic stress disorder (PTSD). Some researchers have proposed that they are variants of the same disorder. In one study, approximately one-third of people in the community with BPD were found to meet criteria for PTSD.

REFERENCES

1. Bateman A, Fonagy P: Treatment of borderline personality disorder with psychoanalytically oriented partial hospitalization: An 18-month follow-up. Am J Psychiatry 2001;158:36–42.
2. Dreissen M, Hermann J, et al: Magnetic resonance imaging volumes of the hippocampus and amygdala in women with borderline personality disorder and early traumatization. Arch Gen Psychiatry 2000;57:1115–1122.
3. Gunderson JG, Sabo AN: The phenomenological and conceptual interface between borderline personality disorder and PTSD. Am J Psychiatry 1993;150:19–27.
4. Gurvits IG, Koenigsberg HW, Seiver LJ: Neurotransmitter dysfunction in patients with borderline personality disorder. Psychiatr Clin North Am 2000;23:vi.
5. Linehan MM, Armstrong HE, et al: Cognitive-behavioral treatment of chronically parasuicidal borderline patients. Arch Gen Psychiatry 1991;48:1060–1064.
6. McLean L, Gallop R: Implications of child sexual abuse for adult borderline personality disorder and complex posttraumatic stress disorder. Am J Psychiatry 2003;160:369–371.
7. Zanarini MC, Frankenburg FR, et al: Axis I comorbidity of borderline personality disorder. Am J Psychiatry 1998;155: 1733–1739.

Jean Kim, MD

PATIENT 20

A 49-year-old man with anxiety

History of Present Illness: A 49-year-old man with a history of hypertension and obesity presents to the medical emergency department (ED) during the evening. He complains of a bad headache, shortness of breath, and mild chest pain and is found to have a blood pressure of 185/120 mmHg with a pulse rate of 95 beats/min but normal respirations. He receives clonidine for hypertension, which resolves without incident. The patient describes feeling worried and upset about his blood pressure, which is high again even though he takes his medications and visits his primary physician regularly. The doctor in the ED suggests speaking to a psychiatrist about his anxiety.

The psychiatrist on call consults with the patient. Over the past year, the patient reports worsening anxiety since being diagnosed with hypertension. He has started exercising and dieting and has reduced his cigarette habit to only one cigarette per day. Continued hypertension at regular visits to his internist causes him to worry even more. He fears that he will never regain control of his health and that he may even die. He experiences significant stress about salt and fat in his diet and feels that these thoughts constantly occupy his mind. He also worries about other issues in his life aside from health concerns, such as driving his car safely and completing details at work. He says that he ruminates about these issues almost all of the time and sometimes has trouble sleeping at night as a result. He reports never feeling fully rested during the day and at times describes aches and pains in his body.

Lately he has felt even more tense and irritable at work, leadng to some arguments with coworkers. He states that, beginning 1 month ago, he began to experience moments of intense panic and fear, wondering whether he may die. He has these feelings and thoughts a few times a week. Generally he reports wishing to live his life to the fullest and strongly denies any suicidality. He has a depressed mood at times, however, related to his medical problems and stress, and wonders if his health will ever improve.

Past Psychiatric History: The patient has never seen a psychiatrist before. He states that he has been a somewhat "high-strung person" his whole life but has never felt this kind of anxiety until last year. He denies heavy alcohol or illicit substance abuse. He has no history of psychiatric hospitalizations or suicide attempts. He denies any family history of psychiatric illness or substance abuse. He lives with his wife and two preteen boys.

Mental Status Examination: The patient is a moderately obese man who appears his stated age. He is pleasant and well related with good eye contact and is cooperative with the interview. He lies calmly on a stretcher but is slightly restless. He describes his mood as "worried," and his affect appears somewhat constricted and anxious. His speech is normal in both rate and rhythm with a mildly anxious tone. His thought process is linear, logical, and goal-directed. He is preoccupied with the status of his health and blood pressure, although he is somewhat relieved that his blood pressure responded to the administration of clonidine. He denies any suicidality, homicidality, hallucinations, or delusions. He is fully alert and oriented and appears to have good insight and judgment into his condition with good impulse control.

Physical Examination: Unremarkable except for obesity.

Laboratory Examination: Complete blood count and electrolytes are within normal limits, TSH is normal, and cardiac enzymes are not elevated. Urinalysis and toxicology screen are negative.

Diagnostic Testing: Electrocardiogram shows nonspecific S-T abnormalities and no acute changes.

Questions: What is the diagnosis? How might this patient be treated?

Diagnosis: Generalized anxiety disorder (GAD).

Discussion: According to the DSM-IV-TR, GAD is characterized by persistent, excessive anxiety and worry for more than 6 months, leading to clinically significant distress or impairment in the patient's daily life. The worry is difficult to control and is associated with a constellation of symptoms, including at least three of the following: restlessness/edginess/hypervigilance, easy fatigability, difficulty with concentrating/mind going blank, irritability, muscle tension, and sleep disturbance (including trouble falling or staying asleep or feeling poorly rested afterward).

As this patient demonstrates, people with GAD tend to be constantly fearful and worried even over relatively trivial matters and typically expect the worst of possible outcomes. Symptoms may exacerbate during periods of stress. People with GAD often present to primary care doctors with somatic complaints related to motor tension and autonomic hyperactivity, such as muscle stiffness and pain, headaches, restlessness, palpitations, excessive sweating, and gastrointestinal complaints (e.g., chronic diarrhea). Patients tend to seek help only after a long period of having symptoms because usually there is no discrete precipitating event. Typically only 14% to 33% of patients with GAD eventually seek professional treatment, and one study has noted that only 4% consult mental health professionals.

GAD affects from 4% to 6% of Americans, tends to be more common in people aged 25 and older, and occurs twice as often in women, especially women over age 45. Being separated, widowed, divorced, or a homemaker is also correlated with higher rates of GAD. GAD is quite common in the elderly and is often comorbid with medical illness. Of course, GAD may occur in children and adolescents as well, and in such cases it tends to present in more chaotic family environments and to have a more deleterious course. The symptoms of GAD are quite persistent, with only one-third of patients experiencing spontaneous remission.

The etiology of GAD remains unknown. A genetic component may be present because the risk of developing GAD is increased in family members, and twin studies have demonstrated higher rates in monozygotic compared with dizygotic twins. Biological theories focus on the regulation of neurotransmitters. One area of investigation suggests that GAD is partly due to catecholamine dysregulation in the sympathetic nervous system. In fact, patients with GAD under stressful conditions have been shown to secrete excessive catecholamines compared with control subjects. Other areas of investigation involve the regulation of GABA receptors. This theory gains support from the fact that benzodiazepines effectively target anxiety symptoms in patients with GAD. Still other investigators are examining central nervous system serotonergic receptors, since antidepressants act on serotonin and also effectively treat symptoms of anxiety. Some studies have also shown EEG abnormalities that appear specific to GAD, implying a neurophysiologic basis.

The psychological theories of GAD come mainly from psychoanalytic and cognitive-behavioral approaches. Freud studied anxiety from a variety of perspectives. At one point in his career, he described anxiety as resulting from conflict over the discharge of libidinal impulses. In another instance, Freud suggested that anxiety operates as a signal based on a memory trace from a previous traumatic experience to protect the person against engaging in a particular behavior or emotion. This anxiety signal leads to the use of defense mechanisms to prevent intolerable thoughts and feelings from coming into awareness. Another psychodynamic theory describes impaired integrity of childhood attachment with the primary caregiver as the focal point around which later anxiety develops. Still other psychodynamic theories focus on issues of inferiority or undischarged aggressive impulses. Cognitive-behavioral theories, in contrast, suggest that anxiety is the result of conditioning, in which the cognitive misinterpretation of harmless affects or stimuli becomes linked to an autonomic anxiety response.

Psychopharmacologic treatments for GAD include tricyclic antidepressants (TCAs), selective serotonin reuptake inhibitors (SSRIs), atypical antidepressants, buspirone, and benzodiazepines. Antidepressants and benzodiazepines have been found to be equally effective overall, but antidepressants seem to address more effectively the negative thinking and affects (i.e., cognitive symptoms) associated with GAD, whereas the benzodiazepines have better addressed the somatic and motor tension symptoms. According to one study, benzodiazepines seem to have a faster effect (i.e., within a few hours to days) that tapers over time, whereas antidepressants tend to become more effective with time (i.e., 1 month or more). Because benzodiazepines can lead to physiologic dependence and sedation, some studies support their use acutely until an antidepressant takes effect. Longer-acting formulations of benzodiazepines such as clonazepam may be preferable to shorter-acting formulations, which are associated with an increased risk of rebound anxiety and abuse. Some studies have shown buspirone (a partial serotonin agonist) to be as effective as benzodiazepines in treating GAD, with fewer side effects and less addictive potential, although, like antidepressants, buspirone takes several weeks to reach full effect. Anecdotal evidence suggests that beta and alpha blockers, gabapentin, and pregabalin may be of some utility as well.

In addition to medication, there are many effective psychotherapeutic treatments for GAD. Cognitive-behavioral therapy can be used to extinguish maladaptive conditioned behaviors and to address cognitive schemas of crisis and worry. Classical psychodynamic psychotherapy is directed toward uncovering unconscious conflicts to work them through to resolution. Supportive psychotherapy can help reassure and educate patients in distress. Meditation and biofeedback also have been used to help patients gain control over their symptoms and to learn relaxation techniques. No definitive research studies have demonstrated which of these treatments or combination of treatments is best for GAD.

The present patient was diagnosed with GAD based on chronic symptoms of anxiety and worry and the presence of sleep disturbance, hypervigilance, irritability, and motor tension. It is possible that he has a comorbid diagnosis of panic disorder, given the history of panic-type symptoms. However, his anxiety does not appear simply to signal anxiety related to the possibility of future attacks alone; thus, GAD is the most appropriate diagnosis. His symptoms also have occurred apart from his episodes of hypertension, and his medical lab tests and examination were otherwise within normal limits; thus, a diagnosis of anxiety due to general medical condition is not warranted. Because of his nicotine addiction, it is important to consider the possibility of nicotine withdrawal, although his symptoms occurred before he started to cut down on his smoking. He denies other substance abuse, which is important to rule out because drugs and alcohol can contribute to generalized anxiety in some patients. He does worry excessively, but his worries are not limited to specific intrusive core thoughts, which are more typical of obsessive-compulsive disorder. He mentions some depressed mood but does not otherwise meet criteria for major depression. The patient was referred to an outpatient psychiatrist for further evaluation and treatment.

Pearls

1. GAD is often present with another psychiatric disorder, most frequently major depression, panic disorder, social phobia, or substance abuse.
2. Newer antidepressants such as the SSRIs and venlafaxine are becoming first-line treatments for GAD. Benzodiazepines, beta blockers, and buspirone are other pharmacologic therapies that can be effective alone or as an adjunct to antidepressants.
3. Many patients with GAD present initially to medical (nonpsychiatric) doctors with somatic complaints related to motor tension and autonomic hyperactivity.
4. Directions for future research include uncovering the biological etiology of GAD with respect to serotonin or GABA modulation in specific areas of the brain and the regulation of the autonomic nervous system's response to stress via catecholamines.

REFERENCES

1. Hollander E, Simeon D, Gorman J: Anxiety disorders. In American Psychiatric Association Textbook of Psychiatry. Washington, DC, American Psychiatric Association, 1999, pp 567–589.
2. Kaplan HI, Sadock BJ (eds): Synopsis of Psychiatry, 8th ed. Baltimore, Williams & Wilkins, 1998, pp 623–628.
3. Lepine J: The epidemiology of anxiety disorders: Prevalence and societal costs. J Clin Psychiatry 2002;63(Suppl 14):4–8.
4. Mojtabai R, Olfson M, Mechanic D: Perceived need and help-seeking in adults with mood, anxiety, or substance use disorders. Arch Gen Psychiatry 2002;59:77–84.
5. Rickels K, Rynn M: Pharmacotherapy of generalized anxiety disorder. J Clin Psychiatry 2002;63(Suppl 14):9–16.
6. McLean L, Gallop R: Implications of child sexual abuse for adult borderline personality disorder and complex posttraumatic stress disorder. Am J Psychiatry 2003;160:369–371.
7. Zanarini MC, Frankenburg FR, et al: Axis I comorbidity of borderline personality disorder. Am J Psychiatry 1998;155: 1733–1739.

Alex Kolevzon, MD

PATIENT 21

An 18-year-old man with grandiose delusions

History of Present Illness: The patient is an 18-year-old man who is brought to the emergency department by his sister after stealing her car, filling it with all of his possessions, and then withdrawing 600 dollars from her checking account. These events occurred in the context of the World Trade Center attack, which took place 4 days before the current presentation. The patient attends high school in lower Manhattan and, on the evening of the attack, was required to remain in school until 10 PM for safety. He is now convinced that he is on a mission from god to make peace in New York City. He likens himself to Martin Luther King, Jr. and describes messages from the television directing him to "help people." He intended to donate his belongings, the car, and the money to the relief effort. Since the attack he has not been sleeping but nevertheless describes increased energy. He states that thoughts are racing in his head and may include other people's thoughts because he can read minds. When asked about substance abuse, the patient says that he smokes marijuana almost daily but denies any alcohol, cocaine, or heroin use.

Past Psychiatric History: The patient has no past psychiatric history. He has never been hospitalized, has never received psychiatric medicine, and saw a psychiatrist only once after his mother died 7 years ago. He denies any history of depressive, manic, or psychotic symptoms. The patient's sister describes him as social, athletic, and a consistent honors student. She notes that he has always had a great deal of energy and managed "to do many things at the same time." The patient denies any history of suicide attempts.

Mental Status Examination: The patient is a well-groomed, tall, thin young man with long hair and a baseball hat. He appears his stated age and is dressed in a basketball jersey, shorts, and sneakers. He is well related, with good eye-contact, and cooperative with the interview. His psychomotor behavior is agitated, and he frequently stands to demonstrate what he is saying. Speech has increased rate and volume at times, but there are no noted abnormalities in the rhythm. He describes his mood as "humble," and his affect is euphoric, expansive, and labile. He appears quite happy, smiling to himself and laughing inappropriately throughout the interview. His thought process is pressured and tangential, with occasional flights of ideas if he is allowed to speak without interruption. His thought content is disturbed by ideas of reference, grandiose delusions, and feeling as though he can read minds. He denies auditory, visual, or command hallucinations. He denies suicidal ideation. He is alert and oriented and appears intelligent with a good fund of knowledge and capable of abstract thinking. His judgment and insight are clearly impaired because he identifies lack of sleep as his only problem and does not understand why his recent behavior is of concern to his sister.

Questions: What is the diagnosis? What disorders should be considered among the differential diagnoses?

Diagnosis: Bipolar I disorder, single manic episode.

Discussion: Bipolar disorder is characterized by mood cycling between discrete episodes of mania and depression. It occurs in approximately 1% of the population and affects men and women equally. The etiology of bipolar disorder is unknown, but abnormal regulation of the biogenic amines serotonin, norepinephrine, and dopamine, is thought to contribute to its pathogenesis. Clear genetic factors are also involved in developing bipolar disorder, and first-degree relatives are significantly more likely to be affected.

The diagnosis of bipolar disorder is based on the history or presence of one manic episode. A manic episode is characterized by 1 week of symptoms such as pressured speech, decreased sleep, grandiosity, hypersexual or hedonistic behavior, increased goal-directed activity, increased distractibility, and racing thoughts. Patients with mania can be extremely excited, agitated, and hyperactive. Their speech is rapid, and attempts to interrupt them often result in hostility and anger. Their affect may appear euphoric or irritable and is often labile with rapid switches from laughter to tears.

Psychotic symptoms can occur during manic episodes, and patients may experience ideas of reference or feeling that they have special powers, such as mind-reading in the present patient. Psychotic symptoms are more likely to be mood-congruent and nonbizarre as compared with psychotic disorders, so that patients with heightened self-esteem may have grandiose delusions or auditory hallucinations telling them to save the world. In the natural course of mania, symptoms eventually resolve and give rise to a major depressive episode. Patients tend to enjoy the symptoms of mania and lack insight into the need for treatment. The symptoms of depression are intolerable, however, and patients may become suicidal and seek help; thus most patients are in the depressed phase when they first present to a psychiatrist. Bipolar disorder is also commonly associated with comorbid substance abuse. Patients may self-medicate with alcohol or illicit drugs to attempt to relieve the feeling of mood instability. The presence of comorbid substance abuse greatly increases the risk of suicide.

There are many differential diagnoses to consider in the present patient. For example, he may be experiencing a brief psychotic disorder or reactive psychosis in response to the stress he endured during the World Trade Center attack. These symptoms are also consistent with the beginning of a long-term psychotic illness such as schizophrenia, and the recent stress may have simply exacerbated an underlying psychotic process whose prodrome had previously gone unnoticed. In considering the presence of a bipolar mood disorder, it is important to distinguish between mania and hypomania. Hypomania is a less severe form of mania that is not accompanied by psychotic symptoms and does not require hospitalization. It is possible that hypomania may occur in the progression to mania, but some patients also experience mood cycling between periods of major depression and hypomania. This entity is known as bipolar disorder, type II. A third cycling mood disorder, called cyclothymia, is defined by chronic fluctuations between dysthymia and hypomania over the course of 2 years as opposed to the discrete episodes characteristic of bipolar I and II disorder. The fact that the patient smoked marijuana should also raise suspicion of a possible substance-induced psychosis. Although substance-induced psychotic symptoms are less likely with marijuana, illicit drugs are far from reliable or pure in the form sold on the street. Psychotic symptoms are more common with substances such as cocaine, amphetamines, and phencyclidine (PCP), and there have been reports of "lacing" marijuana with such drugs. However, given the patient's grandiosity, decreased sleep, pressured speech, and increased goal-directed activity, the most likely diagnosis is mania and therefore bipolar I disorder.

Bipolar disorder typically follows a chronic course and requires lifelong prophylaxis with mood stabilizers. The treatment of *acute* mania is often accomplished with a mood stabilizer; if psychotic symptoms are present, an antipsychotic is typically added. Benzodiazepines can also be used as adjunctive treatment for sedation in acute mania. According to the Expert Consensus Guidelines on Medication Treatment of Bipolar Disorer, the first-line choices are lithium and divalproex; carbamazepine and lamotrigine are generally considered as the leading alternatives. Newer anticonvulsants, such as gabapentin, oxcarbazepine, tiagabine, and topiramate, are considered second- or third-line agents. In a recent placebo-controlled study, lamotrigine was found to be effective for relapse prevention in bipolar disorder. In addition, with the exception of lithium, lamotrigine is the only mood stabilizer with a large randomized controlled trial to support its efficacy in bipolar *depression*. In cases of bipolar depression, most clinicians consider adding antidepressants, such as, buproprion, venlafaxine, or selective serotonin reuptake inhibitors (SSRIs) for short periods. Other recommendations may include adjunctive treatment with thyroid hormone or psychostimulants. In psychotic depression associated with bipolar disorder, in cases of refractory mania, or in mania during pregnancy, electroconvulsive therapy (ECT) is an effective option with considerable evidence to support its use.

Lithium has the most randomized controlled trials to support its efficacy in the maintenance treatment of bipolar disorder, but a narrow therapeutic window and potential lethality in overdose are often prohibitive factors that limit its use (see Table 1). One of the biggest challenges in treating patients with bipolar disorder is their initial lack of insight and hesitancy to take medication. They may feel extremely productive during manic phases and complain of medication side effects such as cognitive slowing and difficulty concentrating. Psychotherapy is important to help the patient develop insight into and cope with chronic illness. A recent study compared the use of cognitive therapy to placebo in patients on mood stabilizers and found that cognitive therapy in conjunction with mood stabilizers significantly reduced the number of relapses and improved social functioning compared with the use of a mood stabilizer alone.

Table 1. Effects of Lithium Toxicity

Lithium Level (mEq/L)	Side Effects
< 1.2	Generally nontoxic: sedation, nausea, diarrhea, cognitive clouding, polyuria, polydipsia, weight gain, psoriasis, and tremor.
1.2–1.5	Borderline toxicity: increased nausea/diarrhea, polyuria/dipsia, tremor, cognitive symptoms, mild ataxia, and fine hand tremor.
1.5–2.0	Mild-to-moderate toxicity: coarse hand tremor, dizziness, vomiting, severe diarrhea, ataxia, and confusion.
2.0–2.5	Moderate-to-severe toxicity: delirium, abnormal EEG, abnormal renal function, cardiac arrhythmias, and risk of coma. > 2.5 Severe toxicity: acute renal failure, seizures, and death.

The present patient was started on divalproex, and the dose was quickly titrated upward to 750 mg twice daily until the blood level was 96 μg/ml. Olanzapine was added because the patient remained delusional and for the advantage of its sedating properties. After approximately 2 weeks, the patient's mood approached euthymia; he was sleeping 8 hours each night and convincingly denied psychotic symptoms. He was referred to an outpatient psychiatry clinic for ongoing medication management and to group psychotherapy to address issues of coping with mental illness.

Pearls

1. The presence of psychotic symptoms during a major depressive episode in adolescence may predict the eventual development of bipolar disorder.
2. Recent studies have supported the efficacy of olanzapine in the treatment of acute mania. Likewise, evidence has also been accruing to support the use of risperidone and quetiapine for acute mania. However, long-term studies are needed to determine the effectiveness of atypical antipsychotics in preventing relapse.
3. Neuroimaging studies have implicated the dorsolateral prefrontal cortex as an anatomical site of dysfunction in bipolar disorder.
4. Structural changes have also been found in the amygdala and may affect an hypothesized neural pathway that is thought to regulate mood in bipolar disorder. This pathway has been proposed to run from the amygdala through the thalamus to the prefrontal cortex.

REFERENCES

1. Bowden CL, Calabrese JR, Sachs G, et al: A placebo-controlled 18-month trial of lamotrigine and lithium maintenance treatment recently manic or hypomanic patients with bipolar I disorder. Arch Gen Psychiatry 2003;60(4):392–400.
2. Goldberg JF, Harrow M, Whiteside JE: Risk for bipolar illness in patients initially hospitalized for unipolar depression. Am J Psychiatry 2001;158:1265–1270.
3. Lam DH, Watkins ER, Hayward P, et al: A randomized controlled study of cognitive therapy for relapse prevention for bipolar affective disorder: outcome of the first year. Arch Gen Psychiatry, 2003;60(2):145–52.
4. Sachs GS, Printz DJ, Kahn DA, et al: The Expert Consensus Guidelines Series: Medication Treatment of Bipolar Disorder. Postgrad Med 2000;Apr:1–104.
5. Tohen M, et al: Olanzapine versus placebo in the treatment of acute mania. Am J Psychiatry 1999;156:702–709.
6. Rajkowska G, Halaris A Selemon LD: Reductions in neuronal and glial density characterize the dorsolateral prefrontal cortex in bipolar disorder. Biol Psychiatry 2001;49:741–752.
7. Strakowski SM, et al: Brain magnetic imaging of structural abnormalities in bipolar disorder. Arch Gen Psychiatry 1999;56:254–260.

Michael A. Rapp, MD, PhD

PATIENT 22

A 51-year-old man with disruptive behavior

History of Present Illness: A 51-year-old man is brought to the psychiatric emergency department by emergency medical services after exhibiting sexually inappropriate behavior toward staff and attacking a roommate in his nursing home. The patient was noted to have become increasingly paranoid over the past months, often remaining isolated in his room and refusing visits from family. He accused staff of trying to "lock him up" and began to have violent outbursts with difficulty in controlling his behavior. Before his placement in the nursing home, the patient's wife reported that he had become verbally and physically aggressive and frequently appeared to cry unpredictably. For several years he had exhibited cognitive decline and psychomotor agitation. The patient is also described as very depressed, with difficulty in sleeping and poor energy.

Past Medical History: The patient first presented to a neurologist at age 39 for general clumsiness and unsteady gait. Over the following 6 years his motor symptoms worsened, with continued unsteady gait, frequent falls, sudden dropping of objects, and uncontrollable movements of the upper and lower extremities. Although the patient's wife cared for him initially, he was eventually transferred to the current nursing home because of potential safety risks. Since his placement in the nursing home, the patient has slowly lost his verbal abilities, and now speech is restricted to moaning sounds. Recently he has developed difficulty with swallowing as well.

Family History: The patient's parents died early of an unknown cause. His 31-year-old son recently developed restlessness, sudden uncontrollable movements, and a subtle memory deficit.

Mental Status Examination: The patient is a tall man who looks older than his stated age. He cannot maintain eye contact and lies on a mattress in a fetal position, showing continuous, involuntary, writhing movements of both legs and arms. His speech consists of repetitive moaning sounds. His mood may be described as irritable, and his affect is labile with rapid changes from dysphoria to severe irritability. The patient's thought process and content cannot be formally assessed due to impaired speech. He is currently denying suicidal ideation, but the severity of the reported physical attacks, in addition to poor impulse control, suggest possible homicidal tendencies. The patient responds only to simple commands and can be redirected at times.

Physical Examination: General cachexia. Pupils are equal, round, and reactive to light. The neck is supple. The patient demonstrates constant writhing facial contortions. Motor strength bilaterally is 4+/5. Choreiform movements are present in both arms and legs. Deep tendon reflexes bilaterally are 2. Babinski sign is negative bilaterally.

Diagnostic Testing: No pertinent findings in routine laboratory, EKG, and chest x-ray. CT of the head is negative for bleeding or mass effect.

Questions: What is the diagnosis? Discuss its etiology, pathophysiology, and clinical course.

Diagnosis: Huntington's disease.

Discussion: Huntington's disease was originally described by George Huntington in 1872. The prevalence rate is estimated to be approximately 4–7 per 100,000. Huntington's disease is associated with a single autosomal dominant gene mutation on chromosome 4. Genealogic studies of cases in Massachusetts and Connecticut have traced the disease back to 17th century immigrants from England. The characteristic gene mutation manifests as a triplet repeat of a cytosine-adenine-guanine sequence near the end of the gene on chromosome 4. The disease is confirmed, therefore, through genetic testing. Huntington's disease results from an unstable trinucleotide repeat sequence (CAG) on chromosome 4. It is transmitted in an autosomal dominant pattern with complete penetrance. Damage occurs through neuronal loss in the caudate nucleus and putamen by a mechanism that remains unknown. Several studies have shown hypometabolism in the caudate nucleus years before diagnosis in at-risk persons. Recent theories include mitochondrial dysfunction that results in neurotoxicity by the neurotransmitter glutamate. Other leading theories involve proposed abnormalities of protein metabolism and transcriptional dysregulation.

The onset of Huntington's disease is quite variable. Most patients develop symptoms around the age of 40. Approximately half of patients initially present with neurologic symptoms and half with psychiatric symptoms. Early neurologic symptoms include the characteristic choreiform movements, twitching, transient facial grimaces, and slight dysarthria. Early psychiatric manifestations may include memory impairment, impulse control problems, depression, paranoid ideation, and personality changes. In the present case, the initial manifestation was neurologic rather than psychiatric. However, a number of patients may also present with psychiatric symptoms alone. A greater number of trinucleotide repeats is correlated with more severe neuronal loss, earlier age of onset, and lower cognitive performance. A juvenile form of Huntington's disease also exists, with a greater degree of motor impairment earlier in the course of the illness and a more rapid rate of disease progression.

Over the course of the disease, the neurologic symptoms become more severe, with abrupt, jerky, uncontrollable movements, constant facial contortions, and myoclonus. Unsteady gait develops into a broad, dance-like gait that is accompanied by bizarre choreiform movements of the head and arms. This picture gave the cardinal symptom its name (*chorea* = Greek for dance). Psychiatric manifestations of the disease can range from episodes of depression to severe agitation and irritability. Dementia is also a prominent feature of Huntington's disease. Memory deficits progress slowly and are typically preceded by apathy and personality changes. Patients show features characteristic of subcortical dementia, with early impairments in recognition and implicit memory; later in the process, they show significant deficits in explicit memory and orientation. The disruptive behavior seen in this case is typical for later stages of the disease but may also be aggravated by the possible presence of pneumonia or electrolyte imbalance. Pneumonia and electrolyte imbalances are common in later stages due to increased difficulty with swallowing, as with this patient.

There is no cure for Huntington's disease. Genetic counseling has shown some effect in reducing its prevalence, but clinicians must follow strict ethical guidelines to protect confidentiality among family members. However, because parents may die at young ages and because the disease manifests only late in reproductive age, genetic counseling may not reach all families carrying the gene mutation. Thus, as in the present case, the parents' diagnosis may often be unknown to the patient and his siblings. The emerging symptoms in the patient's son, together with genetic testing, confirmed the clinical diagnosis in this case.

The treatment is symptomatic and aims at ameliorating both disruptive behavior and choreiform movements. High-potency neuroleptic agents have demonstrated some value in reducing disruptive behavior, but controlled clinical trials are still lacking. Given the high prevalence of episodes of depression and anxiety, case series have also reported some success with anxiolytics and antidepressant agents in Huntington's disease. Behavioral interventions, such as treatment in skilled nursing facilities, may be of benefit, especially in later stages of the disease.

Pearls

1. Huntington's disease is an autosomal dominant disorder affecting the caudate and putamen. It manifests in midlife with both psychiatric and neurologic symptoms.
2. Metabolic hypoactivity in the caudate and putamen may be an early marker for the development of Huntington's disease.
3. The number of CAG-triplet repeats on chromosome 4 has been shown to correlate negatively with the age of onset of Huntington's disease.
4. A stimulating environment has recently been shown to postpone the age of onset of symptoms of Huntington's disease in mice carrying the genetic defect.

REFERENCES

1. Harper PS: A specific mutation for Huntington's disease. J Med Genet 1993;30:975–977.
2. Huntington G: On chorea. Med Surg Rep 1872;26:307–321.
3. Mazziotta JC, Phelps ME, Pahl JJ, et al: Reduced cerebral glucose metabolism in asymptomatic subjects at risk for Huntington's disease. N Engl J Med 1987;16:357–362.
4. McHugh PR, Folstein MF: Psychiatric symptoms of Huntington's chorea. In Benson DF, Blamer G (eds): Psychiatric Aspects of Neurologic Disease. New York, Grune & Stratton, 1975, pp 469–493.
5. Van Dellen A, Blakemore C, Deacon R, et al: Delaying the onset of Huntington's in mice. Nature 2000;404:721–722.
6. Vessie RP: On the transmission of Huntington's chorea for 300 years. J Nerv Ment Dis 1932; 6:553–573.

Asher B. Simon, MD

PATIENT 23

A 23-year-old man with chest pain and shortness of breath

History of Present Illness: A 23-year-old man in his second year of law school presents to a psychiatric office practice complaining that "there's something wrong with me, but no one can seem to figure it out." He describes having gone to multiple emergency departments as well as several general practitioners for such divergent complaints as shortness of breath, palpitations, tingling in his fingers, sharp pains in his chest on the right side, and a severe sense of dizziness. All of these symptoms are associated with an unwelcome sensation described as an "out-of-body experience." These events seem to arrive out of the blue, beginning with shortness of breath and then following a fairly stable progression to the feeling of impending death, all lasting approximately 10–15 minutes. As the doctor begins to focus her inquiry on these reported symptoms, the patient becomes exasperated, stating, "Everyone has checked all this out. I've had all the tests. That's why they sent me to you. They don't know what's going on with me. Is it in my head?" The patient complains that he is unable to get his school work done because he is so preoccupied with preventing these seemingly unprecipitated episodes. He is essentially paralyzed and fears not being able to predict when another episode will occur. As such, he feels that the time when he is not "symptomatic" is in fact the worst. "You've never felt anything like this. I mean, those times are awful. But just waiting for them to happen and not knowing, that's just incapacitating."

He describes his first such episode as occurring 1 year ago as he was sitting in his favorite professor's office, mentally preparing for an oral exam. All of a sudden, he felt the room spinning and put his head between his knees without relief. He really became scared when this physical feeling was joined by a sensation that he was "going out of my mind." Fearing potential misunderstanding by his professor, he tried to maintain his composure; failing that, he started a volitional coughing fit and was excused from the room. His symptoms resolved after 10 minutes. "But I was marked. All I could do was to fear another of these." His fear was borne out, as he experienced an average of 1 episode each week over the next 12 months; some were precipitated by thoughts of pending papers and exams, while others came out of the blue. Fearing a medical cause, his internist and other medical colleagues provided a "million-dollar work-up." After 6 months without relief, they suggested that he see a psychiatrist. He balked initially, influenced by personal and familial stigma. The current presentation to a psychiatrist comes after he exhausted all other resources and is precipitated by an increase in the frequency of symptoms after having received lower scores this semester than he had hoped. "Maybe I am crazy," he states, putting his head in his hands.

Past Psychiatric History: The patient has never been to a psychiatrist, nor has he taken any psychiatric medications. "In fact, my family doesn't believe in you guys." He also denies any history of psychiatric illness in his family. "They're healthy like horses….They never complain."

Past Medical History: "I had lots of colds as a kid, but otherwise I'm fine." The patient denies any significant past medical illness and denies taking any medication on a regular basis.

Substance Use: No heroin, cocaine, cannabis, or other hallucinogens. No cigarettes. Less than 5 drinks of alcohol per week, and not all on 1 night. The patient describes being more likely to socialize and better able to cope with the fear of having an "episode" if he uses alcohol.

Social History: He was born and raised in the Northeast United States, attended boarding school, and graduated Phi Beta Kappa from a small liberal arts college. Currently he is in his second year at an Ivy League law school. He describes always being successful in school, love, and play, although not currently in a relationship. "Just at the time when it's all about to pay off, I can't seem to hold it together."

Mental Status Examination: The patient is a well-groomed and handsome man, although he appears fatigued. He is initially apprehensive with the interview but becomes increasingly more cooperative. Eye contact is appropriate. There is evidence of mild psychomotor restlessness, wringing hands, and sitting bolt upright. Speech is of normal rate, rhythm, and volume, without an increase in latency or signs of pressure. Mood is anxious. Affect is full range, generally neutral but with some intermittent nervousness, and is congruent to mood and appropriate to content. Thought process is linear and goal-directed without evidence of a formal thought disorder. Thought content is appropriate to the setting. Of note, however, he is fairly uncomfortable when initially describing his symptoms and appears rather shameful; no delusional or obsessional material is elicited. No suicidal or homicidal ideation is present. The patient has no hallucinations or illusions and does not appear to be preoccupied with internal stimuli. Insight is fair, as is judgment. Impulse control is good. Cognition is intact, with no deficits in attention, concentration, or orientation.

Laboratory/Imaging Studies: Physical exam, serum chemistries, blood counts, thyroid/liver function tests, electrocardiogram, esophagogastroduodenoscopy, and brain MRI are within normal limits in the past year.

Questions: What is the diagnosis? Which treatments are considered most effective?

Diagnosis: Panic disorder without agoraphobia.

Discussion: Panic disorder is a fairly common anxiety disorder that is often first encountered in a medical setting such as an emergency department or internist's office. Panic disorder is the fifth most common problem (medical and psychiatric) seen in primary care offices and confers the same degree of disability as major depressive disorder. Epidemiologically, panic disorder has a lifetime prevalence of 1.5–2.5% of the population, although this figure may be much higher in specialized medical clinics. It has a bimodal age distribution with peaks both in late adolescence and again in the late 30s. Women are afflicted twice as often as men. Additional risk factors include limited education, early parental loss, physical and sexual abuse, death of a spouse, divorce, and urban living. Of note, the majority of cases (60–96%) first manifest in the context of a separation or loss, relational problems, or development of new responsibility. The etiology of panic disorder is currently a topic of intense research, specifically on genetic, biochemical, neuroanatomic, and psychological fronts. A full review of the etiologic theories, differential diagnoses, course, and directions for future research is covered in case 51.

The diagnosis of panic disorder is wholly clinical. Although panic attacks may occur in nearly all anxiety disorders, the specific symptoms surrounding these attacks distinguish panic disorder. First, only in panic disorder are the attacks spontaneous and not bound to any particular situation. Two spontaneous panic attacks must occur for a diagnosis of panic disorder, although future attacks may become situationally bound. Panic attacks are characterized by discrete periods of fear and discomfort, and in order of frequency symptoms consist of palpitations, tachycardia, diaphoresis, trembling, shortness of breath or a feeling of being smothered, choking, chest pain, nausea, abdominal pain, dizziness, unsteadiness, faintness, derealization and depersonalization, fear of losing control, fear of dying, paresthesias, and hot and cold flashes. Patients frequently anticipate catastrophic outcomes from these symptoms. Symptoms typically crescendo to a peak at approximately 10 minutes and can occur during wakefulness or sleep. Within an individual patient and between patients, there may be different combinations of symptoms, differing levels of severity, and different time courses of attacks. "Full" panic attacks occur at an average of 1–2 per week in panic disorder, although the presence of "limited-symptom" attacks is common as well, especially during and after treatment. In aiding diagnosis and assessing treatment options, it is often helpful to have the patient keep a diary of his/her symptoms.

Critical to the diagnosis of panic disorder is a 1-month period of persistent anxiety concerning the recurrence or implications of the attacks or a change in behavior in response to the attacks. Patients become afraid of the consequences of not being able to escape or receive help if a panic attack occurs. This concept is termed "anticipatory anxiety." Thus, trains, buses, auditoriums, and other public places may be avoided because the person fears losing control or other consequences of an attack. Agoraphobia, or a pathologic fear of open or public spaces, is quite common in panic disorder and may be present in 33–50% of community-based and 75% of clinic-based samples.

The treatment of panic disorder is fairly well established and may take a variety of forms, following the different etiologic conceptualizations (see case 51). Crucial to treatment is the psychoeducation of the patient, especially concerning the etiologic, therapeutic, and prognostic factors concerning the disorder. Many patients are demoralized, feeling resigned or psychologically "weak," and need to be reassured. Of the therapies available, both pharmacotherapy and cognitive-behavioral therapy have equivalent efficacy, and each has its advantages and disadvantages for particular patients. Other less well-studied therapies include psychodynamic psychotherapy and "panic-focused psychodynamic psychotherapy."

Antidepressants of the tricyclic (TCA), monoamine oxidase inhibitor (MAOI), and selective serotonin reuptake inhibitor (SSRI) classes have been studied and found to be effective. Although SSRIs and TCAs have roughly equivalent efficacy, the safety and reduced side-effect burden of the SSRIs make them first-line treatment. Although certain SSRI's have been FDA-approved for panic disorder, theoretically all should be effective. MAOI's are usually third-line agents given their increased potential for side effects and the requirements of a tyramine-free diet. In initiating treatment with any of the antidepressants, it is important to begin with about half of the usual starting dose; patients may be hypersensitive to drug side effects because they typically have catastrophic interpretations of somatic sensations. Antidepressant medications themselves may also have initial panicogenic effects in about one-third of patients. Occasionally, physicians prescribe low doses of a benzodiazepine during the initiation of antidepressant therapy both to counter the initial activating effects and to immediately treat the disorder's anxiety symptoms. Benzodiazepines work immediately, whereas antidepressants may take up to 6–8 weeks for effect. Antidepressant doses should be titrated not only to full resolution of panic attacks but also (and almost more importantly for quality of life) to resolution of anticipatory anxiety and phobic avoidance. Patients should be treated with antidepressants for 12–18 months before a taper is initiated. Benzodiazepines can also be used alone to treat panic disorder, but they may have more side effects than antidepressants (e.g., sedation, slurred speech, amnesia, ataxia), are more difficult for the patient to taper, and do not treat comorbid depression. If a benzodiazepine is used, one with a longer half-life is preferred to minimize interdose rebound of symptoms.

Cognitive-behavioral therapy (CBT) is based on a theory that patients with panic disorder interpret physical symptoms in a catastrophic way, activating their fight-or-flight response system inappropriately. In adaptive stress reponses, there is usually a specific threatening stimulus, but panic attacks come out of the blue; thus, the fear response itself may become the focus of attention and concern. Panic attacks come with a firing of the alarm reaction in which patients react with catastrophic thinking, experiencing heightened arousal that furthers their anxiety and again discharges the alarm reaction. Thus a vicious cycle forms: vigilance to bodily sensations ensures that additional sensations are noticed. The hallmark of CBT in panic disorder is the identification and altering of automatic dysfunctional thoughts, modifying maladaptive behaviors, and learning relaxation techniques. It may include graded exposure to disturbing stimuli that eventually prevents the patient's usual pathologic responses. Patients undergo breathing exercises, record their cognitions, and confront fearful situations. This therapy may include family and significant others who may be critical in the patient's return to functioning, as well as for his/her psychoeducation. Cognitive behavioral treatment usually lasts for 3 months. Advantages of CBT are its shorter duration than pharmacotherapy, the fact that gains are usually maintained for years after completion of therapy, and the fact that the patient is directly involved in his/her treatment, allowing a greater sense of agency.

Psychodynamic psychotherapy has not been well studied, but anecdotal reports are positive. A specific type, called "panic-focused psychodynamic psychotherapy," has been developed and shows promise. Like CBT, it consists of 3 months of therapy. It may be more effective for patients with comorbid personality disorders, especially for those with dependent, fearful, and unassertive traits and with cold, controlling, critical, and unsupportive parents.

The present patient was diagnosed with panic disorder without agoraphobia based on the presence of discrete, recurring panic attacks and significant anticipatory anxiety. Although he was not overly avoidant, he did show some symptoms of reclusiveness. This patient does not fit in either age peak for the typical age of onset, but the clinical picture is nevertheless wholly consistent with the diagnosis. As with most patients with panic disorder, his symptoms were first precipitated by a stressful situation, and only later did he experience spontaneous panic attacks. He also was quite overwhelmed by anticipatory anxiety, as he stated that he found this "not-knowing-when" quality to be more noxious than the attacks themselves.

Perhaps the most striking feature about this patient's symptomatology was his attitude toward his symptoms. His lack of insight regarding any psychological significance is fairly usual in panic disorder, especially given his family's distrust of psychiatry. While he did seem aware of some psychological component to his symptoms, his degree of demoralization and stoicism prevented it from gaining any foothold. His family's and his appraisal of his symptoms as physical was the catalyst for his receiving such a thorough medical work-up. Not until long into the course of his illness did a physician mention to him that panic disorder was a likely diagnosis. He may not have listened to such a doctor, but if the suggestion was made in an empathetic and educational manner, this patient may have been spared the excessive symptoms that he experienced. In the psychiatrist's office, he was provided with a simple explanation regarding the neuropsychiatric, genetic, and psychological mechanisms that are proposed to underlie panic disorder. Such an understanding allowed the patient to overcome his demoralization, his feeling of "weakness," and his fear of relaying more of his symptoms to his family. He reported feeling a big weight lifted off his shoulders.

A choice between the treatment options of CBT and pharmacotherapy was offered. This patient chose to use medication only, reporting that it felt like it was more of a "real" treatment. He was started on sertraline, 25 mg/day, and was instructed to call the doctor if he felt any immediate discomfort or increased frequency of panic attacks. His dose was titrated slowly to full effect, reached at 150 mg/day. He also received supportive therapy and psychoeducation during follow-up medication management sessions. The patient was given the option to involve his family in the discussion of his case for their education, but he was reluctant and declined.

Pearls

1. In assessing outcome of treatment for panic disorder, the number of panic attacks should be considered equally important to avoidant symptoms, quality of life, and degree of functional impairment.

2. It is highly therapeutic to reassure patients that their symptoms reflect real physiologic events (e.g., tachycardia) and are not dangerous to their health in the acute setting.

3. The best-studied treatments (CBT, pharmacotherapy) target specific symptoms, but the physician must treat the patient as an individual. Therefore, less well-studied therapies such as psychodynamic psychotherapy may be the treatment of choice in certain clinical situations (e.g., comorbid personality disorders or psychosocial stressors).

4. It is considered normal to experience panic attacks for several weeks following discontinuation of any substance of abuse, especially central nervous system depressants such as alcohol, benzodiazepines, and barbiturates.

REFERENCES

1. American Psychiatric Association: Diagnostic and Statistical Manual of Mental Disorders, Fourth Edition, Text Revision. Washington, DC, American Psychiatric Association, 2000.
2. American Psychiatric Association: Practice Guideline for the Treatment of Patients with Panic Disorder. Washington, DC, American Psychiatric Press, 1998.
3. Ballenger JC: Panic Disorder and Agoraphobia. In Gelder MG, Lopez-Ibor JJ, Andreasen NC (eds): New Oxford Textbook of Psychiatry. Oxford, Oxford University Press, 2000, pp 807–822.
4. Gelder M, Mayou R, Cowen P: Shorter Oxford Textbook of Psychiatry. Oxford, Oxford University Press, 2001.
5. Gorman JM, Kent JM, Sullivan GM, Coplan JD: Neuroanatomical Hypothesis of Panic Disorder, Revised. Am J Psychiatry 2000;157:493–505.
6. Lydiard RB, Otto MW, Milrod B: Panic Disorder. In Gabbard GO (ed): Treatments of Psychiatric Disorders, 3rd ed, vols. 1 & 2. Washington, DC, American Psychiatric Press, 2001.
7. Swoboda H, Amering M, Windhaber J, Katschnig H: The long-term course of panic disorder—an 11 year follow-up. Anxiety Disord 2001;17:223–232.

Malaika E. Berkeley, MD

PATIENT 24

A 22-year-old college student approaching graduation

History of Present Illness: A 22-year-old woman currently in her senior year of college is brought to the psychiatric emergency department by friends because she has become progressively more withdrawn in the past month and has not left her bed in the past 3 days. The patient reports that she had been looking forward to graduating but was concerned about her upcoming finals and finding a job after graduation. As graduation approached, she became increasingly anxious about not finding a job. She reports withdrawing from her friends and refusing their invitations to social events. She also describes significant difficulty with sleeping; she awakens after only 4 hours and is unable to return to sleep. The patient found herself unable to concentrate on classes, and her grades began to suffer. Over the past few days, she reports feeling too sluggish to get out of bed or even to eat. She has also been missing classes for the first time since starting college. The patient describes thoughts about death and a pervasive feeling that life may not be worth it. She denies any specific plan, however. She also denies any history of manic symptoms, psychosis, or significant anxiety beyond concerns about finding a job after graduation.

Past Psychiatric History: The patient denies any prior psychiatric contact but reports feeling exceedingly sad for several days after graduating from high school. She admits to drinking alcohol socially on the weekends but denies symptoms of abuse or dependence.

Past Medical History: None; no medications.

Family History: The patient initially denies the presence of psychiatric illness in any family members, but on further questioning she reports that her mother has taken antidepressants in the past.

Mental Status Examination: On presentation to the emergency department, the patient was alert and fully oriented. She had poor eye contact and was slouched in her chair with little spontaneous movement. Her voice was barely audible and monotonous with no spontaneous speech and considerably increased latency. She reported her mood to be "not so good" and appeared depressed and tearful. Her affect was constricted to the dysphoric range but congruent and appropriate. She denied hallucinations, delusions, or obsessions, but her thoughts were centered on feeling hopeless about her future. She reported suicidal ideation without a plan or intent but no homicidal ideation.

Laboratory Examination: Complete blood count, chemistry, thyroid function tests, vitamin B12, folate, and urine toxicology are within normal limits.

Question: What is the diagnosis?

Diagnosis: Major depressive disorder (MDD).

Discussion: MDD is characterized by 2 weeks of sustained depressed mood and/or anhedonia along with several other symptoms that are severe enough to cause impairment in social or occupational functioning. Anhedonia is defined as the loss of interest in or withdrawal from regular and pleasurable activities. The diagnosis of MDD can be made if patients exhibit 5 of 9 symptoms over a 2-week period, including either (1) depressed mood or irritability or (2) anhedonia. The other symptoms may include (3) a change in sleep patterns, (4) guilt, hopelessness, or helplessness, (5) anergia (lack of energy), (6) impaired concentration, (7) change in appetite or weight, (8) psychomotor agitation or retardation, or (9) thoughts of death and suicidal ideation.

MDD has a general prevalence of 15% with a twofold greater prevalence in women. The mean age of presentation is approximately 40 years, with a range from 20 to 50 years. There are, however, reports of childhood and late-onset depression, and recently the prevalence in the elderly has been reported to have increased to 25–50%. There are no reported differences in the incidence of MDD based on socioeconomic status or race; however, one source indicates that clinicians may misdiagnose mood disorders as schizophrenia in patients from different cultural backgrounds.

The exact etiology of depression remains unclear, but it is generally thought to be an interaction between genetic, biological, and psychosocial factors. Genetic studies indicate that first-degree relatives of patients with depression are at 2–3 times greater risk of developing depression than the general population. Twin studies also indicate greater concordance rates in monozygotic compared with dizygotic twins. Biological studies show some possible neuroanatomic changes in the caudate nuclei and frontal lobes, while neurochemical theories propose a dysregulation in the levels of norepinephrine (NE), serotonin (5HT), or dopamine (DA) in the brain as a contributing factor. The current thinking about depression places serotonin at the center, based largely on the efficacy of serotonin reuptake inhibitors in the treatment of depression. In considering the fact that it takes several weeks for serotonergic medications to take effect, earlier theories that posited a low level of serotonin have been superceded by dysregulation theories. It has also been noted that stressful life events more often precede a first episode than subsequent episodes, and some authors have suggested that the stress of an initial major depressive episode may cause neuronal or synaptic changes that predispose individuals to subsequent episodes.

Symptomatology in major depression is quite variable. Although up to 50% of patients may not recognize their depressed mood, they may exhibit withdrawal and other signs of anhedonia. In patients who do report depressed mood, half say that the depression is worse in the morning than in the afternoon (i.e., diurnal variation). Sleep is also disturbed, and studies indicate that 80% of patients suffer from insomnia, which in depression more frequently manifests as early morning awakening or interrupted sleep. Anergia has been reported in up to 97% of cases. Typically, patients also report a decrease in appetite and weight loss, but in atypical depression increased appetite and weight gain can be seen. Suicidal thoughts and behavior are common in major depression. Studies indicate that two-thirds of patients contemplate suicide and that 10–15% actually commit suicide. Although not listed in the criteria for major depression, anxiety and somatic complaints are also common presenting symptoms.

Psychomotor retardation is a common sign of depression, although in the elderly psychomotor agitation is frequently seen instead. As with this patient, many people suffering from depression may exhibit stooped posture and poor eye contact. Other signs include decreased rate and volume of speech, using single-word answers, and showing delays or latency of speech. Psychotic symptoms such as delusions and hallucinations are also sometimes seen in severe episodes of major depression. The delusions in particular tend to be congruent with the patient's mood. For example, a delusion that may occur in psychotic depression is that internal organs are rotting-the content of the delusion is concordant with the depressive mood state. Patients' thoughts also tend to be negativistic with ruminations about guilt, loss, suicide, and death. Cognition is also often impaired in depression and may be evident in the inability to attend to tasks and to concentrate, as in the present patient. Patients are generally oriented to person, place, and time, but impaired concentration and forgetfulness may present a dementia-like picture commonly called pseudodementia.

It is important that all patients with depression receive a thorough medical history and physical exam as well as routine blood tests, including complete blood count, blood chemistries, thyroid function testing, and vitamin B12 and folate levels to rule out medical etiologies. Urine toxicology screens are done to rule out depressive symptoms resulting from drug use. The differential diagnosis of depression should always include adrenal and thyroid dysfunction, especially in patients with weight changes. HIV must be ruled out in high-risk individuals. It is also important to remember that many medications can induce depression, including antihypertensives, analgesics, and antiparkinsonian drugs. A thorough neurologic examination should be conducted since several neurologic conditions can also be associated with depression (e.g., epilepsy, Parkinson's disease, cerebrovascular accidents, cardiovascular disease, neoplastic disease). In the elderly, it is especially important to rule out dementia of the Alzheimer's type.

A thorough psychiatric history is also essential, as other psychiatric diagnoses need to be ruled out, including bipolar disorder, dysthymia, and cyclothymia. Personality disorders can often account for many of the symptoms of depression, and a complete social history should be obtained to investigate this possibility. Substance abuse and substance-induced mood disorders should also be considered, along with psychotic illnesses (e.g., the negative symptoms of schizophrenia), eating disorders, anxiety disorders, and adjustment disorders.

A complete treatment plan must address not only a patient's immediate treatment to obtain remission but also long-term mental health to reduce the risk of relapse. Patient safety is the most acute and primary goal, and the physician often must decide on the need for hospitalization. If the patient indicates a potential danger to self or others or is debilitated to the extent that self care is compromised, hospitalization is warranted. Once the patient's safety is ensured, the focus of treatment generally becomes a combination of medication and psychotherapy.

Specific pharmacologic treatments have been available for four decades. Pharmacologic treatments include selective serotonin reuptake inhibitors (SSRIs), tri- and tetracyclic antidepressants (TCAs), monoamine oxidase inhibitors (MAOIs), and newer, atypical antidepressants. All antidepressants seem to alter the concentrations of norepinephrine, serotonin, and/or dopamine at the synaptic cleft, although different compounds tend to act uniquely on each of these neurotransmitters. Most antidepressants have been shown to have similar efficacy in the treatment of depression, and medication is therefore chosen largely on the basis of side effects. Because of their relative safety and tolerable side-effect profile, SSRIs are often considered the first line of treatment (see Table 1).

It is important to tell patients that antidepressants may take up to 4–6 weeks to exert their full effect. Medications should be raised to maximum effective doses and maintained for at least 4–6 weeks before concluding that the medication trial has been unsuccessful. In the event that any one antidepressant fails, augmentation strategies include lithium, thyroid hormone supplementation, or l-tryptophan. Some clinicians also use combinations of antidepressant medications to take advantage of differing mechanisms of action. Failing these alternatives, electroconvulsive therapy (ECT) remains a safe and viable option, especially in elderly or pregnant patients, for whom it is often considered a first-line treatment.

Most mental health practitioners believe that a combination of psychotherapy and pharmacotherapy is the most effective treatment for patients with major depression. Recommended modes of psychotherapy include short-term cognitive, behavioral, and interpersonal therapies. Behavioral therapy has not been well studied but hypothesizes that maladaptive behaviors lead to negative feedback and rejection; therefore, teaching more adaptive behavior should result in positive reinforcement and reduction in depressive episodes. Cognitive therapy is based on the idea that depression is at least partly the result of an individual's negative view of self, others, and the world. Cognitive therapists, therefore, seek to identify and correct this distorted thinking to provide symptomatic relief of depression. Interpersonal therapists suggest that unsatisfactory social bonds promote depressive symptoms. In their view, if interpersonal relations can be strengthened and communication improved, symptoms should resolve. Some mental health practitioners also recommend long-term psychoanalytic therapy. Psychoanalytic theories of depression have developed over time, and multiple hypotheses are associated with different subgroups of psychoanalysis. That said, depression is largely understood by the psychoanalytic community as relating to childhood conflicts that revolve around self-esteem and internalized hostile impulses. In psychoanalytic therapy, patients work through these issues, studying them as they recur in the relationship between the patient and analyst, a phenomenon called transference.

Untreated depression can last from 6 to 13 months, although with antidepressant treatment the episodes tend to be significantly shortened. Premature withdrawal of antidepressants often results in return of symptoms. Antidepressants, therefore, should be maintained for at least 6 months from the point of remission. With each major depressive episode, relapses tend to occur more frequently, last longer, and be more severe. Prophylactic psychopharmacologic treatment tends to lower the relapse rate, and some patients may need to be treated prophylactically on an ongoing basis.

The present patient presents with a first episode of major depression. She may have also suffered some form of a depression after graduating from high school, although it was not severe enough to come to the attention of a clinician and resolved on

Table 1. Some Common Antidepressant Medications

Class	Medication	Proposed Method of Action	Major Side Effects	Risk in overdose
TCA	Tertiary amines Amitriptyline Clomipramine Doxepin Imipramine Trimipramine Secondary amines Desipramine Nortriptyline Protriptyline Tetracyclics Amoxapine Maprotiline	All tri-and tetracyclics increase the concentration of 5HT and NE by inhibiting their reuptake into the presynaptic neurons.	Dry mouth, dizziness, blurred vision, constipation, urinary retention, orthostatic hypotension, sedation	Doses in excess of 1 gm may be fatal. Death is generally the result of hypotension, seizures, or QRS prolongation leading to cardiac arrythmias
SSRI	Fluoxetine Paroxetine Fluvoxamine Sertraline Citalopram Escitalopram	Selectively inhibits reuptake of 5HT into presynaptic serotonergic neurons.	Nausea, diarrhea, anxiety, headache, sexual dysfunction	Relatively safe in overdose due to lack of ardiotoxic effects.
MAOI	Phenelzine Tranylcypromine	Increases the availability of 5HT, NE, and DA by inhibiting the enzyme monoamine oxidase, which is responsible for their degradation.	Hypertensive crisis, orthostatic hypotension, insomnia, dizziness, somnolence, sexual dysfunction.	Death may result from CNS depression, renal failure, seizures, and cardiac arrythmias
Atypical	Venlafaxine	Inhibits the reuptake of 5HT and NE.	Nausea, anxiety, insomnia, dizziness, hypertension, sexual dysfunction	Generally similar to the SSRIs
	Bupropion	Inhibits the reuptake of NE and DA.	Nausea, insomnia, anxiety, anorexia, seizures, psychosis	Seizures may occur in doses higher than recommended and in acute overdose.
	Nefazodone Trazodone	Inhibit the reuptake of 5HT and act as an antagonist at the 5HT2 receptor	Nausea, headache, dry mouth, dizziness, sedation, priapism with trazodone, liver failure warning with nefazodone	Generally considered safe in overdose but has potential for cardiac arrythmias
	Mirtazapine	Antagonizes the NE, 5HT2 and 5HT3 receptors	Sedation, dry mouth, confusion, increased appetite and weight gain, neutropenia	Relatively safe in overdose

5HT = serotonin, NE = norepinephrine, DA = dopamine, TCA = tricyclic antidepressant, SSRI = selective serotonergic reuptake inhibitor, MAOI = monoamine oxidase inhibitor.

its own. However, the current episode is severe enough to affect social and academic functioning. The episode was characteristically preceded by stress of examinations, graduation, and a significant life transition into adulthood and independence. The diagnosis was based on the symptoms of anhedonia, insomnia, anergia, poor concentration, poor appetite, and suicidal ideation. Signs of depression are also evident in the patient's mental status examination, which indicated psychomotor retardation, soft, monotonous speech, dysphoric affect, poor concentration, and thoughts of hopelessness. The patient reported thinking about suicide but had not conceived of a plan. Given the patient's thoughts of death and potential risk to herself, she was hospitalized on an inpatient psychiatric unit. Despite the absence of any active suicidal plan, a brief inpatient stay was useful to ensure her safety, initiate treatment, and provide a therapeutic atmosphere in which outside stressors were temporarily held at bay. Escitalopram, 10 mg/day, was started, and the patient was soon after discharged to outpatient psychiatric care for medication management and brief cognitive therapy.

Pearls

1. Mood is defined by some authorities as the patient's reported internal emotional state, whereas others describe mood as the objectively observed internal sustained emotional state. Affect, on the other hand, is defined by some authorities as the external expression of present emotional content, whereas others describe affect as the moment-to-moment fluctuations in emotional tone. Most consider either convention as correct.

2. Always determine suicidality because the patient's safety is of utmost importance. Expressions of suicidality must always be taken seriously, and patients who express suicidal intent are strong candidates for hospital admission.

3. In assessing the patient with depressive symptoms, always rule out bipolar disorder because of the significant treatment implications. In fact, treating patients with bipolar disorder with antidepressants has been known to induce a manic episode.

4. Recent research has focused on assigning more specific roles to the serotonergic receptor system based on subclasses and locations of these receptors. The hypothalamic-pituitary-adrenocorticoid axis is also receiving renewed attention. Researchers are investigating the role of chronic corticoid activation in utero and childhood as a risk factor as well as the role of life stressors that put strain on this system.

REFERENCES

1. Kaplan, Sadock: Synopsis of Psychiatry. Philadelphia, Lippincott Williams & Wilkins, 1998.
2. Kendler K, Thornton L, Gardner C: Genetic risk, number of previous depressive episodes, and stressful life events in predicting onset of major depression. Am J Psychiatry 2001;158:582–586.
3. Lewinsohn P, Rohde P, Seeley J, et al: Natural course of adolescent major depressive disorder in a community sample: predictors of recurrence in young adults. Am J Psychiatry 2000; 57:1584–1591.
4. Muller-Oerlinghausen B, Berghofer A: Antidepressants and suicidal risk. J Clin Psychiatry 1999;60(Suppl 2):94–99.
5. Pezawas l, Stamenkovic M, Jagsch R, et al: A longitudinal view of triggers and threshold of suicidal behavior in depression. J Clin Psychiatry 2002;63:866–873.

PATIENT 25

A 73-year-old woman with agitated behavior

History of Present Illness: A 73-year-old Caucasian woman is brought to the psychiatric emergency department by her daughter after she yelled at her family, throwing plates at her son-in-law and smearing food all over her clothes. The patient has lived with her children in a suburban home since the death of her husband 4 years ago. The daughter describes her as pleasant, friendly and energetic most of the time, but for the past 3 weeks she has noted several episodes of confusion. The patient has been forgetful, misplacing items in the house and also sleeping significantly less at night without evidence of daytime sleepiness. The patient's son-in-law describes worsening irritability over these past weeks and frequent arguments despite the fact that their relationship is usually quite good. One week before the current presentation, the patient told her daughter that her husband was committing adultery and may not be the honest person that everybody thinks he is. In addition, the patient's grandson has noticed his grandmother shaking more when drinking her coffee during their breakfasts together.

Past Psychiatric History: After the sudden death of her husband, the patient saw a psychiatrist for 2 years. She was treated with citalopram and received counseling by a social worker for complicated bereavement for about 1 year. The symptoms subsided after she moved in with her family, and the pharmacotherapy and counseling were discontinued. No other significant past psychiatric history is evident.

Past Medical History: The patient's daughter reports a longstanding history of cardiac disease, including coronary artery disease and two past episodes of atrial fibrillation. The patient has also suffered from osteoporosis since age 62. She takes aspirin, isosorbide dinitrate, and calcium carbonate on a regular basis.

Mental Status Examination: The patient is a very thin woman who looks slightly older than her stated age. She appears to be sweating and repeatedly complains about the heat in the examination room. Her eye contact is limited, and she seems distracted from the interview, at times appearing to have fluctuations in consciousness. There is some psychomotor restlessness and a continuous tremor of about 10 Hz. Speech is incoherent at times, with increased rate and volume. Her mood appears to be irritable, with labile affect and rapid shifts to anger. Thought process is tangential and disturbed by perseveration; when asked about problems with everyday activities, she repeatedly replies: "There is something wrong with my son-in-law." Her thought content is preoccupied with paranoid ideation toward her son-in-law, who allegedly convinced her daughter that she is a "bad woman" who "needs to be taken care of." She denies perceptual disturbances and suicidal and homicidal ideation. She is not consistently alert and is oriented to person only, but not to place or time, and is altogether unaware that she is in a hospital. Her attention span is impaired (digit span of 2), as is her short-term memory (immediate recall is 1/3), although her long-term memory is preserved. Impulse control is impaired as evidenced by violent behavior. Her insight is limited, and her judgment is impaired.

Physical Examination: General cachexia. Slight exophthalmos. Mucous membranes moist. Chest is clear to auscultation bilaterally. Heart rate = 153 beats/min, irregularly irregular. Abdomen benign. Bilateral hyperreflexia. Tremor. Babinski's signs negative.

Diagnostic Testing: The EKG shows tachycardia and atrial fibrillation (see figure, p. 89). The EEG shows a generalized beta rhythm with occasional delta waves and rare sharp waves. A CT scan of the head is negative. The laboratory tests show a thyroid-stimulating hormone (TSH) level less than 0.02.

Questions: What is the diagnosis? What is the underlying cause?

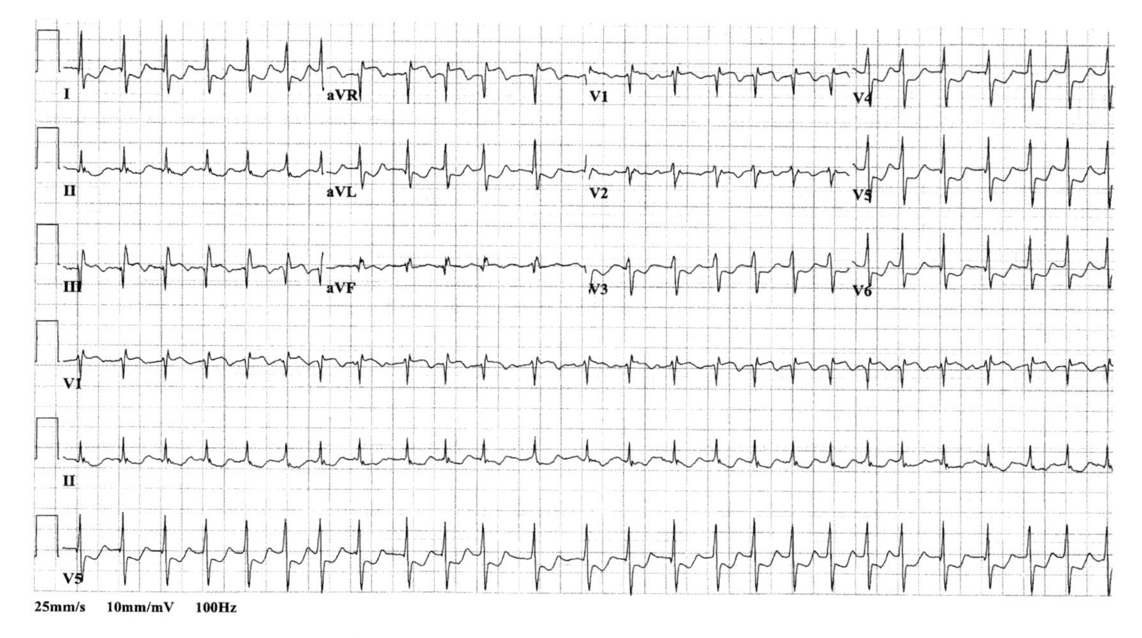

Atrial fibrillation with rapid ventricular response.

Vent. rate	153	bpm
PR interval	*	
ARS duration	84	ms
QT/QTc	304/485	ms
P-R-T axes	* 44	185

Diagnosis: Delirium due to hyperthyroidism.

Discussion: Delirium is usually easy to recognize but difficult to define. Delirium can be distinguished from mania and psychosis by its course (usually acute onset), its stability (usually fluctuating with "waxing and waning" of consciousness), and its global nature. In this patient, the diagnosis of delirium was based on the presence of decreased attention, fluctuating levels of consciousness, and impaired concentration. Although symptoms of psychosis (e.g., paranoid ideation) and mania (tangentiality and perseveration of thought) were present in this patient, the diagnosis rests on the global changes in mental status (i.e., the presence of disturbances of attention and memory as well thought process and content), accompanied by fluctuating levels of consciousness.

Once a syndromal diagnosis of delirium is established, the identification of the underlying cause is of paramount importance. Delirium is associated with substantial mortality, since many of its causes (e.g., stroke, myocardial infarction, electrolyte imbalances) are potentially life-threatening and frail people are more prone to developing delirium. Following guidelines for the treatment of delirium, the management in this patient should be interdisciplinary. Although many drugs, especially psychoactive substances, can cause delirium, in this patient drug-induced delirium could be ruled out given the benign medication regimen. Rather, hyperthyroidism emerged as the cause of delirium.

The general psychiatric manifestations of hyperthyroidism may include restlessness, agitation, decreased sleep, hyperactivity, and irritability. Short-term memory may also be impaired in hyperthyroidism, as in this patient. The diagnosis was based on the presence of multiple physical signs of hyperthyroidism, such as exophthalmus, tremor of 8–12 Hz, wasting, heat sensitivity, and brisk reflexes. Atrial fibrillation is also a common consequence of hyperthyroidism, especially in new onset thyrotoxicosis (see figure, p. 89). Other causes of atrial fibrillation, such as myocardial infarction and hypertension, must also be ruled out in this patient. The EEG findings in hyperthyroidism are often nonspecific, although systematic analyses point to an increase in sharp waves and a predominant beta rhythm. Beyond general psychiatric symptoms, many patients also exhibit more specific disturbances of mood and thought. Classical case series report mood disorders in up to 30% of patients with hyperthyroidism and psychotic symptoms in up to 11% of cases. The subtle paranoid symptoms in this patient may well be interpreted in that context.

The acute treatment of thyrotoxicosis requires the collaboration of endocrinologists and psychiatrists. In this case, cardiologists were also of particular importance because of the presence of atrial fibrillation. Attempts to quickly revert the patient to a euthyroid state can have fatal consequences on the cardiovascular system, especially in cases of long-standing hyperthyroidism. Symptomatic treatment should include neuroleptic agents for agitation and benzodiazepines for anxiety. Constant monitoring of cardiovascular function is also typically indicated.

The prognosis for thyrotoxicosis is generally good. Psychiatric manifestations can be expected to cease when a euthyroid state is attained. Adjunctive treatment with psychotropic agents is helpful symptomatically but may not affect prognosis, which depends primarily on cardiovascular functioning. When symptoms of depression are present, patients may also benefit from a limited course of antidepressant treatment.

Pearls

1. Delirium is distinguished from mania and psychosis by the acuity of onset, fluctuations in consciousness, and a global change in mental status.
2. Hyperthyroidism may be present in hospitalized geriatric populations at a rate of up to 14%. It affects females more commonly than males (6:1), and the risk for developing hyperthyroidism increases with age.
3. In contrast to hyperactive delirium, apathetic delirium in a hyperthyroid patient may be a hallmark of impending myxedema and coma.

REFERENCES

1. Abend WK, Tyler HR: Thyroid disease and the nervous system. In Aminoff MJ: Neurology and General Medicine. New York, Livingstone, 1989, pp 509–536.
2. Bursten B: Psychoses associated with thyrotoxicosis. Arch Gen Psychiatry 1961;4;267–273.
3. Dunlap HF, Moersch FP: Psychic manifestations associated with hyperthyroidism. Am J Psychiatry 1935;91;1215–1238.
4. Lishman A: Organic Psychiatry. London, Blackwell 1998.
5. Whybrow PC, Prange AJ, Treadway CR: Mental Changes accompanying thyroid gland dysfunction. Arch Gen Psychiatry 1969;20;48–63.

PATIENT 26

A 38-year-old woman who fears that something is wrong with her body

History of Present Illness: A 38-year-old, single, unemployed woman without a formal psychiatric history was referred to an outpatient psychiatric clinic by her primary care doctor. On initial presentation she complains, "I don't know why I'm here. My problem is that no one can tell me what's wrong with me; they all say I'm crazy. Maybe they're right; nothing they give me works. The problem is that they think I'm making it all up." Even before the psychiatrist can start a structured interview, the patient launches into a detailed history of her symptoms and the work-up to date.

Her symptoms first crystallized 3 years ago in the context of both her father's death from a heart attack and her sister's diagnosis with systemic lupus erythematosus. She describes her sister as "just like me, always sick, always with some pain or illness. We both get everything that's going around." She reports that her sister was initially misdiagnosed and did not get treatment for the illness early in its course. She fears that this may be happening to her and imagines a slow and painful deterioration of her body. Although she has always felt that something is wrong with her body, only in the past few years has she been unable to think of anything else. She also describes feeling increasingly frustrated with doctors who cannot find any tangible malady to diagnose or treat.

The patient reports first going to her doctor 3 years ago for evaluation of right upper quadrant pain without other associated symptoms. This pain was unrelenting and severe, and the patient feared she had hepatitis, learning of the condition from one of the books in her library of medical texts. The doctor performed a physical exam and reassured her that nothing was out of the ordinary. The patient nevertheless insisted on blood tests before leaving the doctor's office. Despite the fact that all results were found to be normal the next week, the pain would not abate, and she presented again for an unscheduled appointment. This time the doctor referred her for an abdominal sonogram, which was normal. She continued to call his office, every week or so, reasserting her original complaint. The doctor continued to order more and more tests, including an abdominal CT scan and endoscopy. All results were normal. Still she was not satisfied with the results and became distrustful of this doctor's methods and thoroughness; feelings of resentment grew, as he would send her for tests without agreeing to see her for yet another unscheduled visit.

Gradually, the patient's preoccupation with right upper quadrant pain receded, but soon after concerns began about occasional feelings of breathlessness and fatigue. She feared emphysema. She referred herself to a pulmonologist, and again a full work-up was negative. This symptom constellation relieved itself in about 1 month and was succeeded by a feeling of "tiredness in my eyes when I read for a long time." She immediately thought of going blind. Her ophthalmologist diagnosed her with convergence insufficiency and gave her "eye muscle exercises" to perform every night. The exercises relieved her symptoms for about 3 weeks, although all the while she maintained underlying fears of hepatitis, occasionally of emphysema, and increasingly, as of late, of a brain tumor. "I have a headache. I can't read so well anymore. Something has got to tie all this together." She eventually returned to her initial primary care physician, but "he was not happy to see me. He told me it was all in my head and refused to do anything for me until I saw a psychiatrist."

She denies any change in mood and denies any worries about money, friends, or anything else not related to her health. She is able to acknowledge, ever so briefly, that there may not be a physical ailment to account for her symptoms but greatly minimizes this suggestion. She reports thoughts about having various illnesses "popping into my mind, and then I have to examine the parts of my body involved, or check with a friend." She denies the presence of panic attacks but states that occasionally her heart beats quickly, sometimes her hands feel numb, and often she feels dizzy. She fervently denies suicidality, "I'm trying to find out what's wrong with me, to prevent my pain and death. Again, a doctor doesn't understand me!"

Past Psychiatric History: The patient has never before seen a psychiatrist and has never taken any psychiatric medications. She describes herself as an anxious person, however.

Past Medical History: The patient reports having "many colds" as a child. Throughout her life, she frequently presented to her primary care doctor with complaints of throat pain and redness and always insisted on taking antibiotics. She was never admitted to the hospital and has no known medical problems beyond those described in the history of present illness.

Social History: The patient was born and raised in the Midwest United States and graduated from college with a degree in visual arts. She worked for an advertising firm until 3 years ago, when she took off time to mourn her father's death as well as to help her sister with her new illness. She never went back to work as her own symptoms grew in intensity. In her mid 20s, she became divorced after a 4-year marriage and has no children. The patient says that her marriage ended because "he thought I was too neurotic and would say that I was always negative." She is not currently sexually active or involved in a relationship.

Mental Status Examination: The patient is a well-groomed and attractive woman. She feels her pulse while leaning back in the office chair, occasionally taking deep breaths, appearing to concentrate on her body. She alternates between attitudes of being condescending and submissive during the interview. There are no psychomotor changes, and she maintains good eye contact. Her speech is fluent, with normal rate, rhythm, and volume. Mood is remarkable for mild anxiety. Affect is full range, slightly nervous, and congruent with mood and appropriate to content. Her thought process is linear and goal-directed, although she is preoccupied with her history of poor medical care and returns each new topic of conversation to this theme. There is no evidence of delusional material, suicidality or homicidality, or hallucinations. Insight is poor. Judgment is fair. Impulse control is intact. Cognition is intact; she is alert and oriented to person, place, and time with intact attention and concentration.

Questions: What is the diagnosis? How would you treat this patient?

Diagnosis: Hypochondriasis.

Discussion: Hypochondriasis is classified as a somatoform disorder by the current edition of the American Psychiatric Association's DSM (IV-TR). While historically it has been one of the most durable disease concepts, experts disagree about the accuracy of its conceptualization as an axis I illness and whether it is a personality trait, personality disorder, or a dimension of some other pathology. What is clear, however, is that it is quite disabling with significant morbidity. Many patients have significantly impaired physical functioning and work performance and frequently use a disproportionate degree of medical services. Multiple epidemiologic reports have found that 1–5% of the general population and 2–7% of patients seen in general medical clinics suffer from hypochondriasis. Many patients are referred to psychiatrists with a label of hypochondriasis based solely on the exclusion of a physical disorder rather than on the presence of specific psychological symptoms and processes. An initial psychiatric formulation should demonstrate evidence of a specific underlying psychological process, including the presence of etiologic and maintenance factors.

The specific etiology of hypochondriasis is unknown at present, but a number of theories have been presented. Developmental theorists propose that early childhood adverse environments, such as abuse, and the presence of severe illness in childhood are potentially contributing factors. Cognitive-behavioral theorists, on the other hand, posit that faulty cognitive appraisals attribute otherwise normal bodily sensations to a pathologic process, thereby creating symptoms of anxiety and resultant autonomic hyperactivity. Patients may subsequently show selective memory and attention to medical information and physical changes that support the diagnosis of a particular illness while ignoring contradictory information. Sociocultural factors in the etiology of hypochondriasis include assuming the sick role, in which care is elicited from others and the afflicted individual may be exempt from responsibility and blame for the illness. In some cases, the presentation of symptoms as physical may serve to minimize the stigma associated with psychiatric illness. Hypochondriasis may also be partially iatrogenic in origin, as physicians make alarming statements, order anxiety-producing tests, and tell patients that nothing is wrong despite their symptoms. However, these sociocultural issues may play a maintaining role in the presence of hypochondriasis rather than contribute to its initial etiology.

Clinically, hypochondriasis exists along a spectrum of severity. Although 60–80% of healthy persons have unexplained physical symptoms in any given week and 10–20% of healthy persons experience intermittent worry over the same period, they can usually be reassured by others. Hypochondriacs, however, cannot be reassured for long. The essential feature of hypochondriasis is a morbid preoccupation with and a sense of vulnerability concerning one's body. Patients are preoccupied with fears of having or developing a serious medical illness. Their minds become filled with images and ideas of a disabling or disfiguring illness, up to and including death; one or more organ systems may be affected. These intrusive thoughts are typically accompanied by a sense of conviction and become overvalued. The patient's attention is narrowly focused on his or her body, specifically its functions (e.g., heartbeat, respiration, peristalsis), minor abnormalities (e.g., bumps, small sore), and vague or diffuse sensations (e.g., poor concentration, fatigue). In response to the intrusive thoughts, patients often engage in checking behaviors, examining their bodies, poking and prodding, seeking reassurance from others, and consulting medical texts. They frequently experience alarm when reading or hearing about a disease or when someone whom they know has become sick with a serious illness. Patients often have limited insight into the nature of their symptoms, although their fears of illness never quite reach delusional proportions. Patients are often quite self-absorbed, and others frequently find that all conversations revolve around the patient's physical health or lack thereof. Social relationships may also become strained because patients often expect friends and family to provide them with special treatment. In general, hypochondriasis has three key components: bodily preoccupation, fear of disease, and disease conviction. These symptoms must be present for at least 6 months and must not be better explained by an anxiety disorder, a major depressive disorder, another somatoform disorder, or a psychotic disorder.

In the psychiatric setting, the most efficacious therapeutic modalities include cognitive behavioral therapy (CBT) and pharmacotherapy, although there is still only minimal evidence for each. The hallmark of CBT is the identification and altering of dysfunctional beliefs about health and disease, modifying maladaptive behaviors, and learning relaxation techniques. It may include graded exposure to disturbing stimuli to prevent pathologic responses (exposure-response prevention). Cognitive behavioral treatment also includes an educational component—namely, that an organic illness is not the only reasonable explanation for a patient's symptoms. Some authors have mentioned that CBT should be reserved for times in the course of the illness when the patient has a greater degree of insight.

Psychopharmacologic treatment for hypochondriasis consists of antidepressants of the selective serotonin reuptake inhibitor (SSRI) class and a few from the tricyclic (TCA) class. Again, only limited studies are available. On initiation of pharmacotherapy, it is important to explain to the patient that these medications work at the level of the brain, citing a central nervous system pathology that accounts for their symptoms. One also must start at smaller doses than usual, because patients tend to be highly sensitive to side effects. The final effective dose may often be in the highest range for the particular medication, and response time may be longer than usual, similar to the treatment of obsessive-compulsive disorder. Medications should be continued for at least 1 year. Anxiolytic therapy (benzodiazepines) may also be used for temporary relief. Any and all comorbid psychiatric illnesses must be treated, and nearly two-thirds of patients with hypochondriasis have a comorbid psychiatric disorder: the lifetime prevalence of major depressive disorder is 40%; of panic disorder, 16%; and of obsessive-compulsive disorder, 5–10%. Personality disorders occur 3-fold more often in people with hypochondriasis than in controls in a general medical clinic. The presence of such comorbidities often complicates the course of illness.

The differential diagnosis of hypochondriasis includes specific phobia, panic disorder, generalized anxiety disorder, obsessive-compulsive disorder, major depressive disorder, somatoform disorders, delusional disorder, and the presence of a general medical illness that explains the symptoms. The current patient was diagnosed based on her persistent fear of having an underlying illness despite all evidence to the contrary. As is typical in hypochondriasis, this patient's symptoms began in the context of psychosocial stressors. Her father died, and her sister, a close family member with whom the patient identifies, was diagnosed with a serious illness. It is curious and unusual, however, that this patient did not present with a fear of lupus at any time in her history. She nevertheless followed a highly characteristic path for the development and psychological conceptualization of symptoms in hypochondriasis. With each new symptom, she believed an additional serious illness was developing, well out of bounds of normal interpretation. She felt that no one understood her, especially her doctors; as a result, she shopped around continuously. With each new doctor, patients possess a small degree of hope as well as significant apprehension. The present patient's presentation may call on the physician's therapeutic zeal, and this patient seemed able to get each of her physicians to embark on a crusade to find her correct diagnosis. Many doctors faced with such a patient may become frustrated and want to provide a hasty diagnosis or simply tell the patient that "it is all in your head," as was the case here.

The eventual psychiatric treatment of this patient began by first providing an explanation for the psychosomatic nature of her symptoms, which she appeared to absorb with a modicum of acceptance. She was not fully convinced, however, and retained a degree of apprehension. She was also given a prescription for fluoxetine, 10 mg/day, which was to be titrated to effect. Although she was initially pleased with the possibility of a medication to treat her distress, she remained hesitant and stated that she would have to read about the medication before filling the prescription. She also stated that she wished to be followed by her primary care doctor instead of the psychiatrist. The following treatment guidelines were provided for her physician: (1) schedule regular weekly or biweekly appointments and do not reinforce symptom-driven visits; (2) use reassurance sparingly with repeated explanations of symptoms; (3) employ a nonconfrontational approach when new symptoms arise; (4) validate symptoms but limit the number of tests and treatments; (5) permit dependence initially to allow the development of a trusting relationship; (6) eventually encourage independence to avoid regression; (7) always set limits; (8) do not ask about the symptoms if she does not present them; and (9) remember that the doctor-patient relationship is the most important therapeutic modality.

Hypochondriasis generally follows a waxing-and-waning course. Just as the initial presentation can be precipitated by stressful life events, course exacerbations may also occur in the same context and be superimposed on a baseline of chronic symptoms. Approximately two-thirds of patients show some improvement but continue to meet diagnostic criteria 5 years later. The remaining third of patients have persistent, albeit fewer symptoms. Only on occasion do patients spontaneously experience full recovery. Good prognostic indicators include the presence of a comorbid serious medical illness (multiple theories without conclusive explanation have been given for this factor), lack of other psychiatric illnesses, absence of neurotic personality traits, and shorter duration of illness. Some studies have shown overall rates of improvement of 70–80% with pharmacologic intervention or CBT, although no standardized measure of remission exists.

Pearls

1. Using objective measures of visceral interpretation, no differences have been found between subjects with hypochondriasis and normal controls. However, subjects with hypochondriasis score consistently higher on scales of somatic amplification, a measure of an increased subjective belief in the presence of pathology.
2. Despite improvement with treatment or even with spontaneous improvement, patients' scores on scales of bodily sensation amplification do not change. This finding may reflect the trait-like nature of this construct and certainly confers a high vulnerability to relapse.
3. The doctor-patient relationship is crucial in hypochondriasis and involves the recognition that the physician's approach alone may be the most powerful therapeutic tool.
4. Patients may develop a regimen of compulsive behaviors designed to minimize their symptoms of fear and anxiety.
5. The clinical picture of hypochondriasis is heterogeneous, and subtypes may be differentiated by the degree of disease fear and disease conviction. Anxiety may be more likely to occur in patients with severe disease fear, whereas disease conviction manifests more frequently with increased somatic symptoms.

REFERENCES

1. American Psychiatric Association: Diagnostic and Statistical Manual of Mental Disorders, 4th ed., Text Revision. Washington, DC, American Psychiatric Association, 2000.
2. Barsky AJ: The patient with hypochondriasis. N Engl J Med 2001;345(19):1395–1399.
3. Fallon BA, Feinstein S: Hypochondriasis. In Phillips KA (ed): Somatoform and Factitious Disorders. Washington, DC, American Psychiatric Press, 2001, pp 27–65.
4. Lipsitt DR: Hypochondriasis and body dysmorphic disorder. In Gabbard GO (ed): Treatments of Psychiatric Disorders, 3rd ed, vols 1 & 2. Washington, DC, American Psychiatric Press, 2001.
5. Magarinos M, Zafar U, Nissenson K, Blanco C: Epidemiology and treatment of hypochondriasis. CNS Drugs 2002;16(1):9–22.
6. Noyes R: Hypochondriasis. In Gelder MG, Lobez-Ibor JJ, Andreasen NC (eds): New Oxford Textbook of Psychiatry. Oxford, Oxford University Press, 2000, pp 1098–1106.
7. Warwick HMC: Assessment of hypochondriasis. Behav Res Ther 1995;33(7):845–853.

PATIENT 27

A 31-year-old woman with symptoms of anger and irritability

History of Present Illness: A 31-year-old woman presents with her boyfriend to the psychiatric emergency department with complaints of depressed mood and thoughts that her life might not be worth living. She was in her usual state of good mental health until 2 weeks ago when her investment advisor informed her that she had lost the bulk of her retirement fund in a stock market crash. Since then, she has had several days when she feels tired and irritable and has been staying up watching late-night television until the early hours of the morning. Friends and coworkers have complained to her that she has been unusually short-tempered and curt recently. Her boyfriend has also found her teary-eyed a few times. During those episodes, she told him that she was upset with herself for not having been more careful with her money. Despite all of this, she still manages to enjoy watching television every Thursday night to see her favorite sitcoms. She also continues to eat a healthy balanced diet and, until a few days ago, she went to the gym five days per week on average. Her boyfriend insisted that she be evaluated after she mentioned that her life might not be worth living.

The patient has no history of substance abuse, but she does have an occasional glass of wine when socializing with friends on the weekends. She reports a highly supportive network of family and friends with whom she interacts on a regular basis. The patient has been working as a successful architect but has been unable to go to work for the past few days.

Past Psychiatric History: The patient has no significant past psychiatric history. She denies any history of depressive, manic, or hypomanic episodes. She has no history of suicidal ideation or attempts and denies any family history of psychiatric disorders or suicide.

Mental Status Examination: The patient is a healthy-looking woman who appears younger than her stated age. Her eye contact is limited, and she occasionally gets teary-eyed. She appears internally preoccupied with a delay in response to questions. She is cooperative but not very engaging. Her psychomotor behavior is neither agitated nor retarded. Her speech is of normal rate, volume, and tone. She describes her mood as "horrible" and appears moderately depressed. Her affect is mood-congruent and stable. Her thought process is perseverative; she insists on talking about how she could have prevented her financial loss. Her thought content is focused on her financial situation with no magical thinking and no delusions. She denies any plan or intent to kill herself but thinks that she might be better off if she just "didn't wake up." She denies any homicidal ideation, paranoid ideation, or perceptual disturbances. Her insight and judgment are fair, and she is in good control. She is alert and oriented, and her concentration is within normal limits.

Diagnostic Testing: Urine and serum toxicology are negative for substances. Chemistries, liver function tests, complete blood count with platelets, and thyroid-stimulating hormone levels are within normal limits. Vitamin B12, folate, and syphilis testing were also unremarkable.

Question: What is the diagnosis?

Diagnosis: Adjustment disorder with depressed mood, acute.

Discussion: Adjustment disorder is characterized by the development of maladaptive behavior or emotional disturbances that begin in the context of a defined stressor. The stressor is usually a common event rather than a life-threatening or catastrophic one. The patient's reaction must be out of proportion to the intensity of the stressor, or the symptoms should cause impairment in social or occupational functioning. If the presenting symptoms are consistent with a more specific axis I disorder, the patient should receive that diagnosis instead. Patients who already have a psychiatric disorder can still be given the diagnosis of adjustment disorder if there are new symptoms in response to a stressor as long as the response is not a simple exacerbation of an already present axis I or II disorder.

There are two forms of the disorder-acute and chronic. Most cases are the acute form, in which the symptoms start within 3 months of the acute stressor and resolve within 6 months of the termination of that stressor or when the patient is able to adapt to it. The chronic specifier is used if symptoms persist for more than 6 months following the removal of the stressor, or if the stressor has enduring consequences.

When the diagnosis of adjustment disorder is considered, other psychiatric disorders must also be ruled out, such as bipolar disorder, major depressive disorder, dysthymia, bereavement, mood disorder secondary to a general medical condition, and substance-induced mood disorder. Because the present patient reports no history of signs or symptoms consistent with mania or hypomania, bipolar disorder is unlikely. Although she currently has depressed mood and poor sleep and reports that she occasionally feels tired, this pattern does not occur on most days, as would be expected in a major depressive disorder. In addition, her guilt about losing her money is not excessive or inappropriate. As a result, despite the presence of passive suicidal ideation and several neurovegetative symptoms, she does not meet criteria for a major depressive episode. Dysthymic disorder is also unlikely because her depressed mood has only been present for a few weeks; she does not meet the time course criterion (2 years). And given that the patient's lab results were normal in conjunction with the absence of any past medical history, she does not appear to have a mood disorder secondary to a general medical condition. Finally, the patient's urine toxicology was negative, and she denies drug use; thus, there is no evidence for a substance-induced mood disorder. In considering the patient's normal functioning prior to the stressor of losing her money and the significant impact that it has had on her mood and social functioning, she meets criteria for an adjustment disorder with depressed mood, acute.

There are six different subtypes of adjustment disorder (see Table 1): (1) with depressed mood; (2) with anxiety; (3) with mixed depressed mood and anxiety; (4) with disturbance of conduct; (5) with mixed disturbance of emotion and conduct; and (6) unspecified. According to several epidemiologic studies, adjustment disorder with depressed mood is the most common subtype. The present patient best fits into the subcategory "with depressed mood" because she is depressed, does not have anxiety as a prominent symptom, and does not demonstrate behavior that violates the rights of others or that goes against societal norms (with disturbance of conduct).

Adjustment disorder has a broad definition as a "maladaptive reaction" that makes it hard to distinguish from depressive disorder not otherwise specified (NOS) or anxiety disorder NOS. Often, the tentative diagnosis of adjustment disorder is confirmed by the outcome of the case because patients tend to recover quickly and return to their previous level of functioning. Adjustment disorder may not be a stable diagnosis in the hospital setting, however, and one study noted that 40% of patients given this diagnosis on admission were given a different diagnosis on discharge. It has also been suggested that the diagnosis of adjustment disorder might be overused because it is perceived to be less stigmatizing for the patient than other axis I or II diagnoses. However, this idea remains speculative. The overall prevalence of adjustment disorder is also unclear; rates vary from 4% to 20% according to the study.

Suicide is a concern in patients with adjustment disorder; therefore, it is always important to assess

Table 1. Subtypes of Adjustment Disorder

Subtype	Salient Features
With depressed mood	Symptoms of mild depression
With anxiety	Anxiety is the prominent symptom
With mixed depressed mood and anxiety	Combination of a mild depression with anxiety
With disturbance of conduct	Behavior that violates the rights of others or goes against societal norms
With mixed disturbance of emotion and conduct	Mood disturbance with behavior that violates the rights of others or goes against societal norms
Unspecified	The adjustment reaction does not clearly fall under any of the above categories

the patient's risk of suicide when this diagnosis is contemplated. In comparison with patients with major depressive disorder, patients with adjustment disorder tend to be younger, less likely to have had previous psychiatric contact, and more likely to have comorbid psychoactive substance use disorders. Importantly, patients with adjustment disorder are also less likely to convey suicide intent to health care providers. Several studies found that suicide attempts in adjustment disorder are more likely to be associated with alcohol abuse compared with major depressive disorder. It is also hard to assess the risk for suicide in this patient population because patients with adjustment disorder often commit suicidal acts in an impulsive manner. They do not typically have a history of previous suicide attempts; they are less likely to create a plan or write a note and less likely to discuss their intent with health care providers compared to suicidal patients with major depressive disorder. A history of alcohol abuse and impulsive behavior are important markers of risk in making a suicide assessment in patients with adjustment disorder.

The two main goals in treating a patient with adjustment disorder are (1) to address the patient's symptoms and (2) to assess the risk for suicide. There is no clear guidance on the use of pharmacotherapy in the management of adjustment disorder; no controlled studies have confirmed the benefits of antidepressants or anxiolytics. That said, patients are generally treated for their symptoms with antidepressants and/or anxiolytics, depending on presentation. One study reported that patients who have adjustment disorder with depressed mood benefit from treatment of depressive symptoms as much as patients who suffer from depressed mood in the context of other diagnoses. Accordingly, prescription rates for anxiolytics and antidepressants for adjustment disorder have been found to be the same as for other axis I and II disorders when examined in an inpatient consult-liaison setting. Furthermore, some authors have argued that patients with adjustment disorder with depressed mood might actually be suffering from subthreshold depression and therefore benefit from an early start in treatment. Although no solid evidence supports this notion, the benefits of beginning treatment probably outweigh the risks in most cases.

Psychotherapy is also recommended as a treatment, and a variety of modalities have been suggested, including, but not limited to, counseling, supportive therapy, cognitive behavioral therapy, and psychodynamic therapy. The focus of the treatment, regardless of orientation, tends to be to help the patient gain insight into the nature of his or her reaction to the stressor.

The present patient was considered for hospitalization because of the extent of her depressed mood and the presence of suicidal thoughts accompanied by the additional risk factor of alcohol use. However, her alcohol use probably did not reach proportions of abuse or dependence, and she had no history of suicidality or poor impulse control. In addition, at the time of the evaluation, she was denying suicidal ideation and had good social support. Instead of hospitalization, the patient was referred to outpatient treatment with a psychiatrist who initiated brief supportive psychotherapy in addition to a selective serotonergic antidepressant medication. Within several weeks, she reported significantly improved mood and continued to deny suicidal ideation. Over the course of the following month, the patient's depressive symptoms abated altogether, as is appropriate in adjustment disorder, and the brief treatment and medication regimen were discontinued after 6 months.

Pearls

1. Adjustment disorder is a diagnosis of exclusion. Other disorders, including bipolar disorder, major depressive disorder, and bereavement, should be carefully ruled out.
2. Suicide risk in patients with adjustment disorder appears to be driven by impulsivity and/or substance abuse; a thorough history to assess both factors is therefore critical.
3. Preliminary studies have suggested that in patients with adjustment disorder who attempt suicide, platelet monoamine oxidase (MAO) activity may be lowered and maximal binding capacity of platelet serotonin-2A receptors may be elevated. These findings, if replicated, suggest potential indicators of suicidality in patients with adjustment disorder and are consistent with earlier studies of suicidality in the context of other psychiatric disorders.
4. One of the more interesting arguments in the literature revolves around the limitations of the DSM in distinguishing between major depression and adjustment disorder because of the rigid nature of the diagnostic criteria. Many researchers argue that DSM diagnostic criteria are oversimplified and that clinicians should not apply a cookbook approach to the field.

REFERENCES

1. Casey P, Dowrick C, Wilkinson G: Adjustment disorders: Fault line in the psychiatric glossary. Br J Psychiatry 2001;179: 479–481.
2. Greenberg WM, Rosenfeld DN, Ortega EA: Adjustment disorder as an admission diagnosis. Am J Psychiatry 1995;152:459–461.
3. Isometsä E, Heikkinen M, Henriksson M, et al: Suicide in non-major depressions. J Affect Disord 1996;36:117–127.
4. Jones R, Yates WR, Williams S, et al: Outcome for adjustment disorder with depressed mood: Comparison with other mood disorders. J Affect Disord 1999;55:55–61.
5. Polyakova I, Knobler HY, Ambrumova A, Lerner V: Characteristics of suicidal attempts in major depression versus adjustment reactions. J Affect Disord 1998;47: 59–167.
6. Rao ML, Hawellek B, Papassotiropoulos A, et al: Upregulation of the platelet serotonin 2A receptor and low blood serotonin in suicidal psychiatric patients. Neuropsychobiology 1998;18: 84–89.
7. Snyder S, Strain JJ, Wolf D: Differentiating major depression from adjustment disorder with depressed mood in the medical setting. Gen Hosp Psychiatry 1990;12:159–165.
8. Strain JJ, Smith GC, Hammer JS, et al: Adjustment disorder: A multisite study of its utilization and interventions in the consultation-liaison psychiatry setting. Gen Hosp Psychiatry 1998;20:139–149.
9. Tripodianakis J, Markianos M, Saratidis D, Leotsakou C: Neurochemical variables in subjects with adjustment disorder after suicide attempts. Eur J Psychiatry 2000;15:190–195.

PATIENT 28

A 35-year-old man with ataxia and cognitive impairment

History of Present Illness: A 35-year-old man is transferred to a tertiary care facility from a chronic psychiatric hospital because of a change in mental status. When the patient is interviewed, he cannot remember the year or the name of the hospital where he has lived for more than 10 years. He is unable to give a reasonable account of his psychiatric history, answering most questions with either, "That's a good question," or "I don't remember." He spends the entire interview wandering in a circle around the edges of the room, clinging to the wall for support and guidance, despite attempts to get him to sit down. The psychiatrist walks the room with him, conducting the interview. When the patient's passage is obstructed by a chair, he stops abruptly, shrieks, and begins to cry. When the chair is removed, he stops crying just as suddenly and resumes his walking.

The patient states that he used to hear voices many years ago, but he has not heard voices for a "long time." When asked to clarify, he states, "Years." He denies any history of visual hallucinations. And although the reliability of his answers is low, he denies suicidal and homicidal ideation.

Vital signs reveal normal blood pressure, heart rate, respirations, and temperature. Pulse oximetry shows 100% saturation on room air.

Past Psychiatric History: A chart review is initiated, spanning his 15-year hospitalization history. Apparently he originally presented at age 17 with auditory hallucinations that were largely a running commentary on his own thoughts and behaviors. He had two episodes of catatonia early in the course of his illness. He was hospitalized multiple times over the first few months of his illness, and eventually, because of increasingly disorganized and bizarre behavior, he was institutionalized at a state hospital, where he has been since age 20. The chart describes a man with auditory hallucinations, disorganized behavior, and inappropriate affect that appeared unresponsive to antipsychotic medications. Eventually the patient was placed on clozapine, and his symptoms appeared to diminish somewhat—he no longer reported auditory hallucinations and his affect appeared less strange. His disorganized behavior persisted, however, and seemed to worsen slowly with time. He began to have significantly long periods when he would not speak, and a return of his catatonia was repeatedly suspected.

He seemed to be stable for a time, without recurrence of a full-blown psychotic state but with significant residual thought and behavior disorganization. Then, a few months ago, he began to deteriorate and developed a tremor, which was originally thought to be the result of years of antipsychotic use. His gait changed—he started walking with a wider stance and seemed unsteady on his feet. He began to become more impulsive and uninhibited. He started to expose himself in the dayroom of the unit and had to be escorted back to his room during these times because he seemed unable to comply with requests that he "zip up." He quickly became agitated and angry at staff when he did not get his way, and recently he had struck staff members on two separate occasions.

Corroborative History: Corroborative history was obtained from the patient's mother. She gave the account of his early life and educational history. He apparently had a "normal" childhood, reaching developmental milestones without delay or difficulty. He had been a good student until age 17 when he began to have significant trouble at school. He would often be found staring out the window during class, making strange gestures apparently to no one, and laughing to himself without explanation. His grades began to slip quickly. He was unable to concentrate on tasks and his work during this time revealed a remarkable falling off of performance. When he began to talk to himself, the mother brought him to the emergency department, where the history of his hospitalizations began. The rest of her history coincides with the information found in the chart.

Mental Status Examination: This 35-year old man appears significantly older than his stated age. He is dressed in a hospital gown that is worn with the opening toward the front, and he has allowed this part of the gown to remain open, exposing his genitals. He is poorly related and inattentive, requiring the evaluating doctor to repeat questions several times before he responds. He has a fine tremor that appears to be present both at rest and with intentional movement; however, no oral-buccal movements are observed. His speech is sparse and nonspontaneous. Besides the few answers that he does give to questions, he largely makes shrieking noises when frustrated. He is unable to describe his mood, but he appears mildly agitated. His affect is somewhat labile; he can switch from playful interest in a spot on the wall to frustrated crying in a matter of seconds. Thought process and content are difficult to ascertain given his inability to converse coherently, but he does say "no" to questions about auditory or visual hallucinations, paranoia, and obsessions. In rare instances, he is able to provide a somewhat coherent statement in response to a simple question. He does not appear to be responding to internal stimuli. He is unable to attend to a formal assessment of his cognitive status with the mini-mental status examination. Insight and judgment are markedly impaired.

Physical Examination and Diagnostic Testing: A physical examination reveals abnormalities only in his neurologic exam. Specifically, he appears to have some lateral nystagmus, pronounced frontal release signs, ataxia, impaired ability to perform repetitive movements, tremor, and some mild spasticity throughout his proximal and distal flexors and extensors in both upper and lower limbs. No clonus is observed, and no cogwheel rigidity is elicited. Deep tendon reflexes are symmetrical and equivocally increased.

Computed tomography (CT) of the head reveals markedly dilated ventricles and increased sulcal markings, consistent with global atrophy. No space-occupying lesions or hemorrhage is noted. Magnetic resonance imaging (MRI) of the brain reveals global, diffuse white matter hyperintensities throughout the frontal and parietal lobes (see figure).

A series of laboratory tests are performed, including a lumbar puncture, heavy metal screen, vitamin B12, folate, rapid plasma reagin, and thyroid function tests. All are within normal limits.

Question: What is the most likely diagnosis?

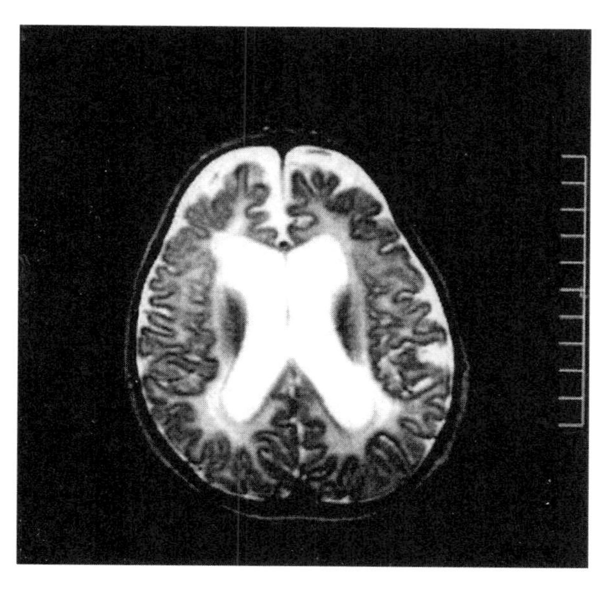

MRI of a 10-month-old patient with MLD. Note the hyperintense changes in deep white matter (areas surrounding the ventricles) along with cerebral atrophy (pronounced sulcal enlargement around the perimeter of the cortex). Even though this patient has the infantile form, findings in the adult form of the disorder show a similar distribution of periventricular white matter demyelination and atrophy. (From Sener RN: Metachromatic leukodystrophy: Diffusion MR imaging findings. Am J Neuroradiol 2002;23(8):1424–1426, with permission. Copyright 2002 by the American Society of Neuroradiology [www.ajnr.org].)

Diagnosis: Metachromatic leukodystrophy (MLD), late onset.

Discussion: MLD is an autosomal recessive disease caused by defects in arylsulfatase A (ASA) or its sphingolipid activator protein B (saposine-B). Either defect leads to accumulation of sulfatides in both central and peripheral nervous systems, with consequent demyelination. There seems to be no gender, racial, or ethnic preferences in distribution of the disorder. Thus far, 87 mutations in ASA have been identified with varying degrees of disease severity; five mutations in saposine-B have been identified as well.

There are three subtypes of MLD defined by age of onset: infantile, juvenile, and late onset (adolescent to early adulthood). MLD in infancy occurs between 18 and 24 months of age, and children first present with a gait disturbance of ataxia or weakness along with hypotonia. The disease progresses rapidly over 12 months to hypertonia, spasticity, abnormal involuntary movements, and intellectual deterioration. Peripheral neuropathy is sometimes also present. Survival is limited, and most patients do not survive past 8 to 10 years of age, although some patients may persist in a vegetative state into their teens.

Juvenile MLD usually presents between 4 and 10 years of age. The disease usually begins with poor school performance and bradykinesia with unsteady gait. This form is usually more insidious in progression, with patients developing similar symptoms to the infantile form, but over a much longer period. Patients can live 20 years or longer.

When the disease begins in adolescence or young adulthood, which is quite rare, it often presents like and is misdiagnosed as schizophrenia. In fact, up to 53% of patients who present with MLD at this time have psychotic symptoms; in contrast, patients with childhood-onset MLD do not present with psychosis. This disorder is rare enough that the clinical features remain described primarily in case reports, and the typical description of such patients includes auditory hallucinations, difficulties with concentration, inappropriate affect, and either catatonia or bizarre gesturing. The present patient had most of these symptoms at some time in the course of his illness. Some cases have been described with primarily negative symptoms of schizophrenia (e.g., amotivation, alogia, flat affect). These psychotic symptoms coincide with the time during the illness when the demyelination is confined to the frontal lobes. As the demyelination spreads through the brain, psychotic symptoms tend to disappear and are replaced by neurologic symptoms (disorders of movement and posture) and a mixed frontal and white matter-related dementia. In the present patient, it is possible that the disappearance of active psychotic symptoms (in particular, auditory hallucinations) was not a result of clozapine treatment but rather due to progression of his disease.

In later stages of the illness, symptoms are primarily cognitive; remarkably, they have a great deal of overlap with the cognitive symptoms of schizophrenia. Patients with MLD have deficits in executive functioning, attention, recall, nonverbal reasoning, working memory, new learning, and problem solving. And although not confirmed by large-scale investigations, all of these cognitive domains are purportedly impaired in schizophrenia. The present patient has progressed to a level of dementia beyond these moderate cognitive symptoms; thus, formal neuropsychological testing is unlikely to be informative.

The differential diagnosis of late-onset MLD depends on when the disease first presents. If the patient presents during the early stages of the illness, schizophrenia, schizoaffective disorder, and other psychotic disorders are high on the differential list. In fact, patients may be misdiagnosed with schizophrenia for years or a lifetime if they present during this stage of the illness, just as the present patient was misdiagnosed. Some patients are correctly diagnosed only at autopsy, when extensive areas of demyelination are discovered. Although rarely described in the literature, patients with MLD at this stage can demonstrate mood lability that may lead to a misdiagnosis of schizoaffective disorder. If the disease presents later in its course, it is likely to be confused with a frontal dementia. In addition, at this late stage neurologic symptoms become prominent, and the appearance of these neurologic symptoms sometimes provokes a neuroimaging work-up that eventually leads to the correct diagnosis. Definitive diagnosis is through a demonstration of arylsulfatase A activity in either leukocytes or urine with accompanying increased urinary sulfatides (to exclude a pseudodeficiency).

On CT scan, it is likely that the changes at this early stage of the disease would not have been detectable with the technology of 15 years ago, and MRI was not used clinically in psychiatry with any regularity until the 1990s. Even so, it is not clear to what degree the early changes in MLD would be observable on regular MRI. As demyelination becomes more prominent, however, these changes appear on MRI quite clearly (see figure).

A relatively new form of MRI called diffusion tensor imaging (DTI) has been applied to X-linked adrenoleukodystrophy (X-ALD), a disease closely related to MLD. DTI provides a measure of the vectors of water diffusion within axons or myelin sheaths. This measure represents the anisotropy of the tissue—the coherence of structures within a given region. High anisotropy measures correspond to tissue that is oriented along a similar axis, whereas low anisotropy is observed in cases in which tissue is less uniform or more disorganized. This imaging modality has been directed against white matter structures in the brain. Patients with X-ALD have been found to have decreased anisotropy with zones of myelination proceeding in levels of gradation. Of interest, DTI has also been directed against white matter structures in the brains of schizophrenia patients, where decreased anisotropy has also been found.

With regard to treatment, hematopoietic cell transplant has been shown to slow the progression of MLD-related central nervous system dysfunction and intellectual impairment, although this finding is contested by some authorities. This treatment has been applied to patients with infantile MLD with better results, and its success appears to be associated with earlier intervention, while neuropsychologic functions are still relatively intact. No established treatments exist for the other forms of MLD. Treatment is directed at overt symptoms, usually with the hope of controlling dangerous or grossly inappropriate behavior. Antipsychotics are used with mixed effect, as are mood stabilizers. The present patient was eventually admitted to the nursing home section of the chronic psychiatric hospital as his symptoms became progressively more consistent with dementia and less consistent with a psychotic process.

Pearls

1. Patients with their first psychotic break are often given an MRI of the brain to look for gross pathologic abnormalities. This practice is not universal and constitutes a point of controversy in the management of the first presentation of psychosis. Given the rarity of late-onset MLD, large-scale investigations that examine when MRI findings first appear have not been performed.
2. Diffusion tensor imaging, a special type of MRI that measures the organization of white matter tracts in the brain, may be a useful tool for investigating demyelinating diseases. Schizophrenia has also been shown to have abnormalities in diffusion tensor imaging modalities.
3. Schizophrenia-like symptoms that present with neurologic signs, are refractory to treatment, or progress to dementia should be re-examined for diagnostic accuracy.
4. The infusion of allogenic mesenchymal stem cells, as evaluated by Koc et al., led to improvements in nerve conduction velocities in MLD, but no observable improvement in the patients' overall health was noted.
5. The finding of arylsulfatase A activity in umbilical cord blood has raised the possibility of using unrelated hematopoietic stem cells in the transplantation treatment of MLD.

REFERENCES

1. Alves D, Pires MM, Guimaraes A, Miranda MC: Four cases of late onset metachromatic leukodystrophy in a family: clinical, biochemical and neuropathological studies. J Neurol Neurosurg Psychiatry 1986;49(12):1417–1422.
2. Berger J, Moser HW, Forss-Petter S: Leukodystrophies: Recent developments in genetics, molecular biology, pathogenesis, and treatment. Curr Opin Neurol 2001;14:305–31.
3. Davis KL, Stewart DG, Friedman JI, et al: White matter changes in schizophrenia: Evidence for myelin-related dysfunction. Arch Gen Psychiatry 2003;60(5):443–456.
4. Finelli PF: Metachromatic leukodystrophy manifesting as a schizophrenic disorder: Computed tomographic correlation. Ann Neurol 1985;18(1):94–95.
5. Hageman ATM, Gabreels FJM, de Jong JGN, et al: Clinical symptoms of adult metachromatic leukodystrophy and arylsulfatase A pseudodeficiency. Arch Neurol 1995;52:408–413.
6. Hyde, TM, Ziegler JC, Weinberger DR: Psychiatric disturbances in metachromatic leukodystrophy: Insights into the neurobiology of psychosis. Arch Neurol 1992;49:401–406.
7. Koc ON, Day J, Nieder M, et al: Allogenic mesenchymal stem cell infusion for treatment of metachromatic leukodystrophy (MLD) and Hurler syndrome (MPS-IH). Bone Marrow Transplant 2002;30(4):215–222.
8. Peters C, Steward CG: Hematopoietic cell transplantation for inherited metabolic diseases: An overview of outcomes and practice guidelines. Bone Marrow Transplant 2003;31(4):229–239.
9. Shapiro EG, Lockman LA, Knopman D, Krivit W: Characteristics of the dementia in late-onset metachromatic leukodystrophy. Neurology 1994;44(4):662–625.

Jennifer Petras, MD

PATIENT 29

A 9-year-old girl who threatened her teacher

History of Present Illness: A 9-year-old girl is brought to the psychiatric emergency department from school for evaluation because the school counselor reports that the patient's behavior has become increasingly out of control. Today the patient threatened to harm her teacher, stating, "I will get you, just you watch," after she was asked to climb down from the classroom windowsill. The girl is described as disrespectful toward this teacher and other school staff, frequently yelling, arguing, and cursing at them. Any limit-setting, such as being told to complete one task and move on to the next task, seemingly triggers these disruptive episodes. She is described by the school counselor as "sneaky and full of excuses," always quick to blame others for her behaviors. Her mother reports that at home the patient is disrespectful and rarely follows the rules, explaining, "Everything is an argument." The mother also reports that it seems as though the patient "really knows how to push my buttons" and seems at times to be deliberately annoying her. The mother denies that the patient has threatened or become violent toward her. There is no history of stealing, fire setting, hurting animals, or destruction of property. The patient is sleeping and eating well and is reported to be able to focus during activities that interest her.

Past Psychiatric History: Since the age of 4 years, the patient has exhibited disruptive behaviors, noted first as an inability to follow the rules of bedtime routine. The patient attended regular education classes until 1 year ago, when she was changed to special education because of behavioral problems. She has been seeing the school counselor for almost 2 years. Despite the school's recommendation that the patient be evaluated by a psychiatrist, until now no evaluation has not been done. The patient's biologic father is currently incarcerated for assault, and the patient has had sporadic, minimal contact with him throughout her life. Her mother is a single parent with three other children who currently live with their grandmother out of state. The mother recently got a new government clerical job, leaving the patient under the supervision of a neighbor after school.

Past Medical History: The patient was born full term; there were no complications of pregnancy or delivery. She achieved all developmental milestones on time. During routine screening at age 2 years, she was noted to have an elevated lead level and microcytic anemia. After treatment with iron supplementation, monitoring of lead levels, and home inspection for sources of lead, the problem resolved and no further treatment was needed.

Mental Status Examination: The patient is a well-groomed, pleasant, well-related girl who appears her stated age. She makes good eye contact and answers all questions in a matter-of-fact tone. Her mood is reported as good, and her affect is full-range and mood-congruent but inappropriately bright at times. She sits calmly in her chair, playing with her hair throughout the interview. She denies any suicidal thoughts or perceptual disturbances. She reports that she no longer wants to harm her teacher and denies any other homicidal thoughts. She is alert and oriented. When asked simple computational math problems, she became frustrated, her affect appeared angry and her tone was disrespectful as she told the interviewer that these questions and the interviewer were "stupid."

Diagnostic Testing: Neuropsychiatric testing from the school records reveals a normal IQ. Routine laboratory screening tests (complete blood count, chemistry, and thyroid function tests) are within normal limits.

Questions: What is the diagnosis? What are the challenges in studying it and the treatment options?

Diagnosis: Oppositional defiant disorder (ODD).

Discussion: ODD is described by the DSM-IV-TR as a recurrent pattern of negativistic, defiant, disobedient, and hostile behavior toward authority figures, leading to disturbances in one of three domains of functioning: academic, social, or occupational. Specifically, at least four of the following eight criteria must be present over the prior 6 months: (1) often loses temper; (2) often argues with adults; (3) often actively defies or refuses to comply with adults' requests or rules; (4) often deliberately annoys people; (5) often blames others for his or her mistakes or misbehavior; (6) is often touchy or easily annoyed by others; (7) is often angry and resentful; (8) is often spiteful or vindictive. The patient must also not meet criteria for conduct disorder or antisocial personality disorder (if older than 18 years). The patient described above clearly meets at least five of these criteria.

ODD is part of a larger category of disruptive behavior disorders (DBD) that also includes conduct disorder (CD). CD is distinguished from ODD by a more persistent pattern of behavior in which the basic rights of others or major age-appropriate societal norms or rules are violated. These behaviors include destruction of property, deceitfulness or theft, serious violations of rules, and aggression toward people and animals. Although causes, comorbidities, and treatments of the disruptive behavior disorders have been well researched, studies often look only at specific behaviors, such as aggression, delinquency, or violence, and place all subjects into a single generic category. Most studies that use strict diagnostic criteria focus primarily on patients with CD. The relationship between ODD and CD is controversial and poorly understood, and it is unclear whether CD research can apply wholly to patients with ODD. The fact that most research relevant to ODD has examined overlapping constructs, and not ODD alone, is one of the biggest challenges to understanding and treating ODD.

The limited amount of specific research available on ODD is surprising, considering that ODD is quite common, with a point prevalence in the range of 2-10%. The average age of onset is about 6 years. The diagnosis is more common in boys in the prepubertal age group, after which the gender difference decreases significantly. It is also more likely to occur in families of lower socioeconomic status. The case described above is atypical in these aspects because the patient is a prepubertal female whose mother works full-time at a fairly well-paying government job.

ODD is frequently found to be co-morbid with attention-deficit hyperactivity disorder (ADHD) and other disorders, such as major depressive disorder, dysthymic disorder, and early-onset bipolar disorder. Anxiety disorders, especially separation anxiety disorder, can present with behavioral problems and should always be considered in the differential of ODD. The high frequency of comorbidity has important implications for prognosis and treatment. For example, it has been observed that patients with ODD and comorbid ADHD have a poorer prognosis than patients with ODD alone when prognostic outcome is future development of CD. Yet some studies indicate that patients with ODD and a comorbid depressive disorder show improvement in oppositional behavior with treatment of the depression.

Although the diagnosis of ODD is based on a cluster of behaviors, biologic elements that may help to understand and treat the symptoms are thought to underlie the associated behaviors. There is no genetic marker for ODD, but initial twin and family studies have found somewhat higher prevalence rates of ODD in the families of affected members compared with the general population. The strength of these findings depends on the source of information (observer vs. parental sources) and therefore requires further study. Children with ODD have difficulties regulating their emotions, which is most probably a function of the frontal brain regions. Electroencephalographic (EEG) studies of oppositional children without comorbid conditions have found atypical activation patterns in these frontal brain regions. Such changes are hypothesized to be a biologic substrate of the negative affective style or approach to the environment that oppositional children frequently exhibit. Studies of physiologic markers have also found lower baseline heart rates and higher post-experimentally induced frustration heart rates in boys with ODD vs. controls. The hormone cortisol has been studied in ODD and is known to play a part in the physiologic response to stimulation and stress. Low salivary cortisol levels have been associated with ODD. These findings suggest a biologic hypothesis that patients with ODD experience physiological underarousal, which may lead to more stimulating, risky, and disruptive behaviors. Lead and other environmental toxins are also known risk factors for disruptive behavior disorders, and high levels of lead as measured in bone are associated with increased aggression. In the present case, the effect of prior increased serum lead levels is not clear, but lead exposure may be one of multiple possible etiologies for the patient's oppositional and defiant behaviors.

Despite preliminary investigations into the biologic elements underlying ODD, the evidence is insufficient to guide specific treatment interventions. The current treatments for ODD include behavioral (family, parent, and school) interventions and pharmacologic options. Parent-child interactional training (PCIT) has been shown in randomized studies to result in clinically significant improvement in children with ODD. PCIT involves two components of training for parents. First, parents are trained in child-directed interactions and are taught through play skills how to improve the quality of their interactions with the child. Second, parents are trained in parent-directed interactions that improve parenting skills by teaching them how to use time-outs, ways to give praise, and how to give clear instructions. In one study, parents were trained with a receiver in their ear, allowing them to hear coaching from trainers as the interactions between parent and child were observed. PCIT has been shown to be particularly effective with younger children. In general, parent management training strategies are among the most effective techniques for treatment of disruptive behavior disorders.

Multimodal interventions that address many risk factors in a comprehensive way are under long-term evaluation in two large studies, the Fast Track Program and the LIFT intervention. These studies are focused on prevention of conduct problems beginning with high-risk first graders in the fast track study and high-risk first and fifth graders in the LIFT intervention. Both use multiple interventions, including a combination of classroom social skills, communication between parents and teachers, home visits, parental skills training, anger control training, academic tutoring, and a playground behavior program. Initial findings have been positive, with reductions in problem behaviors in the intervention group compared with other high-risk children without the intervention.

Although these behavioral interventions have shown some success, pharmocologic interventions have also been studied. Patients with ODD have been included in only two randomized, double-blind, placebo-controlled trials. Both looked at the treatment of aggression. One study found divalproex to be more effective than placebo, and the other found methylphenidate to be more effective than placebo. Open-label clinical trials for the treatment of aggression have been conducted in mixed populations that included ODD and have found that clonidine, citalopram, droperidol (studied for acute aggression only), risperidone, and divalproex are effective. However, the total number of subjects represented in the above-mentioned studies is less than 200. No study focused exclusively on ODD; all were combination studies. Current clinical practice in the treatment of ODD often employs atypical antipsychotics, although this approach is not strongly supported by the literature. On the other hand, significant evidence supports the fact that pharmacologic treatment of comorbid disorders improves outcome in ODD. In addition, in patients with comorbid ADHD and ODD, aggressive behavior has been found to respond to stimulant medication.

The present patient was treated with risperidone, 1 mg twice daily, and referred to an outpatient psychiatrist for medication management. The mother was educated about her daughter's diagnosis and taught methods of limit-setting and appropriate discipline at home. In addition, the patient's school setting was changed to a therapeutic day treatment program, and an intensive case manager was assigned to coordinate outpatient care and make home visits to assist the family in setting up and complying with a more structured home setting.

ODD is a complex disorder of childhood with multiple causes and possible treatments. For a disorder that is so prevalent, the available research is minimal. Perhaps further research will help make strides in our understanding of this disorder and its relationship to conduct disorder and other related problems.

Pearls

1. Understanding normal child development is crucial to making an accurate diagnosis of oppositional defiant disorder because oppositional behavior is part of normal development. For example, coercive behavior occurs normally around 2 to 3 years old and again in early adolescence. Temper tantrums around the ages of 2 to 4 years can also be part of normal development.
2. The course of progression from oppositional defiant disorder to the more severe conduct disorder and ultimately to antisocial personality disorder is a debated topic. The relationship among these disorders is complex, with factors such as psychiatric comorbidity and substance use clearly playing a role.
3. The treatment of children with oppositional defiant disorder should be multimodal, using both behavioral and psychopharmacological therapies. Yet, at this time, the Food and Drug Administration has approved no medication for treatment of oppositional defiant disorder.

REFERENCES

1. Baving L, Laucht M, Schmidt M: Oppositional children differ from healthy children in frontal brain activation. J Abnorm Child Psychol 2000;28(3):267–275.
2. Burke J, Loeber R, Birmaher B: Oppositional defiant disorder and conduct disorder: A review of the past 10 years. Part II. J Am Acad Child Adolesc Psychiatry 2002;41(11):1275–1293.
3. Greene RW, Biederman J, Zerwas S, et al: Psychiatric comorbidity, family dysfunction and social impairment in referred youth with oppositional defiant disorder. Am J Psychiatry 2002;159 (7):14–1224.
4. Loeber R, Burke J, Lahey B, et al: Oppositional defiant disorder and conduct disorder: A review of the past 10 years. Part I. J Am Acad Child Adolesc Psychiatry 2000;9(12):1468–1484.
5. Schuhmann EM, Foote RC, Eyberg SM, Boggs SR: Efficacy of parent-child interaction therapy: Interim report of a randomized trial with short-term maintenance. J Clin Child Psychol 1998;27:34–45.
6. Steiner H, Saxena K, Chang K: Psychopharmologic strategies for the treatment of aggression in juveniles. CNS Spectrums 2003;8(4):298–308.

PATIENT 30

A 29-year-old woman with poor sleep and nightmares

History of Present Illness: A 29-year-old actress presents to the mental health walk-in clinic at a community hospital requesting psychiatric evaluation. During the intake interview, she describes feeling increasingly "sad and nervous, and really sort of hopeless" over the previous 8 to 9 months. She also complains of poor sleep and vivid nightmares during this same period. She has been seeing less of her friends recently and spends most of her time alone in her apartment. Her career has not been thriving, and in the past several months she has rarely attended the auditions that she previously frequented. This isolation has drawn the attention of her mother, who last week wondered aloud why her daughter was not "getting out and around like usual." To allay her mother's concerns, the daughter agreed to seek professional care.

On further inquiry, the patient reveals that she first noticed a change in her mood soon after "a really terrible thing happened" 1 year before her current presentation at the clinic. She was involved in an auto accident. Her boyfriend was driving, and a head-on collision with another car resulted in the deaths of a woman and child in the other vehicle. Neither the patient nor her boyfriend was seriously injured, and they observed at close hand the tragic circumstances in the other car. The patient describes feeling "confused and overwhelmed" in the immediate aftermath of the accident. She is perplexed by feelings of guilt that complicate the intense sadness and shock that she feels are "normal" reactions to the event. Now, 1 year later, the patient feels that the intensity of these emotions has yet to fade.

Past Psychiatric History: The patient denies receiving care from a psychiatrist in the past. However, she recounts an evaluation by a psychologist at age 10 after her mother learned that she had been sexually abused by an uncle. She reports that her mother never brought her back to the doctor for a second visit. When asked about a history of substance abuse, the patient describes alcohol use since the age of 14, with increased consumption in the past year. She estimates that recently she has been drinking two or three glasses of wine at least 3 nights per week, whereas previously she rarely drank on more than 1 night of the weekend. She also details using marijuana once or twice a week over the past 6 months, after having abstained from marijuana for the previous 6 years. She denies remote or recent history of other drugs and does not use tobacco.

Past Medical History: The patient denies any medical problems. Her only medication is a daily multivitamin.

Personal History: The patient is single and has no children. She is currently living alone since separating from her boyfriend 2 months after the accident. She states that her mother gets "panic attacks" and that both her mother and brother have histories of abusing alcohol.

Mental Status Examination: A tall, very slight young woman walks into the clinic office with a slightly stooped and hesitant gait. She looks younger than her stated age and appears physically well. She perches on the edge of the chair and shifts in her seat throughout the interview. Twice she flinches noticeably when doors are slammed shut elsewhere in the clinic. Her speech is remarkable for its soft volume and rapid rate. She reports her mood as "on edge," and her presentation is consistent with this description: her affect is tense and strained and somewhat constricted. She is articulate and speaks in terse, coherent sentences and phrases to describe feelings of isolation and "paralysis" that have troubled her for the past year. She mentions frequent lifelike dreams that "remind me of the accident" and notes that she feels unsettled and fearful for several hours after awakening from these dreams. She denies any perceptual abnormalities when awake. She also denies homicidal or paranoid thoughts. When asked whether she has thoughts of suicide, she describes feeling that "I don't think I'll live a long life. I just can't imagine making it for very long." She adamantly denies any specific thoughts about hurting or killing herself. Based on her decision to seek care, her insight into her illness seems adequate. Her judgment is good, and given her lucid history and excellent communication skills, she appears to be a cognitively intact and intelligent young woman.

Questions: What is the diagnosis? Which other diagnoses should be carefully considered?

Diagnosis: Posttraumatic stress disorder (PTSD).

Discussion: PTSD is characterized by a clinical syndrome of pathologic responses to extreme life stressors that include symptoms of hyperarousal, re-experiencing the event, and avoidant behavior. The illness is categorized as an anxiety disorder according to the DSM-IV-TR and was first delineated over 20 years ago by clinicians caring for Vietnam veterans. Clinicians have long recognized that certain people experience extreme reactions to stressful events. Soldiers have received particular notice, engendering descriptive terms such as "battle fatigue" and "soldier's heart." Over the past 20-plus years, the definition of stressors that have the potential to cause PTSD has expanded, as has the clinical and psychobiological understanding of the illness.

Evidence continues to emerge suggesting that PTSD is one of the most widespread psychiatric disorders in the general population, perhaps ranking only behind depression, phobias, and substance abuse in prevalence among adults. Recent literature suggests that PTSD affects about 1 in 12 adults at some point in their lifetime. Data from surveys of segments of the general population show that approximately 15–24% of people exposed to traumatic events will develop PTSD. Although males tend to have more exposure to trauma, females more commonly develop PTSD. A 2:1 female-to-male lifetime prevalence has been consistently observed. Traumas most commonly associated with PTSD in women are rape and sexual molestation, whereas combat exposure and witnessing trauma to others are more frequent triggers in men. Aside from gender, additional factors that may predict increased risk of PTSD include a preexisting psychiatric disorder, prior history of trauma (especially in childhood), and a family history of anxiety, depression, psychosis, or antisocial behavior. The present patient is noted to possess several of these risk factors: female gender, history of sexual abuse as a child, and family history of anxiety disorder and substance abuse.

It was previously assumed that PTSD was a natural reaction to a profound stressor that represented a pathologic extension of the normal stress response. However, more recent research provides evidence that PTSD reflects a particular type of abnormal adaptation to trauma with neurochemical and neuroanatomic underpinnings. It is also important to note that only a subset of people react to severe trauma by developing PTSD. Investigators have paid special attention to possible dysfunction in the hypothalamic-pituitary-adrenal (HPA) axis, which has long been identified as crucial in the response to stress. Research led by Yehuda and colleagues suggests that in PTSD the HPA axis may be overly sensitized. Although patients have elevated levels of corticotropin-releasing factor (CRF), as is typical in the stress response, their baseline level of cortisol is decreased. In addition, patients seem to have more numerous and more sensitive glucocorticoid receptors, leading to enhanced negative feedback and decreased cortisol secretion. Further research has been dedicated to possible abnormalities in monoamine action in patients with PTSD. Studies have revealed increased catecholamine activity, including an exaggerated norepinephrine response to acute stressors and exaggerated reactivity of alpha-2 receptors.

Investigators have also uncovered growing evidence of neuroanatomic abnormalities that may be hallmarks of PTSD. These findings have centered on the limbic system, the collection of structures and circuits that have a central role in memory formation and in modulating the physiologic and behavioral responses to threatening stimuli. Functional imaging modalities, led by positron emission tomography (PET) and functional magnetic resonance imaging (fMRI), have shown hyperresponsiveness of the amygdala and reduced reactivity of the anterior cingulate and orbitofrontal areas in PTSD. These areas of the limbic system anchor the fear response, which is activated during the hyperarousal states seen in PTSD. In addition, abnormalities in hippocampal structure and function have emerged, which may shed light on memory symptoms in PTSD, including intrusive thoughts and cognitive deficits.

PTSD is defined in the DSM-IV-TR as an abnormal reaction to a severe stressor that is characterized by the coexistence of three symptom clusters—re-experiencing, avoidance, and hyperarousal—that occur for greater than 1 month. **Re-experiencing** refers to the powerful impression of reliving the trauma by means of distressing memories, recurrent distressing dreams (as in the present patient), or so-called flashbacks, in which one feels as though the event were recurring. These sensations are accompanied by profound psychological distress and/or physiologic activation. The present patient is clearly disturbed by the graphic dreams that have troubled her sleep since the accident.

Avoidance describes patients' attempts to minimize their exposure to stimuli that remind them of the trauma; this drive to evade reminders causes patients to shun other stimuli as well and may extend to the avoidance of previously enjoyable activities and lead to social isolation and detachment. In addition, patients typically describe a sense of having a foreshortened future. Again, the present patient fits the profile: over the past year she has been withdrawing socially and specifically described the feeling that "I don't think I'll live a long life."

Finally, **hyperarousal** can be represented by a variety of symptoms, including insomnia, irritability or anger, poor concentration, hypervigilance, and an exaggerated startle response. Based on the mental status exam, we have the sense that the present patient is easily startled and anxious, and she reported many months of poor sleep.

The differential diagnosis of PTSD is complicated by the high rate of psychiatric comorbidity. Concurrent major depression, other anxiety disorders, and substance abuse are frequently seen with PTSD. The hallmark symptoms of PTSD may also overlap with other conditions, most notably depression. Major depression shares a number of symptoms with PTSD, including depressed mood, guilty feelings, suicidality, lack of interest, agitation, loss of libido, anxiety, and weight loss. Investigators have reported comorbid depression in 30–50% of patients with PTSD. Furthermore, a history of major depression may predict more severe posttraumatic illness. Although these two conditions may represent independent disease processes, they may also be acting synergistically to worsen patients' suffering. In the present patient, PTSD is the primary diagnosis, but clinical data suggest that she may suffer from depression as well. This possibility should be pursued further and considered carefully in treatment selection.

Both psychological and pharmacologic approaches are used in the treatment of PTSD but unfortunately tend to produce only partial symptom relief. Cognitive-behavioral therapy (CBT), which involves techniques such as systematic desensitization, flooding, and prolonged exposure treatment, appears to be the most effective psychological technique currently in use. CBT is often supplemented by programs that teach anxiety management techniques, such as deep muscle relaxation and controlled breathing.

A great number of medications have been used to treat PTSD. Antidepressants have been shown to successfully manage symptoms of intrusive thoughts, avoidance, depression, insomnia, and anxiety. Most attention has focused on the selective serotonin reuptake inhibitors (SSRIs), given their ease of use, generally well-tolerated side effects, and safety in overdose. A large randomized controlled trial comparing sertraline with placebo found that sertraline demonstrated significant efficacy in all three major symptom domains of PTSD. To date, the only medications to receive approval by the Food and Drug Administrastion for the treatment of PTSD are sertraline and paroxetine. Other studies have demonstrated that tricyclic antidepressants and monoamine oxidase inhibitors also show promise in treating PTSD, although their respective side-effect profiles should be carefully considered in selecting these medications.

Mood stabilizers may have a role in controlling specific symptoms commonly found in PTSD, such as impulsivity and mood lability. No randomized controlled studies with these drugs have been completed to date, although several are under way. Adrenergic agents may also emerge as helpful in treating and possibly even preventing PTSD. Preliminary reports suggest that use of these agents in the immediate aftermath of a trauma may diminish risk of subsequent PTSD; investigations are ongoing. Although benzodiazepines are frequently used to treat other anxiety disorders, no consistent evidence has documented their benefit in patients with PTSD. Given the high rates of comorbidity of PTSD with substance abuse and dependence, special caution should be taken in prescribing these medications.

The present patient was diagnosed with PTSD based on the diagnostic interview and the absence of any evidence for an underlying medical condition to explain her symptoms. She was noted to have an onset of multiple distressing symptoms and a decline in social and occupational function in the aftermath of a severely stressful life event. By both history and clinical exam, she had prominent findings in each of the three symptom clusters that define PTSD: re-experiencing, avoidance, and hyperarousal. Her symptoms well exceeded the requisite time course of 1 month and showed no signs of improvement in the absence of treatment. The patient was referred to the outpatient psychiatry clinic at a teaching hospital. The diagnosis of PTSD was confirmed by her assigned psychiatrist at the clinic, who believed that the patient's mood and neurovegetative symptoms were largely a consequence of PTSD—not comorbid major depression. The patient was started on an SSRI and enrolled in a CBT program. She was also referred to an alcohol treatment program to address the recent increase in alcohol consumption. She tolerated the medication well and felt that the CBT was helpful, especially with regard to reducing her social isolation and general feelings of nervousness. She continued to experience occasional distressing dreams and still complains of sporadic sleep disturbances. She was able to return to work, however, and recently earned the lead female role in a regional theater production.

Pearls

1. The three diagnostic subtypes of PTSD are based on time course. **Acute PTSD** is diagnosed when symptoms occur for a period of less than 3 months; **chronic PTSD** refers to symptom duration that exceeds 3 months; and **delayed-onset PTSD** is diagnosed when symptom onset occurs at least 6 months after the precipitating event. However, some authors believe that delayed-onset PTSD may simply reflect delayed time to referral or the exacerbation of subclinical PTSD symptoms rather than a new occurrence of symptoms.
2. Given the complex and diverse symptoms of PTSD and the fact that no one treatment has emerged as superior, the best approach to treatment may be a combination of biologic and psychological strategies.
3. A new treatment called eye-movement desensitization may offer significant benefit. Patients engage in coordinated rapid eye movements while recalling images of the traumatic event. However, it is not clear whether the benefit of this technique is derived from the exposure to memories of the event or to the eye movements themselves.
4. N-acetyl acetate, an endogenous molecule that is used as a marker for neuronal density, has been found (via nuclear magnetic spectroscopy studies) to be decreased in the temporal lobes of patients with PTSD compared with matched controls. This finding suggests that an atrophic or degenerative process may be at work in the hippocampi of people suffering from PTSD.

REFERENCES

1. Albucher RC, Liberzon I: Psychopharmacologic treatment in PTSD: A critical review. J Psychiatr Res 2002;36:355–367.
2. Breslau N: Outcomes of posttraumatic stress disorder. J Clin Psychiatry 2001;62(Suppl 17):55–59.
3. Breslau N: The epidemiology of posttraumatic stress disorder: What is the extent of the problem? J Clin Psychiatry 2001;62(Suppl 17):16–22.
4. Brunello N, Davidson JRT, Deahl M, et al: Posttraumatic stress disorder: Diagnosis and epidemiology, comorbidity and social consequences, biology and treatment. Neuropsychobiology 2001;43:150–162.
5. Grossman R, Buchsbaum MS, Yehuda R: Neuroimaging studies in post-traumatic stress disorder. Psychiatr Clin North Am 2002;25:317–340
6. Hageman I, Andersen HS, Jorgensen MB: Posttraumatic stress disorder: A review of psychobiology and pharmacotherapy. Acta Psychiatr Scand 2001;104:411–422.
7. Yehuda R: Post-traumatic stress disorder. N Engl J Med 2002;346(2):108–114.

Patrick Runnels, MD

PATIENT 31

An 80-year-old man with changes in mental status

History of Present Illness: An 80-year-old man is brought to the emergency department by his wife, who states, "Lately, he has not been acting like himself." She reports that for the past 3 or 4 days he has been accusing her and other family members of being members of the Nazi party. Along with these accusations, he has become more agitated toward others and has been seen talking to himself. Sometimes, when he and his wife are the only two people in the room, he has appeared to be speaking to an imaginary person about Hitler and the Third Reich. He has refused meals on multiple occasions because he believed that the food was poisoned. He also locked himself in the bedroom a few times for several hours after accusing his wife of cheating on him. The wife further recounts that he insisted that their daughter stole money from his bank account during her last visit. For many months before the onset of the current symptoms, the wife states that the patient mentioned seeing their deceased dog and his deceased mother but understood that they were not real and did not appear to be bothered by them. He also mentioned difficulty with sleeping for the past few months and is apparently having bizarre dreams.

Past Psychiatric Illness: The patient has no previous psychiatric history, has never seen a psychiatrist in the past, and takes no psychiatric medications.

Past Medical History: Until 1 month ago, the patient's only medical problem was urinary retention secondary to benign prostatic hypertrophy (BPH), for which he has been taking doxazosin for many years. Six months ago the patient started taking levodopa for restless legs syndrome, and the dose has been increased twice since the beginning of therapy. Two weeks ago he had an episode of urosepsis and was hospitalized for 1 week to treat the infection. He was discharged on doxazosin, carbidopa/levodopa, and ceftriaxone and is currently taking these medications.

Social/Family History: The patient is a World War II veteran who owned and ran several gas stations until retiring several years ago. He has been married to his wife for 50 years, and they are currently living together. The patient does not smoke or use unprescribed medications. He has a glass of wine with dinner daily. He and his wife have three female children. The family has no history of psychiatric disorders.

Mental Status Examination: The patient is a well-built, elderly man who remains seated throughout the interview. His eye contact is infrequent, and he appears hostile at times. He is very suspicious toward the examiner, refusing to shake hands or say "Hello." The patient is initially irritable and, when asked about his mood, responds sharply, "Who wants to know?" His affect is congruent and reinforces this sentiment. His thought process is goal-directed and relevant. He denies hearing voices but frequently refers to "the other person in the room." He asks throughout the interview if he is being recorded. Although he is initially resistant to discussing what he is thinking, he eventually reveals that he is certain that Hitler is alive and planning to invade the country. He believes that the hospital is a disguised Nazi concentration camp and that his wife and other members of his family are members of the Nazi party. He is somewhat tearful when discussing an affair that he is certain his wife is having with a neighbor and becomes angry when describing how his daughters are taking money from his bank account in small portions so that they are not caught. He denies suicidal or homicidal ideation but indicates that he will protect himself if attacked. He is alert and oriented, except to place. His memory appears to be intact. He refuses to participate in any tests of cognition, stating, "I refuse to cooperate in my own execution." He has no insight into his condition and poor judgment regarding treatment.

Diagnostic Testing: Blood count: WBC 4800/μl with < 1% bands, 60% neutrophils. Computed tomography of head: diffuse cortical atrophy, no lesions noted.

Questions: What is the diagnosis? What are the treatment options for the patient's symptoms?

Diagnosis: Medication-induced psychotic disorder (levodopa).

Discussion: Psychoses have been long recognized as a side effect of levodopa, a dopamine precursor typically prescribed for patients with Parkinson's disease. Studies suggest that between 5% and 17% of patients without Parkinson's dementia and between 42% and 81% of patients with Parkinson's dementia may develop psychotic symptoms. However, any patient on levodopa is at risk for developing psychotic symptoms, regardless of the indications for which it is initially prescribed. The pathogenesis of levodopa-induced psychosis has not been well characterized, but theories to explain the occurrence of psychotic symptoms come largely from the study of schizophrenia, in which abnormalities in dopamine regulation have been seen as having a modulatory effect on psychotic symptoms.

The psychotic features most commonly induced by levodopa are hallucinations and paranoia. In contrast to primary psychotic disorders, such as schizophrenia, auditory hallucinations are uncommon. Patients are more likely to experience visual hallucinations that are nonthreatening, such as deceased relatives, familiar persons, or pets. The hallucinations often occur at night; they are repetitive and individualized to the particular patient and frequently accompanied by vivid dreams. Early in the course of symptom development, visual hallucinations may be the only manifestation, and at this stage, patients typically have good insight. As the symptoms progress, however, hallucinations may become more threatening, and as delusions develop, insight fades. The most common delusions in patients with levodopa-induced psychosis are paranoid, such as the belief that people are trying to murder them or take their money or that the spouse has been guilty of infidelity. All of these delusions are present in this patient. Negative symptoms and disorganized thought characteristic of schizophrenia usually do not occur (see Case 11).

Psychotic symptoms produced by levodopa can be classified into two broad categories: psychosis with a clear sensorium and psychosis with a cloudy sensorium. Simple levodopa-induced psychoses are not associated with a change in sensorium. Factors that can lead to levodopa-induced psychoses with altered sensorium include underlying infection, metabolic or endocrinologic abnormalities, malnutrition, and dehydration. In patients with Parkinson's disease, treatment medications such as anticholinergics, amantadine, and selegiline can also exacerbate psychoses and lead to delirium. When psychoses develop in patients with advanced Parkinson's disease, the course is more drastic and can include profound changes in consciousness, altered concentration, disturbed sleep-wake cycles, motor symptoms, and autonomic instability.

In cases of levodopa-induced psychotic symptoms, some patients function well for years without using medications to treat the psychosis—often despite the presence of hallucinations. Insight is typically preserved early in the development of psychosis, and the hallucinations are not bothersome. When insight declines, delusions develop, or hallucinations become bothersome, however, medical treatment is necessary. For patients needing medication, atypical neuroleptics are the treatment of choice. Although some sources suggest lowering antiparkinson medications as much as possible to see whether psychotic symptoms subside before attempting to introduce neuroleptics, others believe that this approach exposes patients to unnecessary risks and recommend immediate treatment with an atypical neuroleptic.

In patients with Parkinson's disease, treatment is complicated by the risk of worsening motor symptoms. Currently, the only medication that has demonstrated antipsychotic efficacy in double-blind, placebo-controlled trials without worsening Parkinson's symptoms is clozapine. Risperidone may not be well tolerated by patients with Parkinson's disease due to potentiation of extrapyramidal side effects. Two placebo-controlled, double-blind studies included a total of 167 patients placed on olanzapine. Both found no significant improvement in psychopathology vs. placebo, and both reported significant worsening of motor symptoms (except tremor). Quetiapine may have a lower incidence of extrapyramidal side effects than either risperidone or olanzapine and therefore may be considered as a first-line agent in patients with Parkinson's disease and psychotic symptoms. Although clozapine has not been associated with extrapyramidal side effects in this population, it is generally less well tolerated than quetiapine due to many other adverse effects (e.g., sedation, constipation, sialorrhea).

The literature concerning the efficacy of quetiapine for the treatment of levodopa-induced psychoses has been steadily growing over the past few years. One open-label, retrospective study of 87 patients revealed an 80% resolution of symptoms. Another open-label study that compared quetiapine and clozapine in a sample of 20 patients with levodopa-induced psychoses showed equal efficacy in both groups. A retrospective chart review of 19 nondemented patients with Parkinson's disease and 20 demented patients with Parkinson's disease, all of whom were treated with quetiapine, showed results ranging from 80% improvement to complete amelioration of psychoses in both groups, although motor symptoms were worsened significantly in the group with dementia. Many other open-label studies of small sets of patients and case reports also indicate significant improvement of psychoses with administration of quetiapine.

The present patient was diagnosed with levodopa-induced psychosis based on his past medical history, the characteristic nature of his hallucinations and delusions, and his lack of significant psychiatric history. The diagnosis was confirmed by cessation of symptoms on discontinuation of levodopa. Other possibilities considered were psychosis secondary to systemic infection and very-late-onset schizophrenia. The onset of delusions may have been precipitated by the occurrence of urosepsis or an increase in the medication dosage, although the patient's psychoses completely resolved within 48 hours of discontinuing the levodopa.

The vast majority of patients presenting with levodopa-induced psychoses have Parkinson's disease. Levodopa and other dopaminergic agents, however, are also the treatment of choice for restless leg syndrome (RLS). Although psychosis associated with dopaminergic treatment for RLS is little reported in the literature, this case demonstrates the need to consider the side effects of levodopa in nonparkinson patients as well. RLS can be very disturbing, and this patient continued to have difficulty after cessation of levodopa. In at least one open-label trial of 8 patients, gabapentin showed a beneficial response. In a later double-blind, placebo-controlled trial of 22 patients, it continued to demonstrate efficacy in reduction of symptoms, particularly leg pain. This patient was started on gabapentin with almost complete resolution of symptoms.

Pearls

1. Wolters' theory to explain levodopa-induced psychoses proposes that levodopa causes excessive activation of serotonin receptors, which themselves influence the glutamate-modulated activity of dopaminergic neurons in the paranigral and parabrachial nuclei of the ventral tegmental area. This process results in an overactive mesolimbic system, which may cause the person to assign too much significance to otherwise nonthreatening external stimuli, leading to false beliefs about reality that progress to frank delusions.
2. Any patient taking levodopa is at risk for developing psychotic symptoms, regardless of the indications for which it was initially prescribed.
3. Patients experiencing only medication-induced visual hallucinations often do not require neuroleptic treatment. However, treatment is considered necessary for patients showing evidence of delusional thinking because delusions signal a decline in insight, placing the patient at increased risk for personal harm or harm to others. Regardless, in the case of medication-induced psychotic symptoms, the causative agent should be discontinued if possible.
4. Although risperidone has been shown to cause a significant increase in extrapyramidal symptoms in the general population as well as in some small populations of Parkinson's patients who experience psychoses, several recent open-label trials in small populations of Parkinson's patients experiencing psychosis have shown it to be effective in reducing psychotic symptoms without worsening the motor symptoms of Parkinson's disease. Further studies are needed to resolve this discrepancy.

REFERENCES

1. Adler CH: Treatment of restless legs syndrome with gabapentin. Clin Neuropharmacol 1997;20(2):148–151.
2. Allen RP, Earley CJ: Restless legs syndrome: A review of clinical and pathophysiologic features. J Clin Neurophysiol 2001; 18(2):128–147.
3. Breier A, Sutton VK, Feldmen PD, et al: Olanzapine in the treatment of dopamimetic-induced psychosis in a patient with Parkinson's disease. Biol Psychiatry 2002; 2:438–445.
4. Friedman JH, Factor SA: Atypical antipsychotics in the treatment of drug-induced psychosis in Parkinson's disease. Movement Disord 2000;15:201–211.
5. Garcia-Borreguero D, Larrosa O, de la Llave Y, et al: Treatment of restless legs syndrome with gabapentin: A double-blind, cross-over study. Neurology 2002;59(10):1573–1579.
6. Kuzuhara S: Drug-induced psychotic symptoms in Parkinson's disease: Poblems, management, and dilemma. J Neurol 2001; 248(Suppl 3):III/28–III/31.
7. Reddy S, Factor S, Molho ES, Feustel PJ: The effect of quetiapine on psychosis and motor function in parkinsonian patients with and without dementia. Movement Disord 2002;17:676–681.
8. Tariot PN, Ismail MS: Use of quetiapine in elderly patients. J Clin Psychiatry 2002;63(Suppl 13):21–26.
9. Wolters EC: Dopaminomimetic psychosis in Parkinson's disease patients. Neurology 1999;52(Suppl 3): S10–S13.

Afia A. Hussain, MD
Rajendra J. Daniel, MD
Diane J. Sacks, MD

PATIENT 32

A 48-year-old woman with psychosis

History of Present Illness: A 48-year-old woman is brought to the psychiatric emergency department by emergency medical services (EMS) after her husband called 911. Her husband and 21-year-old son report that the patient was doing fine until 3 weeks ago when she became very disorganized and forgetful. She has not been sleeping well at night and would put herself and her family at risk by leaving the house late at night without locking the front door. She was also described as placing cooking pans in the bathtub, leaving the stove on for hours, and forgetting lit cigarettes in the ashtray. Her husband states that she has become quite frightened of him, refusing to eat any food that he prepares and accusing him of poisoning her. The patient acknowledges this feeling and insists that her husband is turning their children and the whole family against her. At times she has outbursts of anger and may become quite aggressive and loud. At other times she is noted to be laughing to herself.

The family reports that the patient has been trying to contact a person named "Joe," who can save her from her husband. Joe is a construction worker who did repairs in their house about 8 years ago. Although he has had no contact with the patient or her family, she is convinced that he is in love with her. The patient states that she last saw him in her neighborhood a few days ago and that they exchanged "a smile." Over the past several weeks she has increased her visits to a park near Joe's neighborhood, where she sits for hours in the hope of seeing him. On the morning of the current presentation, the patient smelled a gas leak in her basement and began yelling to her son. When he arrived, he found her staring into space and moving her lips in a smacking motion. When he tried to get her attention, she appeared confused, disoriented, and unable to recognize him. At that point EMS was called.

Past Psychiatric History: The patient was first hospitalized approximately 10 years ago. She was working as a secretary at the time and doing well until she started to act strangely. She describes feeling very afraid at the time and apparently wrote a letter to Al Capone, thanking him for his support. Eight years ago she began believing that the construction worker named Joe had fallen in love with her. At that time she was hospitalized on a locked inpatient psychiatric unit and received the diagnosis of schizophrenia. Since then, she has been admitted three times and given the same diagnosis. According to her family, whenever she gets sick, she starts looking for Joe. Eight months ago she filed for divorce after 28 years of marriage and requested an order of protection against her daughter, whom she believed had tried to attack her. The most recent psychiatric admission was 5 months ago for aggressive behavior and outbursts of anger.

Past Medical History: Sixteen years ago the patient underwent surgery with placement of a clip for a ruptured berry aneurysm on the left side of her brain. She was diagnosed with epilepsy approximately 4 years later. She states that just before having a seizure, she experiences a strong smell like burning rubber or plastic as well as confusion and goes into a dreamy, trance-like state. She feels as if "she is sleeping" while she is awake. The family reports involuntary jerky movements of her right arm and sometimes of her right leg, along with lip smacking. The patient states that she had these symptoms on the morning of her presentation and before that about 5 months ago. She has lost consciousness twice in the past. She was started on antiseizure medications but is only partially adherent.

Mental Status Examination: The patient is a Caucasian woman who appears her stated age. She is dressed in street clothes with poor hygiene, and bilateral tremors of the hands are noted. She is uncooperative during the interview and appears to have low frustration tolerance. Her speech is loud, excessive, and pressured. Her mood is angry with congruent affect. Her thought process is tangential. The thought content reveals paranoid delusions that her husband is poisoning her food and fears that the whole family has turned against her. She denies auditory, visual, tactile, gustatory, or olfactory hallucinations currently but admits smelling gas earlier in the morning. She denies suicidal or homicidal ideation. The patient is awake, alert, and oriented to time, place and person. Her recent memory is impaired, as she is unable to recall what happened after smelling gas in the morning. Remote memory also shows lapses. Concentration is impaired, and she is unable to do serial sevens or simple calculations. Proverb interpretation is concrete. Impulse control is impaired, with angry outbursts and frequent banging on the interviewer's desk during the interview. Insight is impaired because the patient denies the presence of psychiatric symptoms. Judgment is also limited due to delusional thinking.

Laboratory Examination: Routine blood work, including urine toxicology, was within normal limits.

Diagnostic Testing: Computed tomography scan of the head: left frontotemporal craniotomy with an aneurysm clip noted within the inferior aspect of the left Sylvian fissure and associated surrounding encephalomalacia. No evidence of a mass, acute hemorrhage, or hydrocephalus. Electroencephalogram (EEG; see figure): abnormal awake recording with left frontal temporal slowing, possibly due to a focal electrical disturbance. Amplitude differences may be a result of the craniotomy. No epileptogenic potentials were seen in the recording, and clinical correlation was advised in considering the presence of a seizure disorder.

Question: Which primary condition accounts for the patient's symptoms?

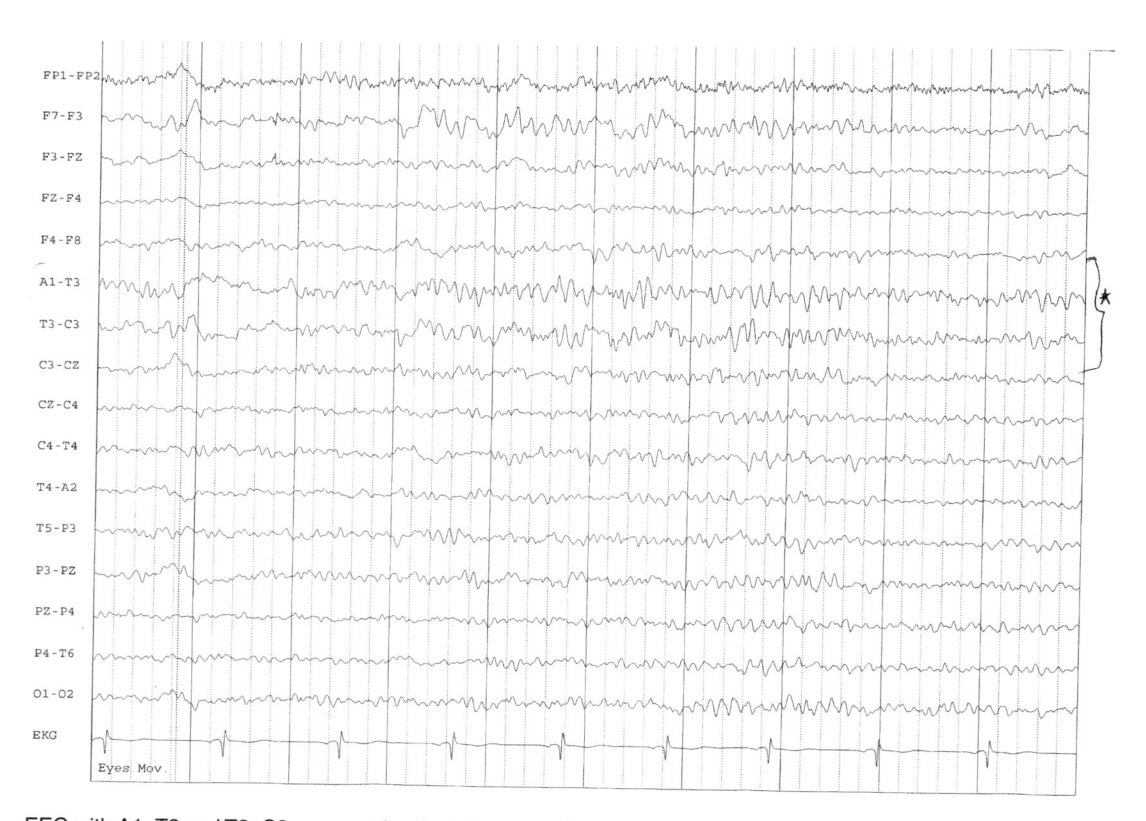

EEG with A1–T3 and T3–C3 representing the left temporal lobe and demonstrating short 5- to 7-Hz wave intermingle (slowing). C4–T4 and T4–A2 represent the right temporal lobe with a normal pattern of 7- to 8-Hz waves. This EEG does not show the classic picture of seizure activity but instead indicates the presence of a structural lesion that can be potentially epileptogenic or previous seizure activity.

Diagnosis: Psychosis due to a medical condition; temporal lobe epilepsy (TLE).

Discussion: TLE was first recognized in 1881 as "uncinate fits" and
the "dreamy state." In 1940 it was described as "psychomotor epilepsy," and in 1985 the International League Against Epilepsy defined the disorder as TLE. The most epileptogenic region of the brain is the temporal lobe. Seizures associated with TLE can be simple partial seizures (without loss of awareness) or complex partial seizure (with loss of awareness). Temporal lobe seizures are accompanied by auras in approximately 80% of cases. Auras consist of altered perceptions, visceral sensations, hallucinations (e.g., olfactory, gustatory, visual, auditory and, rarely, tactile), and autonomic effects, such as, tachycardia, pallor or flushing, cough or shortness of breath, and abnormal epigastric sensations. Patients may have a feeling of familiarity or unfamiliarity (i.e., déjà vu or jamais vu), anxiety or fear, depersonalization, or de-realization. Following the aura, actual seizures consist of oral automatisms, such as, lip smacking, chewing, and swallowing. Repetitive, stereotyped, manual automatisms or unilateral dystonic posturing of a limb can also be observed, or patients may display a wide-eyed stare, with dilated pupils and psychomotor retardation. The duration of auras and automatism is quite short, lasting from seconds to 1 or 2 minutes. The postictal phase may last for several minutes, and amnesia occurs after complex partial seizures because of bilateral involvement of the hemispheres.

There are multiple possible causes of TLE. Trauma may produce hemorrhage or contusions that result in encephalomalacia or scarring. Past infections, such as bacterial meningitis or herpes encephalitis can also produce seizure foci. Tumors, arteriovenous malformations, medial temporal sclerosis, and other idiopathic causes are other potential causes.

The psychosis associated with TLE can be divided into two categories: peri-ictal and interictal. Peri-ictal psychosis is related to the actual seizure episode and occurs during the aura, seizure, and postictal state. Symptoms are usually brief but may be prolonged during temporal lobe status epilepticus. Peri-ictal psychosis is usually associated with autonomic symptoms and perceptual disturbance (i.e., hallucinations) in a setting of altered awareness, especially during the postictal period.

Interictal psychosis is associated with temporal lobe epilepsy but unrelated to the actual seizure event. Patients who develop interictal psychosis usually present with paranoid ideation and hallucinations that appear similar to schizophrenia. Some studies have reported psychosis or a schizophrenia-like picture as a late occurrence in approximately 7% of patients with TLE. Interictal psychosis may be distinguished from schizophrenia by the fact that schizophrenia is typically accompanied by negative symptoms, emotional withdrawal, social deterioration, a family history of the disease, and a chronic, deteriorating course. As in the present patient, psychosis in epilepsy usually develops with a left-sided focus, the presence of foreign body (aneurysmal clip) in this case. Psychosis is also more common in partial complex seizures, left-handed patients, and especially women. It frequently occurs with medial temporal lobe gangliomas and in more severe cases has an earlier age of onset. Many researchers have observed the deterioration of psychiatric status with improved seizure control. Forced normalization, a concept described by Landolt in the 1950s, refers to good seizure control and normalization of the EEG by anticonvulsants leading to worsening of psychiatric symptoms. This phenomenon can be noticed in the present patient. She suffered from interictal psychosis, and her symptoms became worse to the point that she was unable to take her medications as prescribed and had a seizure. The mechanism underlying this phenomenon is not yet understood.

The present patient had a left frontotemporal craniotomy with clip placement after suffering a ruptured berry aneurysm. Four years later she developed seizures, and 6 years after the surgery she developed psychosis that was mistaken for schizophrenia. She presented with paranoid delusions that her husband was poisoning her, and it is likely that seeing "Joe" was a visual hallucination. These symptoms are common in psychosis associated with TLE. The present patient also lacked negative symptoms, and there was no genetic loading for schizophrenia. Bipolar disorder and schizoaffective disorder, bipolar type were also considered in the differential diagnosis because her lack of sleep, behavioral disinhibition, and anger outbursts may have been consistent with mania. In the present case, these findings may be explained by involvement of the amygdala in the seizure activity. The EEG did not reveal seizure activity, but structural lesions (i.e., aneurysm clip) can be potentially epileptogenic. A video EEG was recommended to confirm the strong suspicion of TLE, but the patient refused.

The diagnosis of TLE is made with EEG. Special electrodes, including anterior temporal electrodes or nasopharyngeal leads, may be used to improve recordings from the temporal lobe. In special epilepsy inpatient units, sphenoidal electrodes (wires inserted under the skin of the check) are used to record temporal lobe activity. Video EEG is the gold standard in evaluating patients with seizures and is mostly used in specialized hospital units. High-resolution MRI is used to visualize structural abnormalities such as hippocampal atrophy. If the above tests are normal, positron emission tomography with 18-fluorodoxyglucose (PET-FDG) is a useful tool for seizure localization if surgical intervention is considered for seizures that cannot be controlled with medications. Single-photon emission computed tomography (SPECT) may be an adjunctive imaging technique for surgical candidates. Intracranial EEG with placement of intracranial subdural electrodes can also be done before surgery for localization.

Psychotic symptoms in TLE are treated with antipsychotics. However, most antipsychotics lower the seizure threshold, and clozapine especially should be avoided. Premarketing research studies have shown that clozapine has the highest risk of seizures (5% of cases at doses over 500 mg/day). Olanzapine has a seizure rate of 0.9% at doses up to 20 mg/day, quetiapine has a rate of 0.8% at doses up to 750 mg/day, and risperidone has a rate of approximately 0.3%. This patient responded well to olanzapine, 15 mg/day. Anticonvulsants are also needed to treat the underlying seizure disorder. Approximately 40% of patients with TLE do not respond to antiseizure drugs. This problem may arise in patients with hippocampal sclerosis. In such cases surgical interventions are used, including anterior temporal lobectomy and vagus nerve stimulation. Among the anticonvulsants, some evidence indicates that carbamazepine is of benefit in labile psychotic patients with TLE, although the current patient was restarted on sodium divalproex and titrated to a therapeutic serum level (50–100 μg/ml). During her hospital stay, the patient remained seizure-free.

Pearls

1. Temporal lobe epilepsy is associated with brief peri-ictal psychosis but also predisposes patients to chronic interictal psychosis that can easily be confused with schizophrenia.
2. Additional research is needed to determine the efficacy of neuroleptics in the treatment of psychosis associated with TLE.
3. Temporal lobectomy is performed only in patients with unilateral temporal lobe involvement and patients who are completely unresponsive to high dosages of medication. The seizure disorder should also persist for many years before this treatment is considered; the usual age range for performing this procedure is between 15 and 45 years.

REFERENCES

1. Berzen L: Epilepsy and psychosis. Can Psychiatr Assoc Bull 2002;34(1):11.
2. Kaplan H, Sadock B: Localization of specific brain functions; emotion. In Kaplan H, Sadock B (ds): Kaplan and Sadock's Synopsis of Psychiatry, 8th ed. Philadelphia, Lippincott Williams & Wilkins, 1998, pp 93–94.
3. Kanemoto K, Kawasaki J, Kawai I: Postictal psychosis: A comparison with acute interictal and chronic psychoses. Epilepsia 1996;37(6):551–556.
4. Kanemoto K, Kawasaki J, Mori E: Violence and epilepsy: A close relation between violence and postictal psychosis. Epilepsia 1999;40(1):107–109.
5. Savard G, Andermann F, Olivier A, Remillard GM: Postictal psychosis after partial complex seizures: A multiple case study. Epilepsia 1991;32(2): 225–231.

Nadine Schwartz, MD

PATIENT 33

An 8-year-old girl with worsening school performance

History of Present Illness: An 8-year-old girl is referred to the private office of a child psychiatrist by her pediatrician. It is late March, and the child's grades have decreased significantly, although she is still passing. The child is in a third-grade regular education class and has never been left back. Until late November she was receiving excellent grades, as she also did in the first and second grades. The teacher has reported to the mother that the child is well behaved in the classroom but at times appears to be distracted. The teacher reports no problems with excessive talking or fidgety or restless behaviors or calling out answers out of turn. In fact, the teacher reports that the patient no longer participates much in class, although previously she was an enthusiastic contributor. The teacher has also noted that the girl often withdraws from classmates during recess, although previously she was quite social. The girl's mother says that recently she also noticed that on certain days the patient is not her usual cheerful self. The mother states that this change in mood is not present everyday but about 3 days per week on average. The mother also feels that the child is more "socially anxious" because she frequently cuts short weekend visits with friends even though she used to want to play for hours.

The mother reports that the patient has a normal appetite and at a recent pediatric visit ranked in the 50th percentile for both height and weight. The patient falls asleep readily at 9 PM each night and awakens spontaneously at 7 AM each morning. The mother denies the presence of oppositional behavior, aggression, hyperactivity, tearfulness, or self-injurious or odd behaviors. She states that the patient is primarily responsible for the care of the family's two cats, with whom she is playful and affectionate. She states that the patient has no difficulty in concentrating during the 45 minutes each afternoon that it takes her to complete her homework, but she does seem to struggle more with the work than in the past.

Past Medical History: The mother relates that the patient experiences daytime enuresis 3–4 times per week, both on school days and weekends. The wetting episodes occur at random times during the day, usually no more than one episode in a day. The child is fully continent at night, and before 6 months ago she was fully continent both day and night since just after her fourth birthday. The patient's mother states that the child has recently had a work-up by the pediatrician for this problem, including urine and blood testing, ultrasound, voiding cystourethrogram (VCUG), and a test of bladder capacity. The results of all of these tests were normal. The pediatrician has just prescribed oxybutynin, which the child has been taking for approximately 2 weeks, so far without relief of her symptoms. The patient has no other medical problems and takes no other medications except a multivitamin.

Past Psychiatric History: This child has not previously been referred for psychiatric consultation. She has never taken psychiatric medication.

Social History: The patient is the second child in a kinship of four. Her older brother is 10 years old, her younger sister is 4 years old, and the youngest sister is 7 months old. The patient's mother and father are married, and the mother reports their marriage as stable and the child's relationships with her parents and siblings as emotionally close and affectionate. The mother works part-time as a school librarian and is home every day after school with the children. The patient's father works full-time as a graphic designer. The mother states that in the late autumn, the patient's father took on a part-time job coaching her 10-year-old son's basketball team for supplemental income due to the increased expenses in the household after the birth of the fourth child. Otherwise, the mother cannot identify any stressors or changes in the child's life.

Mental Status Examination: The patient is a neatly dressed child who appears her stated age. She is cooperative with the examiner and readily begins to draw pictures with crayons when they are offered to her. Initially, she makes good eye contact. Her speech is fluent and clearly articulated. She has no unusual movements or stereotypic behaviors and is not restless or fidgety. She initially describes her mood as "all right" and has a full, euthymic affect. She smiles and occasionally laughs when the examiner makes a joke. Her thought process is linear and coherent, and she is able to stick to a storyline without becoming distracted. However, when asked about her school problems and the enuresis, she no longer makes eye contact, her affect becomes constricted and somewhat sad-appearing, and she begins to pick at the hem of her shirt. Her speech becomes quieter and her responses less full. She denies thoughts of ever wanting to hurt herself or others or of seeing or hearing things that other people cannot.

Questions: What single clinical syndrome accounts for all of these symptoms? How might this patient be treated?

Diagnosis: Enuresis.

Discussion: Enuresis is defined by the DSM-IV-TR as repeated voiding in a child older than 5 years at least 2 times per week for at least 3 month or wetting that causes clinically significant distress or impairment in social, academic, or other areas of functioning. Enuresis is further classified by clinicians as primary or secondary. **Primary** enuresis describes the child who has never attained significant continence, whereas **secondary** enuresis describes the child who at one point had been dry for 6 months to 1 year but is now wetting again. **Diurnal** enuresis occurs both during awake and asleep periods, whereas **nocturnal** enuresis occurs only when the child is sleeping. Nocturnal enuresis occurs equally in boys and girls until age 5, at which point cases in boys outnumber those in girls by 2:1. However, diurnal enuresis is more common in girls at all ages. Primary enuresis is also relatively equally common in boys and girls, but secondary enuresis is more common in boys.

Although the DSM-IV-TR criteria define enuresis as pathologic after the age of 5 years, about 15% of all children have not yet achieved nocturnal continence by that age. For each year following age 5, approximately 15% of children who still wet at night will spontaneously remit. As a result, most 5- and 6-year-olds with nocturnal enuresis alone are not treated; instead, parents are reassured by clinicians that most cases resolve spontaneously by around age 8. By late adolescence the spontaneous remission rate approaches zero; thus, enuretic adolescents will presumably remain enuretic as adults. Approximately 1–2% of the adult population has never reached primary nocturnal continence.

The cause of enuresis in most children is not known. Certainly, congenital or neurologic conditions such as urinary tract anomalies, neurogenic bladder, and spinal column pathology (e.g., occult spina bifida) must be ruled out. However, the vast majority of children with enuresis have no demonstrable finding. Parents often believe that affected children, particularly those with nocturnal enuresis alone, are simply deeper sleepers. However, several studies have shown that enuretic children are not harder to arouse from sleep than nonenuretic controls. Still other studies looking at bladder capacity have found no difference between most affected children and controls. A familial predisposition has been demonstrated, however, and a full 70% of children with nocturnal enuresis have a first-degree relative who was also affected with the nocturnal form. In twin studies, a 68% concordance was found in monozygotic twins and a 36% concordance in dizygotic twins.

Is enuresis caused by psychiatric pathology? The answer to this question is more complicated. Again, studies have shown that most cases of enuresis are not primarily psychogenic. Nonetheless, many children with this problem are referred for mental health services. Although **secondary** enuresis is known to be associated with stressful events, such as parental divorce, early hospitalizations, birth of a younger sibling, or head trauma, certainly all children who experience these life stressors do not develop enuresis. One study found that exposure to four or more stressful events in 1 year plus a history of delayed age of nocturnal continence made children more likely to develop secondary enuresis. In other words, experiencing a significant number of life stressors in addition to having some underlying physiologic vulnerability may explain why some children develop secondary enuresis and other children with the same stressors do not. Of note, the child in this case attained continence at a delayed age. In enuretic children, a comorbid psychiatric disorder occurs 2–6 times more frequently than in the general population, especially in children over age 5, those with diurnal or secondary enuresis, and girls. However, the psychiatric disorders found in these children are not limited to a specific type. Furthermore, treatment of the psychiatric disorder does not usually resolve the enuresis, and treatment of the enuresis does not usually modulate symptoms of the psychiatric disorder. However, successful treatment of the enuresis does improve self-esteem in most affected children.

Although enuresis is often comorbid with other psychiatric disorders, the present patient does not fully meet criteria for another psychiatric condition. Children with enuresis frequently experience shame and embarrassment and, like the child in this case, are reluctant to discuss the problem or to be in a setting in which they are likely to be discovered by peers. This pattern explains the moodiness and social withdrawal symptoms of the present patient. Major depression can be ruled out because the mood symptoms are not present every day or even more days than not. In addition, the child is not irritable and has normal appetite and normal sleep patterns. The child's school problems are related to her shame and embarrassment when wet. She does not demonstrate any symptoms of attention deficit hyperactivity disorder with the exception of occasional distractibility, which is actually related to being wet.

Treatment of enuresis is not simple. Many parents and practitioners begin with limiting nighttime fluid intake; yet, this approach is usually ineffective and unpleasant for the child. Caffeinated beverages should be completely eliminated from the child's diet, however. For some children, a simple "star chart" with a reward system for dry nights and/or days can be effective. The most successful treatment for **nocturnal** enuresis involves a classical conditioning model and the use of night alarms. Night alarms are devices with a sensor to detect a few drops of urine; they serve as an unconditioned stimulus and are generally placed in the child's underwear at night. The device then works like a pager with either sound and/or vibration to awaken the child. In this unconditioned stimulus phase, ideally the child wakes, holds the rest of the volume until getting to the toilet, and then completes voiding. After many weeks (16 on average), a conditioned response to the alarm develops, and the physiologic sensations associated with the initiation of voiding cause the child to awaken before actual voiding begins. Alarm systems work in up to 90% of nocturnal cases, although there is a 5–30% relapse rate with discontinuation of the alarm. However, most of those relapses can be corrected with repeat treatment. Although night alarms are most effective in the long term, it takes many weeks for training to become effective. The technique, therefore, is sometimes abandoned too quickly. Night alarms also do not address **diurnal** enuresis unfortunately.

Pharmacologic agents also have drawbacks. Imipramine, a tricyclic antidepressant, was one of the earliest drugs used to treat enuresis. It has multiple effects that might contribute to enuresis control, including weak anticholinergic effects, antispasmodic effects on bladder smooth muscle, and stimulation of antidiuretic hormone (ADH) secretion. Imipramine works in up to 85% of children, but relapse rates are reported to be as high as 60% with discontinuation of the drug and the side effects can be unpleasant. Desmopressin acetate (DDAVP) works in 70% of cases but with a 60% relapse rate after discontinuation. DDAVP is a synthetic analog of ADH and presumably works by decreasing urine output to a volume that is less than the child's bladder capacity. Anticholinergics such as oxybutynin are not effective in enuresis unless a neurogenic bladder or decreased bladder capacity is the underlying cause.

The technique of bladder training has also been described for children with overactive daytime bladder and can be successful in the child with daytime enuresis. A watch with a programmable alarm is set to alarm at fixed intervals for which the child is known to be able to remain dry. Depending on the age of the child, the intervals begin as frequently as every hour. The child then toilets regardless of whether she feels she needs to do so. When a full day of dryness has been achieved, the intervals are increased as tolerated by the child, usually with a maximum interval of 3–4 hours. This technique requires the parents to purchase the watch and set and adjust the alarms daily. In addition, the child must be allowed access to the toilet at each alarm, which can be disruptive to the school day and may draw classmates' attention to the child's problem.

In this case, the child psychiatrist recommended discontinuation of the oxybutynin since neither neurogenic bladder nor decreased bladder capacity had been demonstrated during the pediatric workup. As the child was already consistently dry at night, a night alarm system was not prescribed. Instead, the bladder-training technique was taught to both the child and the parents. In addition, a letter was sent to the child's school explaining the procedure so that the child would be allowed to leave class for the lavatory as needed. The psychiatrist also held a family session for education about secondary enuresis, particularly the role that the birth of a new sibling and the father's increasing work schedule might be playing. The child was able to admit some jealousy about her older brother's extra time with their father at basketball practice everyday. A daily 20-minute session of one-to-one time for this child with either parent was then suggested. At a 1-month follow-up visit, the frequency of wetting episodes had decreased from four to two times per week. At the 3-month follow-up the child had had only one wet day in the preceding 3 weeks.

Pearls

1. Although DSM-IV-TR criteria define enuresis as pathologic after the age of 5, about 15% of all children have not yet achieved nocturnal continence by that age.
2. Children with enuresis are often referred to a psychiatrist or other mental health provider despite the fact that most cases of enuresis are probably not psychogenic in origin. However, children with enuresis are 2–6 times more likely to have a psychiatric disorder than the general population.
3. Nocturnal enuresis has a strong genetic component: 70% of children with nocturnal enuresis have a first-degree relative who has had it, and there is a 68% concordance rate in monozygotic twins (dizygotic twins have 36% concordance).
4. It is important to note that neither punishment nor withdrawal of privileges will help a child overcome enuresis because it is not volitional. Yet these practices remain common among parents of affected children.

REFERENCES

1. Jalkut MW, Lerman SE, Churchill BM: Enuresis. Pediatr Clin North Am 2001;48:1461–1488.
2. Lucas CP, Shaffer D: Elimination disorders. Tasman (ed): Psychiatry. Philadelphia, W.B. Saunders, 1997, pp 731–736.
3. Mikkelsen EJ: Enuresis and encopresis: Ten years of progress. J Am Acad Child Adolesc Psychiatry 2001;40:1146–1158.

Gary P. Katzman, MD

PATIENT 34

A 28-year old woman with auditory hallucinations and depression

History of Present Illness: A 28-year-old woman with a history of familial hypophosphetemic rickets and osteosarcoma diagnosed at age 22 is brought to the emergency department by emergency medical services after she told her parents that she was depressed, no longer wanted to suffer, and had planned to kill herself by taking pills. She reports that since high school she has heard more than 10 voices telling her to hurt herself. Recently, she told her parents that she was receiving aggressive chemotherapy that had suppressed her immune system, leading to secondary leukemia. She said that she did not want treatment because she was tired of battling illness all her life and was getting ready to die. Her parents had respected this desire and flew in from out of town to be with her as she was dying. After two weeks, they became concerned by her overly cheerful demeanor and insisted on speaking with her doctors. It was then that she told them about the voices and said that she was depressed and wanted to end her suffering from the osteosarcoma by killing herself.

The patient says that the voices are "constantly yelling at me" and "always there." She also admitted that she was not receiving chemotherapy but said that the voices had told her to convey this message to her parents. She describes her depression as "unbearable" and says that she feels like she wants to kill herself all the time. She reports the depression as a 10/10, with no periods of relief, just momentary diversions. She says that sometimes the depression "comes over me like a cloud that knocks me unconscious, then passes in 15 minutes." She reports terrible sleep problems (often getting 1–2 hours of sleep per night), decreased appetite ("but I force myself to eat anyway"), decreased energy, decreased ability to concentrate, memory difficulties, almost constant suicidal ideation, and a hopeless feeling about the future.

Past Psychiatric History: This is the patient's first psychiatric encounter.

Past Medical History: As a child, the patient spent much of her time at doctors' offices because of her rickets and received multiple x-rays over the years. Besides moderate bilateral tibia vara (bow-leggedness), she had good musculoskeletal development and functioning. The patient was diagnosed with osteosarcoma at age 22 and had multiple surgeries on both legs as well as on both breasts after metastases were discovered. She also had multiple abdominal laparoscopies for a rare form of endometriosis. With all of these difficulties, she tried to keep a positive attitude, writing songs on the piano for children with cancer, organizing blood drives for the times when she needed transfusions, and "smiling as best as I could." The patient currently lives by herself but has frequent visits from friends, and until her recent confinement to bed, she was active in a local theater program and worked as a part-time research assistant in a hospital. The patient drinks a glass of wine per week and denies the use of any other substances. Her family history is remarkable only for a rather severe form of hypophospetemic rickets in her father. She denies any physical or sexual abuse history.

Mental Status Examination: The patient is a slightly obese woman who appears her stated age. Her eye contact is very good, and she appears cooperative and talkative, eager to tell her story. Her speech is slightly pressured at times. The patient describes her mood as "very depressed and anxious," but her affect is labile and somewhat sexually provocative. Her thought process is circumstantial at times but generally linear and goal-directed. She reports auditory hallucinations, some of which tell her to kill herself, but denies visual hallucinations, ideas of reference, or paranoid ideation. She describes persistent suicidal ideation but denies homicidal ideation, a history of suicide attempts, or self-injurious behavior. She is alert and oriented to person, place, and time. Her insight and judgment are impaired.

Question: What is the diagnosis?

Diagnosis: Factitious disorder with combined psychological and physical signs and symptoms.

Discussion: Factitious disorder is the intentional simulation, production, or exaggeration of physical or psychological signs or symptoms for the sole purpose of assuming the sick role, known as primary gain. There is no apparent secondary gain, such as legal or monetary rewards. This apparent lack of secondary gain is the principal feature that distinguishes factitious disorder from malingering. It is important to note that even though the illnesses in factitious disorder are consciously acted out, the underlying motivations may be unconscious, whereas malingering patients almost always have conscious motivations for their illnesses. At the other end of the spectrum, patients who readily admit to their purposefully destructive behaviors, such as self-mutilation, are not considered to have factitious disorder. Such types of behaviors often fall under the category of personality disorders. The most frequently feigned illnesses include iron deficiency anemia, rash, chronic diarrhea, seizures, fever of unknown origin, renal stones, hematuria, hypoglycemia, cancer, and intestinal bleeding.

The DSM-IV-TR distinguishes three types of factitious disorder: (1) with predominantly psychological signs and symptoms, (2) with predominantly physical signs and symptoms, and (3) with combined psychological and physical signs and symptoms. A fourth subtype has features that do not meet the criteria for any of the other subtypes: factitious disorder not otherwise specified, which includes factitious disorder by proxy. Factitious disorder is often confused and equated with Munchausen syndrome. Munchausen syndrome is an uncommon, severe form of factitious disorder characterized by dramatic illnesses, often with the patient receiving unnecessary surgeries and, when confronted or exposed, traveling from hospital to hospital in pursuit of the sick role.

One component of factitious disorder is that the maintained symptoms are frequently based on kernels of truth, and it is often the case that patients have had some exposure to the medical community. This patient had a genetic form of rickets, for which she was in the sick role as a child. Her bone cancer was a plausible sequela of her numerous x-rays as a child. She also had verified bilateral fibroadenomas, with subsequent excision and breast reduction, which she claimed to be surgery for breast cancer. These creations, termed *pseudologia fantastica*, describe the fact that the stories are not only believable but plausible in the context of previous information. In addition, the stories are often fantastic and grand. The present patient not only had endometriosis; she had a rare form that baffled doctors. She had not one, but both breasts surgically altered.

Patients with factitious disorder do not appear to worry a great deal about their illness. They may verbally complain about their pain or torment but often have labile and inappropriate affect and seem nonchalant when describing their medical condition. Their symptoms may seem vague and not fit the signs and symptoms typically associated with their illness. The symptoms that they describe are often exaggerated and theatrical, as in this patient's dramatic "cloud" of depression. In addition, the signs and symptoms of the illness, physical or psychological, do not typically respond to treatment; if they do respond, they do so in an erratic and atypical pattern.

Most factitious disorders are of the physical type. If a person presents with factitious disorder with psychological signs or symptoms, it is more likely to occur in conjunction with physical complaints. It appears that the present patient initially had factitious disorder of the physical subtype, which was expanded to include symptoms of factitious disorder of the psychological type. The patient's motivation is not entirely clear; however, it can be concluded that this expansion is not a malingerer's attempt to avoid responsibility or explain her behavior once she was confronted. Once she assumed the sick role of a psychotic patient, she settled into that role and has not been "cured" by medication or therapy. She also tried to maintain the facade of her physical illnesses. It is important to note that patients who present with predominantly psychological illnesses tend to have a family history of mental illness and may also have a real psychiatric illness other than factitious disorder or personality disorder. It is not surprising that many patients diagnosed with factitious disorder have comorbid personality disorders. Borderline and histrionic personality disorders are most common, although others may be present.

In 95–98% of cases, factitious disorder by proxy involves a mother who produces signs and symptoms of illness in her child. She is often quick to consent to invasive and exploratory tests. Typically, overt signs of abuse, such as burns or bruises, are absent. Once again, the sick role, this time vicariously, is the principal gain.

Although it is difficult to conduct epidemiologic studies of these patients, it is estimated that the prevalence of factitious physical disorder is between 0.8% and 4%. Factitious psychological disorders are less common (about 0.1–0.5%). In one study, almost 70% of patients hospitalized for factitious disorder had worked in a health-related profession; 36% of them were nurses.

There is no known cause for factitious disorder; however, it is postulated that many patients experienced emotional deprivation in childhood with rejecting parents. Patients, therefore, may have low self-esteem and a poor sense of self, with the need to reinvent themselves as glamorous and important. Alternatively, patients may unconsciously seek from medical professionals the caring and responsive acceptance of which they were chronically deprived in childhood.

At first glance, the present patient may appear to have a primary psychotic illness (schizophrenia or schizoaffective disorder) or a primary mood disorder (major depressive disorder with psychotic features or bipolar disorder, depressive phase). Other diagnoses to consider in this case include either a mood or psychotic disorder secondary to a general medical condition. Her high level of interpersonal and general functioning, in addition to the inconsistent nature of her psychotic symptoms, helps rule out illnesses on the schizophrenia spectrum. Her bizarre descriptions of her depression and their fantastic quality, in light of her inconsistent affect, shed doubt on the veracity of a primary mood disorder. However, it is important to take suicidal ideation seriously. Even when patients are clearly feigning "suicidality," cautious and meticulous risk assessment and aftercare are in order, especially in patients with a history of impulsivity, previous self-destructive behaviors, or poor judgment. It is also conceivable that the present patient has real physical illnesses in addition to rickets. She spent considerable time planning the manifestations of her illnesses. Patients with somatoform disorders, such as conversion disorder, somatization disorder, and hypochondriasis, do not usually fabricate their illnesses consciously, and patients with personality disorders do not usually create illnesses for the sole purpose of assuming the sick role. Malingerers, on the other hand, have conscious intent for gain, such as financial or legal rewards.

Most patients, when confronted, deny feigning illness or subtly withdraw from their sick role. The majority of patients with factitious disorder are not willing to enter treatment. Patients who meet criteria for the severe form, Munchausen syndrome, are usually not amenable to treatment and invariably resume their factitious lifestyle. Some die from accidental miscalculations of their behaviors, whereas others may have morbidity and mortality associated with iatrogenic insults while receiving treatment for the factitious illness.

The goal of treatment is to reduce the factitious behaviors. A nonjudgmental, caring approach, along with techniques and statements that prevent the patient from feeling embarrassment, are used. Medications are used to treat comorbid axis I disorders, and selective serotonin reuptake inhibitors (SSRIs) may be useful in controlling impulsive behaviors. Psychotherapy focuses on teaching the patient to manage life's challenges without resorting to factitious illnesses to fulfill their needs. The present patient was started on sertraline, titrated upward to 150 mg/day, and seen weekly in individual psychotherapy with the intent to support more adaptive coping strategies and to monitor ongoing psychological symptoms.

Pearls

1. Factitious disorder of the Munchausen variety typically occurs in middle-aged, unmarried, and unemployed men. Most other patients with factitious disorder are women in their 20s to 40s.
2. Most patients who present with either physical or psychological factitious disorder have at least an average or above-average IQ.
3. Patients can actually create a real need for medical intervention, such as for adhesions from multiple abdominal surgeries or blood transfusions for factitiously initiated anemia.
4. Patients with factitious disorder are protected under the same rights as other patients; it is recommended that hospital ethics and legal departments should be contacted before room searches or other preventative interventions are done.

REFERENCES

1. Albrecht F: Factitious disorder by proxy. J Am Acad Child Adolesc Psychiatry 2001;40:4–5.
2. Asher R: Munchausen's syndrome. Lancet 1951;1:339–341.
3. Fliege H, Scholler G, Rose M, et al: Factitious disorders and pathological self-harm in a hospital population: an interdisciplinary challenge. Gen Hosp Psychiatry 2002;24(3):164–171.
4. Libow JA: Beyond collusion: Active illness falsification. Child Abuse Neglect 2002;26:525–536.
5. Turner J, Reid S: Munchausen's syndrome. Lancet 2002;359:346–349.
6. Wise MG, Ford CV: Factitious disorders. Primary Care 1999;26:315–325.

Julie Stewart, PsyD
Daniel Stewart, MD

PATIENT 35

A 30-year-old man convinced of the maliciousness of others

History of Present Illness: A caseworker at a shelter asks you to see one of his clients, stating, "This guy is driving me crazy! I have tried a dozen things to get him housing, but every time I set something up for him, he comes back to me describing how the interviewer was against him. A few of the staff have told me that he seems really weird at times, almost psychotic, but I don't see it. I just see a 30-year-old guy who seems to love playing the victim or something. Help!"

When the patient comes to meet you, he is impeccably dressed, formally introduces himself to you, and sits down in a nearby chair. You introduce yourself and ask him, "When did you get to the shelter?" He immediately becomes hostile and says to you, "Listen, I don't like psychiatrists. No offense, but you guys are all stupid. I have had to deal with your type before, looking for an excuse to push your damn pills and make money. Well, let me tell you, I don't need your damn pills. I have taken your pills for 7 years, and they turned me into a damn zombie! I won't take them again, so I don't know what we have to talk about." You spend some time trying to gather a sense of just how his previous psychiatrists treated him and how he felt wronged by them. After you make several significant demonstrations of empathy, he slowly begins to become more open with you.

He denies current psychiatric problems or symptoms of any kind and any history of psychotic, manic, depressive, or anxiety symptoms. He states that he feels "as well as any man can be expected to feel in a shelter," and he begins to discuss how several of the staff seem to have problems with him. It seems that they are jealous of him because he "knows how to carry [himself] and [is] not like these other slobs in here." The patient notes that because he makes the staff uncomfortable, "they must try to treat me like the others in order to keep me from rising above them." When asked about how he is getting along with his caseworker, he replies, "She's just keeping me here so she can collect my Medicaid dollars." When you explain that the caseworkers are on salary at the shelter, he retorts, "Yeah, and where does the money come from to pay that salary? From me."

Past Psychiatric and Social History: You ascertain that he was on haloperidol for 7 years. The drug was started when he was an adolescent "to keep me down." With tremendous effort, you finally get him to reveal that he has been in fights in the past, and this behavior seems to be the basis for treatment with haloperidol. His most recent altercation occurred in the context of his supportive housing program. He reports that a man had decided that he was gay, and the patient told him that he was not. Apparently, the man made a pass at him, which consisted of touching him on the back, and the patient turned and struck the man multiple times. As he tells this story, he makes it clear that this was an affront to his character, and he describes other events in his past of the same magnitude in which he struck out or created a tremendous amplification of some apparently benign remark or gesture. The patient reports being hospitalized psychiatrically after one such incident for a few days, but when the doctors "found nothing wrong with me, they finally let me go." He denies any history of suicide attempts or ruminations, replying, "That type of behavior has never been an option for me, and frankly, I don't understand it."

Mental Status Examination: This well-dressed, thin man appears younger than his stated age. He sits bolt upright in his chair, arms folded in front of him. He is guarded and largely uncooperative until late in the interview, when he becomes more forthcoming. He demonstrates no abnormal involuntary movements, and there is no evidence of psychomotor retardation or psychomotor agitation. His speech is somewhat terse and meticulous, and he often speaks as though he were delivering a speech, with dramatic pauses that are obvious attempts to wait for a response from the interviewer. However, his speech is generally within the normal range of rate, rhythm, and volume. His mood is irritable and angry, and his affect is mood-congruent, appropriate to content, and of moderately increased amplitude but not labile (although he is quick to flash into angry and cutting replies to questions). His thought process is coherent and goal-directed, even if vague. Thought content is devoid of hallucinations, and he has no well-formed delusional system. However, he is markedly paranoid in an all-encompassing way of any event in his life that has not gone his way, and he perseverates on these events, returning to them multiple times over the course of the interview. His insight is poor, and his judgment is limited.

Diagnostic Testing: The patient refuses all laboratory work.

Questions: What is the diagnosis? How does the form of the patient's disorder aid in the differential diagnosis?

Diagnosis: Paranoid personality disorder (PPD).

Discussion: Like all personality disorders, PPD is defined by its pervasive and persistent pattern of behavior across multiple contexts, beginning by early adulthood. According to the DSM-IV-TR, PPD is a pervasive distrust and suspiciousness in which the motives of others are interpreted as malevolent. This distrust manifests in four or more of the following forms: (1) suspicion that others are exploiting, harming, or deceiving him without sufficient evidence for that concern; (2) unjustified preoccupation with the loyalty or trustworthiness of friends or associates; (3) reluctance to confide in others because of concerns that information will be used maliciously, again without a reasonable basis for this concern; (4) reads hidden, demeaning, or threatening meaning into benign remarks or events; (5) bears grudges; (6) perceives attacks on his character that are not apparent to others and is quick to react angrily or to counterattack; and (7) doubts recurrently, and without justification, the fidelity of his sexual partner or spouse. Importantly, the diagnosis requires that these paranoid reaction patterns cannot occur in the context of schizophrenia, a mood disorder with psychotic features, or any other psychotic disorder. Finally, the paranoia cannot be due to the direct effects of a general medical condition. This particular patient has a longstanding history of psychiatric care that began during his adolescence, and he certainly fits enough of the criteria listed above for PPD to be considered high on the differential diagnosis. The difficulty of making this diagnosis lies in ruling out the presence of psychosis, since paranoid patients, regardless of their diagnosis, tend to be guarded and difficult to interview.

Paranoia was originally defined as any delusion (that is, any fixed, false belief that is outside the bounds of the person's culture); however, over the course of psychiatric and lay history, it began to be associated with a particular type of delusion, namely delusions of persecution. The essential feature of paranoia is that it is self-referent; that is, the ideas that make up the delusion refer to the patient himself. A patient does not tend to have a delusion about monkeys planning to take over the earth unless he himself figures prominently in the scenario in some way. Paranoia takes different forms in different disorders, and the manifestations of paranoia can aid in the differential diagnosis.

Some phenomenologists describe a difference between primary delusions and secondary delusions. A **primary delusion** is one that is ultimately not understandable; that is, it has no obvious connection to a person's life circumstances or situation. These types of paranoid delusions are often called bizarre. **Secondary delusions**, on the other hand, are more like over-valued ideas. They have unduly self-referent content, but they are not as well-formed or intricate as primary delusions. These types of delusions are understandable in light of the context of the person's culture, circumstances, or condition. The distinction between primary and secondary delusions is subtle and elusive, creating problems for diagnosticians and students alike. The following discussion describes trends that may aid in diagnosis of paranoid states; however, it does not describe absolutes. As with anything in medicine, there are multiple exceptions to the rules.

The paranoia of schizophrenia tends to be fairly global in scope, often encompassing multiple areas of a patient's life. The paranoia can be bizarre (i.e., aliens have invaded my mind and are controlling my thoughts) in schizophrenia, which delineates it from the global but nonbizarre paranoia of PPD. However, schizophrenic patients can also have nonbizarre delusions of persecution (i.e., the FBI is following me). Schizophrenic paranoia tends to be fairly specific, about a specific agency, person, group, or function, whereas in PPD the paranoia is defined by its ubiquitous if somewhat vague presence in multiple areas of a patient's life. Finally, PPD does not present with the formal thought disorder or hallucinations of schizophrenia. The patient seems to have a particular paranoia about psychiatrists; however, over the course of the interview, this paranoia extends to the staff at the shelter as well. The patient also demonstrates no hallucinations or other symptoms of schizophrenia. As an aside, note that he obviously takes care of himself and tends to personal hygiene. Schizophrenic patients tend to have a great deal of trouble caring for themselves because cognitive and negative symptoms result in more significant impairment.

The paranoia of delusional disorder is fixed in an often elaborate delusional system in which patients feel that they are being malevolently treated in some way. The important element is that the delusion is fixed in both content and scope. In other words, the paranoia does not invade every area of the patient's life but instead remains relatively isolated within the context of the delusional system. In contrast, the patient with PPD usually does not have a fixed delusional system, but rather the pervasive distrust of the present patient. Paranoia in other psychotic disorders, such as those induced by a substance, tend to be accompanied by other markers of psychosis, but more importantly, primary psychotic disorders do not have the long-term, persistent suspicion of malevolence that permeates the entire history of a patient with PPD.

PPD at times can be confused with other personality disorders. Borderline personality disorder can be differentiated based on the fact that patients tend to have tumultuous, passionate, and intense relationships with others, whereas patients with PPD re typically unable to maintain any intense relationships for a sustained period. Patients with schizoid personality disorder do not tend to have paranoid ideas and are withdrawn and aloof rather than angry and confrontational. Antisocial patients tend to have suspicions about the motives of others; however, they also have a long history of criminal or antisocial behavior, which is not typically found in PPD. The present patient's fighting raises the possibility of antisocial personality disorder, but his moralizing presentation argues against it.

PPD is estimated to have a prevalence of 0.5–2.5% of the general population; however, these numbers are dubious because patients with PPD rarely present for treatment. Furthermore, patients with PPD who are forced into evaluation by a boss or partner can often elude discovery during the interview process. Men seem to suffer from PPD more than women. There does not appear to be a familial pattern. However, PPD appears to occur more frequently in families in which a relative has schizophrenia or depression, although results have been conflicting at times. Interestingly, when patients with panic disorder were examined in one study, 54% were found to have comorbid PPD.

Large-scale studies have not been undertaken regarding either the prognosis or treatment of PPD. PPD is sometimes a lifelong character type, and at other times the paranoia can ultimately lead to a psychotic break and schizophrenia. It is not clear whether the latter patients are misdiagnosed in their early presentation or whether PPD predisposes a subgroup of patients to developing schizophrenia. Psychotherapy is considered the treatment of choice for PPD although large-scale trials have not been done. Working with patients with PPD is extremely difficult and requires a confident, empathic, and tactful therapist who is able to judge the patient's comfort level and to adapt accordingly. Therapies in which interpretation plays a prominent role tend to push patients with PPD away since interpretations are generally greeted with the same mistrust and suspicion as the behaviors of other people in the patient's life. Behavioral therapy also tends to be experienced as intrusive by patients with PPD. In general, the best-tolerated therapy includes eclectic approaches, in which the therapist can maintain a professional distance (patients with PPD have trouble with intimacy) and work with the patient's delusional system without making the patient feel criticized. Ultimately, the character of the therapist tends to be as important as the style of therapy for treating patients with PPD.

The present patient was probably misdiagnosed in the past with schizophrenia, paranoid type, given his long history of antipsychotic treatment. Weekly psychotherapy was instituted. However, he was unable to tolerate living in a shelter with so many other people and after two months of treatment disappeared from the shelter and from treatment.

Pearls

1. Paranoid delusions are not only delusions of persecution. Thus, a patient whose delusions are purely grandiose may still be suffering from paranoid schizophrenia.
2. Psychopharmacology, primarily benzodiazepines for anxiety and agitation and antipsychotics for delusions, has been used with mixed results.
3. Freud postulated that paranoia was a defense against homosexual impulses, drawing on examples from his work with patients in whom both were present. It is now generally believed in the psychoanalytic community that paranoia is more likely a projection of intolerable hostile impulses rather than purely sexual impulses.

REFERENCES

1. Kaplan HI, Saddock BJ: Kaplan and Saddock's Synopsis of Psychiatry, 8th ed. Philadelphia. Lippincott Williams & Wilkins, 1998, pp 780–782.
2. Maier W, Lichtermann D, Minges J, Heun R: Personality disorders among the relatives of schizophrenia patients. Schizophr Bull 1994;20:481–493.
3. Reich J, Braginsky Y: Paranoid personality traits in a panic disorder population: A pilot study. Comprehen Psychiatry 1994;35:260–264.
4. Sims A: Symptoms in the Mind, 2nd ed. London, W.B. Saunders, 1995, pp. 128–129; 367–368.
5. Webb CT, Levinson DF: Schizotypal and paranoid personality disorder in the relatives of patients with schizophrenia and affective disorders:A review. Schizophr Res 1993;11:81–92.

Sarah E. O'Neil, MD

PATIENT 36

A 62-year-old woman with paranoid thoughts

History of Present Illness: A 62-year-old woman is brought to the psychiatric emergency department by her daughter because she has been withdrawn, tearful and behaving in an unusual manner. For approximately the past month, the patient has been avoiding people by not returning phone calls and declining social invitations. When her daughter visits, the patient is not interactive but instead paces nervously through the house. She does not bathe, cook, or clean. "Why bother?" she asks tearfully. Over the past week, the patient has appeared fearful and vigilant, at times covering her ears and shaking her head or darting her eyes nervously around the room, as though tracking something. She has drawn her shades and has become suspicious of visitors, opening the door only after much reassurance. She recently told her daughter that she has not slept in a week. Just prior to presentation, the daughter found her mother pacing on the balcony, saying "Stop, stop! Be quiet!" The patient told her daughter that she had been planning to jump from the balcony because "the people are back to kill me." She hears male and female voices criticizing her, and plotting ways to kill her. These people have reportedly been hiding outside her house, trying to get in. She has never seen the people, however, "because they are clever and good at hiding." She instead hears them saying, "Come here," at first in a whisper. But over the past several days they have become louder. She can hear them talking to each other about her activities and how they will break in when she is sleeping to "give her what she deserves".

Past Psychiatric History: The patient acknowledged a past history of depression but denies past suicide attempts or hospitalizations. The daughter adds that her mother has had episodes of fearful, paranoid behavior like this in the past and says that during the paranoid periods her mother would "go somewhere for several weeks and then return back to normal." In retrospect, she believes that these periods were hospitalizations. The patient's daughter also recalls that her mother was taken away twice in an ambulance when she was growing up and wonders whether the incidents were suicide attempts, since her father appeared even more worried than usual while her mother was away. The patient drinks alcohol occasionally but does not use tobacco or illicit drugs. The patient denies medical problems, and any family history of mental illness or substance abuse; she does not currently take any medications. The patient lives alone since her husband passed away several years ago. She is close to her daughter, and neither can think of anything that might have precipitated this episode.

Mental Status Examination: The patient is a slightly overweight, disheveled, and malodorous woman who appears her stated age. She appears exhausted and frightened. She agrees to be interviewed but insists that her daughter remain in the room at all times. Once in the interview room, the patient sits at the wall farthest from the door, grips her daughter's arm, and quietly cries. The patient describes her mood as "terrified." Her affect is congruent, and she is visibly agitated, placing both the examiner and her daughter between the door and her. She repeatedly asks if she is safe here. Her speech is minimal, but she does not appear to have word-finding difficulties. Her thought process is linear. When asked about why she is fearful in the room and of the door, she says that the people followed her here and are on the other side of the door, beckoning her to join them so that they can harm her. She says that she would rather be dead than caught by the people and adds that if she were at home, she would jump from the balcony of her high-rise apartment. She also says that she cannot bear the guilt of avoiding the punishment that she is due. She has no insight that these people may be hallucinations.

Physical and Laboratory Examinations: The patient refuses both but allows assessment of vital signs, which are within normal limits except for mild tachycardia of 105 beats/min.

Questions: What the diagnosis? What questions and lab tests or studies help to clarify the diagnosis?

Diagnosis: Major depressive disorder with psychotic features.

Discussion: Depression with psychotic features is a relatively common form of depression, accounting by some estimates for up to 25% of depressions in the hospitalized population. It is often incorrectly diagnosed as depression without psychotic features, leading to incomplete treatment. To fulfill the diagnosis according to the DSM-IV-TR, a person must meet criteria for depression as well as have delusions or hallucinations during the current episode. The delusions and hallucinations are generally mood-congruent, with themes of criticism, punishment, or impending harm or death of the patient. For example, the delusions are frequently somatic (one's body is rotting or is riddled with cancer), nihilistic (the destruction of the world or one's self is approaching), guilt-ridden (being responsible for misfortune befalling a loved one), or focused on deserved punishment or poverty. Auditory hallucinations, if present, are generally transient and berating toward the patient. Visual and somatic hallucinations are the two other most common types of hallucinations in psychotic depression. Psychotic features that are not clearly related to mood, such as paranoid delusions without the belief that it is deserved punishment, ideas of reference, thought insertion, or thought broadcasting, are less common and predict a poorer prognosis.

Some mental health clinicians believe that depression with psychotic features should be a distinct diagnosis as opposed to a subtype of major depression, and in fact some data indicate that psychotic depression is more similar to schizophrenia than to nonpsychotic depression. Major depressive disorder with psychotic features carries a higher risk of suicide than major depressive disorder uncomplicated by psychosis and constitutes a risk factor for episode recurrence. The depressive symptoms in psychotic depression are distinct from depressive symptoms in nonpsychotic major depression. For example, patients are more likely to have severe psychomotor agitation, more severe depressive symptoms, and more pervasive cognitive deficits than patients with nonpsychotic depression. They are also less likely to have diurnal mood variation. Patients with psychotic depression are more likely to have made suicide attempts in the past and to be actively suicidal compared with nonpsychotically depressed patients. Patients often have a history of cluster A personality traits and a history of past delusions, although not necessarily past depressive episodes. Depression with psychotic features is often viewed as more common in the elderly, but at least one study has shown younger age to be a more common characteristic of psychotic rather than nonpsychotic depression. A recent imaging study comparing patients with schizophrenia, psychotic depression, nonpsychotic depression, and normal controls shows that patients with psychotic depression are more likely to have enlarged ventricles and sulcal volume than patients with nonpsychotic depression, who tend to have preserved white matter.

The differential diagnosis is broad. One must consider nonpsychotic depression, dysphoric mania or hypomania, schizoaffective disorder, schizophrenia, delusional disorder, substance-induced psychosis, and mood disorder caused by a substance or general medical condition. In the above presentation, more information is needed to narrow the diagnostic possibilities. To differentiate dysphoric mania from psychotic depression, for example, clinicians must clarify the need for sleep. The present patient has not slept in 7 days but nevertheless complains of exhaustion, making mania less likely. During hospitalization she reveals that she would like to sleep but is too afraid. She also has no history of other manic symptoms, such as injudicious decisions, racing thoughts, grandiosity, or excessive energy.

The presence of mood-congruent psychotic symptoms, those consistent with the depressive mood, such as hearing critical voices or command hallucinations to kill one's self, is also characteristic of psychotic depression. Even more helpful is the time course of affective and psychotic symptoms. In schizophrenia, the duration of mood symptoms, if present, is brief compared with the total duration of the psychotic episode. In schizoaffective disorder, psychotic symptoms must be present for at least 2 weeks in the absence of mood symptoms. The present patient's presentation differs from delusional disorder in that she has auditory hallucinations and her mood symptoms are a prominent part of her presentation.

The patient is currently too paranoid to permit a medical work-up. The stability of her vital signs and the lack of focal weakness or other gross neurologic findings are comforting. When she permits the work-up, several factors are important to consider. Metabolic disturbances such as hyper- or hypothyroidism can cause mood and psychotic symptoms. Prescribed medications such as steroids can cause a similar picture, and antihistamines can induce a delirium that also resembles the patient's symptoms. The patient's older age makes her more sensitive to the effects of anticholinergic medications, and she also has tachycardia, which is characteristic of anticholinergic delirium (see case XX). Urinalysis should be checked for infection, and urine toxicology should be done to screen for drugs of abuse, especially cocaine, marijuana, amphetamines, and hallucinogens such as PCP or ketamine. A thorough neurologic exam and neuroimaging are indicated, if not previously done or if the current presentation is markedly different from past presentations. Masses, lesions, and ischemic events can sometimes present with psychiatric symptoms similar to those of the current patient. During the hospitalization, the patient consented to a work-up, which was negative. Enlisting the support of a trusted family member was instrumental in gaining the patient's cooperation.

Once the diagnosis is established, treatment should be directed toward both psychotic and affective symptoms. Several antidepressants have been studied. A double-blind European trial comparing sertraline with paroxetine has shown that selective serotonin reuptake inhibitor (SSRI) monotherapy is effective for the clinical improvement of symptoms in 75% and 46% of patients, respectively. The difference in response rates between the two groups was not statistically significant. Among the tricyclics, amoxapine is thought to be most effective due to its D2 and 5HT2 antagonist properties. Other studies show that the combination of antidepressants and antipsychotics is most efficacious. In a multicenter, double-blind, parallel group trial comparing risperidone with the combination of haloperidol and amitriptyline, the combination demonstrated significantly greater efficacy. A recent open trial of olanzapine combined with paroxetine also showed promising results.

It is important to consider that paranoid patients may not be willing to take multiple medications. Olanzapine has been shown to be effective monotherapy in a retrospective study. In a recent review by Schatzberg, atypical antipsychotics are recommended as first-line therapy, with the addition of an antidepressant as the patient's paranoia resolves. However, according to practice guidelines of the American Psychiatric Association (APA), major depressive disorder with psychotic features responds better to treatment with a combination of an antipsychotic and an antidepressant than with either medication alone. Lithium augmentation has also been shown to be helpful in some patients who have not responded to the combined regimen.

Preliminary results of two studies suggest that electroconvulsive therapy (ECT) may be superior to medication for psychotic depression. It is also thought to be a more effective treatment for elderly patients with psychotic depression. According to APA practice guidelines, ECT is highly effective in major depressive disorder with psychotic features and may be considered a first-line treatment.

Once symptoms are controlled, one must decide whether to use maintenance treatment to prevent relapse. Maintenance therapy is generally a continuation of the therapy that was effective during acute and continuation phase treatment. In the APA practice guidelines, psychotic features are not considered as a separate entity with separate treatment recommendations but rather as a risk factor for recurrent major depressive episodes. Maintenance therapy in psychotic depression, therefore, is an important consideration. Use of ECT in continuation or maintenance phase treatment for major depression has not been well studied. It is also not known whether ECT alone is effective in prevention of relapse in psychotic depression or whether antidepressants, antipsychotics, or some combination of the three are best for maintaining remission.

The present patient was hospitalized on a medical psychiatric inpatient unit. She was started on olanzapine at 5 mg and titrated upward to 10 mg per day. Paroxetine was added and titrated to 40 mg per day. Over the course of 2 weeks, the auditory hallucinations disappeared, and shortly thereafter her mood improved as well. Her paranoia resolved with the hallucinations. She tolerated the medication with no complaints of side effects. She was discharged in good condition after 2 weeks on olanzapine,10 mg per day, and paroxetine, 40 mg per day, with follow-up at a community mental health clinic for monitoring of mood and affective symptoms.

Pearls

1. Psychotic depression is a poorly understood and underdiagnosed entity. Patients are undertreated and at higher risk for suicide and symptom recurrence than patients with major depression without psychotic features. Be sure to ask about psychotic symptoms in depressed patients, especially those who have severe depression, marked agitation, or prominent suicidal ideation.

2. Although depression with psychotic features is currently considered a subtype of major depression, several factors indicate that it may be a separate entity. For example, psychotic depression responds differently to antidepressants and ECT from nonpsychotic depression; psychotic depression has a different quality of symptomatology than nonpsychotic depression; it has a poorer prognosis and is marked by declining social function, much like schizophrenia; and it also tends to occur in people who have cluster A personality disorders and a past history of delusions. Patients with psychotic depression may also have MRI evidence of enlarged ventricles and sulci.

3. The best treatment for psychotic depression remains controversial. APA guidelines recommend antipsychotics in conjunction with antidepressants. Also consider ECT early in the course if the patient does not respond to medication; evidence suggests that it may be more beneficial than medication for symptom remission.

4. Some patients with psychotic depression have a markedly abnormal hypothalamopituitary axis. Mifepristone is a potent glucocorticoid receptor antagonist that may be effective in rapidly treating psychotic symptoms. A small, double-blind, placebo-controlled crossover study, an open-label study, and several case reports have shown mifepristone to be effective in early treatment, followed by a switch to antipsychotic-antidepressant combinations.

5. The social and occupational impairment in depression with psychotic features has been hypothesized to be secondary to subtle cognitive deficits caused by the higher cortisol levels frequently observed in these patients.

REFERENCES

1. Flint AJ, Rifat SL: The treatment of psychotic depression in later life: A comparison of pharmacotherapy and ECT. Int J Geriatr Psychiatry 1998;3:23–28.
2. Matthews JD, Bottonari KA, Polania LM, et al: An open study of olanzapine and fluoxetine for psychotic major depression: Interim analysis. J Clin Psychiatry 2002;63:1164–1170.
3. Petrides G, Fink M, Husain MM, et al. ECT remission rate in psychotic versus non-psychotic depressed patients. Journal of ECT, 2001;17(4): 244–253.
4. Rothschild, AJ. Challenges in treatment of depression with psychotic features. Biol Psychiatry 2003;53:680–690.
5. Rothschild AJ, Bates KS, Boehringer KL, Syed A: Olanzapine response in psychotic depression. J Clin Psychiatry 1999;60:116–118.
6. Salokangas RK, Cannon T; Van Erp T, et al: Structural magnetic resonance imaging in patients with first episode schizophrenia, psychotic and severe, non-psychotic depression. Br J Psychiatry 2002;43(Suppl):58–65.
7. Schatzberg A: New approaches to managing psychotic depression. J Clin Psychiatry 2003;64 (Suppl 1):19–23.

PATIENT 37

A 31-year-old woman with delusional thinking

History of Present Illness: A 31-year-old woman is brought to the psychiatric emergency department by her husband, who reports a 4-day history of his wife having "crazy ideas." He notes that earlier in the evening before the current presentation, she was yelling and throwing plates at him and that she has never behaved similarly in the past. He says that for several days she has been pacing the house for most of the night. The patient insists that her husband wants to leave her because she has bad skin and adds that she is certain that he is seeing other women because he locks her out of their bathroom at home. She says that she was throwing plates because of the "wreck that he has made of my life." The patient also reports feeling as though her husband may be responsible for her medical problems. She endorses passive suicidal ideation with no plan. She denies any homicidal ideation or auditory or visual hallucinations.

According to the patient's family, she is mildly anxious but pleasant and sociable at baseline. She is also described as generally affectionate and trusting with her husband. Although she reportedly drinks socially, 1–2 beers a week, she has no history of drug use. She works as a laboratory technician, has been married for 6 years, and has no children.

Past Psychiatric History: This is the patient's first psychiatric hospitalization. She has a history of one major depressive episode (following a miscarriage) that was treated with psychotherapy alone. She has no history of sustained periods of mania and denies the presence of mental illness in family members.

Past Medical History: The patient was diagnosed with systemic lupus erythematosus (SLE) at age 21 and has a history of skin and joint involvement. She had not taken steroids for "years" until 3 weeks before admission when she began oral prednisone at 60 mg/day for proteinuria of 3.4 gm/L, which was noted in routine tests. She has no history of psychiatric side effects from oral steroids but stopped taking them in the past because of concerns about weight gain.

Physical Examination: On neurologic exam, she is alert and oriented to person, place, and time. Cranial nerves 2–12 are intact. No tremors or tics. Strength is 5/5 throughout. Touch and temperature sensation are intact. Standard reflexes are 2+ bilaterally. Babinski reflex is not present. No dysdiadochokinesia or evidence of gait abnormalities; balance is intact. On physical exam: cardiac: regular rhythm and rate, S1, S2, no m/r/g; chest: clear to auscultation bilaterally; abdomen: soft, nontender, nondistended, no organomegaly; extremities: no cyanosis, clubbing, or edema; skin: malar rash on face.

Mental Status Examination: The patient is a thin woman who appears her stated age. Her hair is disheveled, and she wears sneakers with no socks. Her eye contact is limited, and at times she seems distracted. She is cooperative but anxious. During the interview she looks around and several times asks, "Are we almost done?" Speech is quiet but normal in rate and rhythm. The patient describes her mood as "okay," but her affect is irritable and she appears at times on the verge of tears. Thought process is linear and goal-directed but with increased latency. Thought content is notable for paranoid delusions of betrayal. She says that she would not mind being dead but has no plan to kill herself. She denies any homicidal thoughts; she says that she just wanted to make her husband understand her. She is alert and oriented, with intact immediate and delayed recall, and no impairments in attention or concentration. Impulse control is mildly impaired, as evidenced by frequent interrupting. The patient's insight and judgment are limited because she believes firmly in her delusions and feels that her outburst at home was reasonable.

Diagnostic Testing: Complete blood count, chemistry, thyroid function tests, urinalysis, toxicology screen, and rapid plasma reagin test were within normal limits. EKG: normal sinus rhythm at 78 beats/min.

Questions: What is the diagnosis? Discuss the differential diagnosis and its treatment implications.

Diagnosis: Psychotic disorder due to a general medical condition (neuropsychiatric lupus).

Discussion: Neuropsychiatric systemic lupus erythematosus (NPSLE) designates the manifestation of any of a variety of focal and diffuse central and peripheral nervous system disorders in patients with SLE. Among the psychiatric symptoms noted in NPSLE, the most common are anxiety and major depressive symptoms, estimated to occur in 25% and 20% of patients, respectively. Community-based studies estimate the prevalence of psychosis among SLE patients to be around 5%. A recent study noted that the type of NPSLE varied with age, with psychosis having a mean age of onset of 30.4 years and depressed mood having a mean age of onset of 40 years. Nineteen NPSLE syndromes have been defined; psychiatric disturbances (as seen in this patient), headaches, and cognitive dysfunction are the most common. Seizures, polyneuropathies, and cerebrovascular disease are among the other most clinically notable presentations. Many patients present with more than one syndrome.

Differentiating between psychosis due to SLE and corticosteroid-induced psychosis is both challenging and essential, because the treatments for the two entities are entirely different, even contradictory. Put simply, psychosis due to SLE requires an increase in steroid dosage, whereas steroid-induced psychosis necessitates tapering or discontinuation of steroid treatment. Paying attention to the time course may help establish a diagnosis because steroid-induced psychoses tend to occur within 5–14 days of starting therapy. Steroid-induced psychotic symptoms also appear to be dose-dependent. However, it is not unusual for patients to develop psychiatric symptoms from steroids even if the doses are notably lower than what a patient has tolerated in the past. Some researchers have suggested that serum albumin levels may play a role in a patient's susceptibility to steroid-induced psychosis. Since albumin-bound steroids are biologically inactive, steroid psychosis is more likely in patients whose medical conditions cause low levels of serum proteins. If, however, the onset of psychosis is associated with the presence of antiribosomal P antibodies in the serum or other evidence of systemic SLE involvement, the symptoms are probably better accounted for by SLE itself. SLE is also more likely the culprit if cerebrospinal fluid (CSF) levels of IgM, IgA, and IgG are elevated.

In the present patient, the diagnosis at presentation remained uncertain. Antiribosomal P antibodies were not quickly available, and the patient refused a lumbar puncture. Initially the steroid dosage was lowered, and the decision was made not to begin an antipsychotic so that symptoms and the potential response to steroid tapering could be monitored more closely. Since the patient remained psychotic even after the dose was lowered, it was decided that neuropsychiatric lupus was a more likely cause of the psychosis than steroids. The steroid dosage, therefore, was titrated upward and the psychosis resolved. If the patient had not improved with an increase in the steroid dose, it would have been appropriate to consider more seriously the possibility of a primary psychotic disorder unrelated to SLE, such as schizophrenia. Furthermore, in a patient who is immunosuppressed by chronic steroids, as many SLE patients are, one should always keep in mind the possibility of central nervous system (CNS) infection.

Although the patient responded to an increased dosage of steroids, it remains true that current treatment of NPSLE is primarily empirical. Few randomized clinical trials exist. In patients with focal neurologic manifestations and antiphospholipid antibodies, anticoagulation is used with success. For all other patients, including psychiatric patients, corticosteroids continue to be the mainstay of treatment. New studies are examining the benefit and tolerability of intravenous (IV) cyclophosphamide, IV pulse cyclophosphamide, dehydroepiandrosterone (DHEA), and short-term plasmapharesis.

The prognosis of patients with NPSLE syndromes remains an area of active research. The morbidity and mortality associated with any form of lupus has decreased over the years due to use of corticosteroid and immunosuppressive treatments. However, NPSLE events have been shown in prospective studies to be associated with poorer clinical outcome compared with SLE patients without NPSLE events. Recent studies note that 21–47% of patients with NPSLE suffer a recurrence of NPSLE symptoms over a period of 2–5 years.

Pearls

1. Serum antiribosomal P antibodies have been shown to be strongly associated with the development of psychosis and depression in SLE, whereas cognitive dysfunction has been associated with anticardiolipin (aCL) antibodies. A history of persistently elevated aCL antibodies has been linked to greater and sustained cognitive impairment.

2. Although no diagnostic test is sensitive and specific for NPSLE, recent studies have shown that magnetic resonance spectroscopy (MRS) reveals neurometabolic abnormalities that are missed by conventional MRI. These abnormalities are thought to reflect neuronal injury or loss. In addition, although routine electroencephalography (EEG) fails to differentiate NPSLE from SLE without CNS involvement, recently it has been observed that quantitative EEG demonstrates selective involvement of the temporal lobe in up to 85% of patients with NPSLE.

3. Some researchers have hypothesized that cutaneous and articular manifestations of lupus indicate a milder form of the disease overall, with a lower likelihood of NPSLE. However, most of the research looking into risk factors has focused on Caucasian populations, and a more complex picture is emerging as other ethnic populations are increasingly included in studies.

4. The American College of Rheumatology has recently made available specific criteria for NPSLE. Research groups are increasingly using these criteria, thus making possible more meaningful reviews and comparisons between studies.

REFERENCES

1. Brey RL, Holliday SL, Saklad AR, et al: Neuropsychiatric syndromes in lupus: Prevalence using standardized definitions. Neurology 2002;58:214–220.
2. Costallat L, Bertolo M, Appenzeller S: The American College of Rheumatology nomenclature and case definitions for neuropsychiatric lupus syndromes: Analysis of 527 patients. Lupus 2001;10(Suppl 32).
3. Hermosillo-Romo D, Brey RL: Diagnosis and management of patients with neuropsychiatric systemic lupus erythematosus (NPSLE). Best Pract Res Clin Rheumatol 2002;16:229–244.
4. Lopez-Medrano F, Cervera R, Trejo O, et al: Steroid induced psychosis in systemic lupus erythematosus: A possible role of serum albumin level. Ann Rheum Dis 2002;61:562–563.
5. Omdal R: Some controversies of neuropsychiatric systemic lupus erythematosus. Scand J Rheumatol 2002;31:192–197.
6. Sanna G, Khamashta MA: Low-dose pulse cyclophosphamide in the treatment of neuropsychiatric lupus. Lupus 2003;12:1–2.
7. Sirois F. Steroid psychosis: A review. Gen Hosp Psychiatry 2003;25:27–33.

PATIENT 38

A 57-year-old woman with suicidal thoughts

History of Present Illness: A 57-year-old woman is brought to the psychiatric emergency department by police after she was found wandering the streets of a suburban neighborhood. The patient's boyfriend called the police two days earlier to report her disappearance. He also informed the police that she has not been acting like herself lately and that at times she says "strange things." For example, he recalled that about 1 month ago, she told him that the government was trying to communicate with her through the television set. At this time, her boyfriend explained, she began to dress in a slovenly manner and to pay less attention to grooming because she felt that this change in habits would prevent the government officials from identifying her.

The patient is currently unemployed, although previously she has held various jobs as an unskilled employee, including kitchen aide and sanitation worker at local hospitals and schools. She has lived with her present boyfriend for the past year. She is divorced and has had little contact with her former husband or their two children since the divorce 15 years ago. On admission, the patient says that she feels "very depressed" and that she wants to "end it all." She reports that for the past few weeks she has felt "consumed by guilt," yet she cannot explain why. She also describes difficulty with sleeping for 2 weeks prior to admission and little desire to eat. During this time, she thinks that she lost close to 10 pounds. When asked about her concerns regarding government officials, she states that they have been after her for a while and that she knows they were watching her via video cameras in the lampposts as she walked in the streets. The patient denies any alcohol or illicit drug use.

Past Psychiatric History: The patient has had four previous hospitalizations for psychiatric illness. The first occurred when she was 38 years old. She was hospitalized in the general psychiatry unit for seven months after reportedly displaying bizarre behavior, and she was treated with antipsychotic medications, which she discontinued on her own after discharge. The patient states that it was at this time that the government officials began following her. At age 43, age 47, and again five years ago, she was admitted to the general psychiatry unit for treatment of paranoid delusions. She recalls feeling very depressed prior to these admissions, as difficulty coping with the divorce and problems with other relationships in which she later became involved were significant stressors in her life. Between admissions, the patient did not receive psychotherapy or take psychotropic medications that were prescribed for her in the hospital. She felt unable to control her life between admissions in that she had difficulty returning to work and maintaining relationships with boyfriends as well as her children. She reports that the government officials were intrusive during these periods.

Mental Status Examination: The patient is a thin woman who appears her stated age. Her manner of dress suggests little attention to grooming. Her clothing appears dirty, and her hair is poorly brushed. She is cooperative, although her eye contact is variable. At times she seems frightened and distracted when responding to questions. The patient's speech is normal in volume and tone and has a regular rhythm. Her articulation is fair. On occasion, her words are not enunciated clearly but are comprehensible. The patient describes her mood as "depressed," rating it a "2 or 3 out of 10," and her affect is constricted, appropriate, and mood-congruent. Thought process is disturbed sporadically by loosening of associations, although there is no evidence of flight of ideas. The patient has paranoid delusions about the U.S. government, and for the past two months she has been concerned that "senior government officials" were plotting to attack her. She thinks that the government placed video cameras on the streets where she had been walking and that these cameras may also be present in the hospital. When asked to explain the meaning of a proverb, she interprets it concretely. She denies other disturbances of thought content, including auditory and visual hallucinations. The patient admits to having thoughts of harming herself, yet she does not have a suicide plan and denies homicidal ideation. She is alert and oriented to person, place, and time. Her insight and judgment are poor; she cannot explain or understand her behavior for the past two days since her disappearance.

Diagnostic Testing: Mini-Mental Status Examination (MMSE) score: 27/30. The patient recalls 1 of 3 items after 3 minutes. Noncontrast brain MRI: no evidence of infarction; mild cerebral atrophy.

Laboratory Findings: White blood cell count, 7,900/µl; hemoglobin, 13.0 gm/dl; hematocrit, 40.7 gm/dl; platelets, 229,000/µl; sodium, 136 mEq/L; potassium, 4.0 mEq/L; chloride, 100 mEq/L; bicarbonate, 27 mEq/L; blood urea nitrogen, 17 mg/dl; creatinine, 1.0 mg/dl; glucose, 86 mg/dl; calcium, total 9.2 mg/dl; aspartate aminotransferase, 37 U/L; alanine aminotransferase, 20 U/L; vitamin B12, 376 pg/ml; folate, 15 ng/ml; thyroid-stimulatnig hormone, 4.0 µU/ml; rapid plasma reagin test, nonreactive. Urinalysis: yellow in color and clear; specific gravity, 1.015; pH, 5.0. Negative for glucose, ketones, bilirubin, blood, nitrite, leukocyte esterase; no white or red blood cells; no casts or crystals. Urine toxicity screen: negative for amphetamines, cannabinoids, cocaine metabolites, opiates, phencyclidine.

Questions: What is the diagnosis? What other disorders might be considered in the differential?

Diagnosis: Schizoaffective disorder, depressive type.

Discussion: The DSM-IV-TR classifies schizoaffective disorder as a psychotic disorder in which the characteristic symptoms of the active phase of schizophrenia, including bizarre delusions or hallucinations, exist concurrently with a major depressive or manic episode. Subtypes of the disorder include depressive and bipolar, which describe the mood component of the illness. The diagnostic criteria for schizoaffective disorder include the presence of delusions or hallucinations without prominent mood symptoms for at least two weeks of the illness. In addition, the mood disturbance must comprise a substantial portion of both active and residual phases of the psychosis, and patients must meet the full criteria for the mood episode for this diagnosis to be applied. As in schizophrenia, social or occupational dysfunction is also associated with schizoaffective disorder.

People with schizoaffective disorder sometimes have diminished attention and memory. Patients with psychotic disorders in general, particularly schizoaffective disorder and schizophrenia, have been shown to perform more poorly on neuropsychological tests than those with nonpsychotic affective illnesses, indicating that the psychotic disorders may be associated with a greater decline in cognitive function. Neuropsychological tests suggest that people who suffer a depressive episode, including those with the depressive subtype of schizoaffective disorder, major depression, bipolar disorder, or dysthymic disorder, show a similar degree of cognitive impairment compared with healthy controls. The present patient demonstrates some degree of short-term memory loss, based on her performance on the MMSE, although limited evidence suggests cognitive decline.

The lifetime prevalence of schizoaffective disorder is unknown, although most likely it occurs less often than schizophrenia. It may present at any age from adolescence to late adulthood, yet the typical age of onset probably is early adulthood. The depressive type may be found more frequently in older adults, whereas the bipolar type may occur more often in young adults. The disorder appears to be more common in women compared with schizophrenia. Family studies have shown that relatives of patients with schizoaffective disorder are at an increased risk for schizophrenia and bipolar disorder as well as other affective disorders, although psychotic symptoms often accompany affective illness in relatives of schizoaffective patients. In addition, the first-degree relatives of people with schizophrenia or bipolar disorder were found to be at an increased risk of developing schizoaffective disorder.

The diagnosis of schizoaffective disorder is somewhat controversial in that recent studies have questioned its relationship to schizophrenia and affective disorders, with some authors suggesting that it may represent a subtype or a "phenotypic variant" of one of these illnesses or perhaps an "intermediate" on the clinical spectrum between the two diagnoses. Some studies argue that schizoaffective disorder is more similar to schizophrenia than to bipolar disorder, whereas others propose that the disorder is an "intermediate" syndrome between the two. However, there is evidence that schizoaffective disorder is significantly different from either illness. As in the present case, patients with schizoaffective disorder demonstrate more affective and fewer negative symptoms than patients with schizophrenia, yet they have positive symptoms consistent with those seen in schizophrenia. Neuroanatomic and genetic linkage studies of schizoaffective disorder are limited.

The present patient meets the diagnostic criteria for schizoaffective disorder, depressive type in that she has had bizarre delusions and behavior for an uninterrupted period of greater than one month, consistent with criterion A for schizophrenia, and during the same period she also has a major depressive episode. For at least two weeks of the illness, which accounts for a substantial portion of its duration, she experiences a depressed mood, insomnia, poor appetite, and weight loss, along with suicidal ideation and a preoccupation with feelings of guilt, consistent with a major depressive episode. In addition, the patient's psychotic symptoms appear to have been present for at least two weeks in the absence of any mood disturbance, based on the history provided by her boyfriend as well as her narrative.

With regard to the differential diagnosis, it is often difficult to distinguish schizoaffective disorder, depressive type from major depressive disorder with psychotic features or schizophrenia, both of which should be included in the differential for this patient. In psychotic mood disorders, such as major depression with psychotic features, the psychotic symptoms occur only during, and not independently of, the mood disturbance, whereas in schizoaffective disorder delusions or hallucinations exist in the absence of mood symptoms. In schizophrenia, affective symptoms may occur for a brief period of the illness or are not sufficient to meet the criteria for a mood episode.

Dementia should also be considered in the differential diagnosis for an older patient who presents with cognitive impairment. The present patient demonstrates short-term memory loss, social and occupational dysfunction, and an inability to explain her recent actions, and the MRI of the brain indicates mild cerebral atrophy. However, her behavior and poor social function are more likely the result of her delusions and are consistent with the diagnosis of schizoaffective disorder. In addition, there is limited evidence for cognitive decline. People with schizophrenia or major depressive disorder may present with cognitive deficits, which make distinguishing between these diagnoses and dementia more difficult in older patients. In schizophrenia, however, cognitive impairment is less severe than in dementia, and characteristic symptoms suggest this diagnosis over that of dementia. Cognitive decline in major depressive disorder more likely occurs abruptly, accompanying the depression.

Both initial and maintenance treatments of schizoaffective disorder include antipsychotic medications, many of which are reportedly effective. Maintenance therapy with antipsychotic agents prevents relapse in most patients with schizoaffective disorder. Second-generation antipsychotics produce fewer extrapyramidal side effects and for this reason are preferable to first-generation agents in the treatment of patients with psychotic disorders. First-generation antipsychotics, however, may be used in patients who do not respond to second-generation medications. Clozapine is often effective for treatment-refractory schizoaffective disorder. However, it is unclear whether antipsychotic agents alone are effective in treating the psychotic and mood components of schizoaffective disorder or whether thymoleptic medications are also required. Randomized, double-blind clinical trials of treatment options are limited. One such study comparing risperidone and haloperidol found no significant difference in the ability of either drug to reduce psychotic and manic symptoms in patients with schizoaffective disorder, although risperidone led to a greater improvement in depressive symptoms and was better tolerated than haloperidol.

Antidepressants are also often indicated for the treatment of a major depressive episode in patients with schizoaffective disorder, depressive type. Selective serotonin reuptake inhibitors, venlafaxine or mirtazepine, are preferred over tricyclic antidepressants and monoamine oxidase inhibitors because of their greater safety and tolerability. It is recommended that the use of antidepressants in patients with schizoaffective disorder should follow guidelines for the treatment of depressive episodes in bipolar disorder to prevent induction of mania. Mood-stabilizing agents, including lithium and anticonvulsants, are often used in the treatment of schizoaffective disorder as well. Because clinical trials are limited, the presentation of a patient with schizoaffective disorder dictates whether mood-stabilizing medications should be used. In addition, supportive psychotherapy may be beneficial in managing schizoaffective patients. Schizoaffective disorder appears to have a more favorable prognosis than schizophrenia, although its prognosis is worse than that of mood disorders.

Pearls

1. The diagnosis of schizoaffective disorder is somewhat controversial. Some studies suggest that it is more closely related either to schizophrenia or to the affective disorders. Others argue that schizoaffective disorder does not exist as a distinct diagnosis, because a dual diagnosis of schizophrenia and mood disorder accounts for the same clinical presentation. Alternatively, schizoaffective disorder, depressive and bipolar types, may represent misdiagnoses of schizophrenic patients with prominent negative symptoms or pressured speech, respectively.
2. Neuropsychological tests indicate that people with schizoaffective disorder, depressive type have similar impairment in cognitive function after a major depressive episode as patients with major depression, bipolar disorder, and dysthymic disorder compared with healthy controls. However, according to one study, cognitive impairment does not improve when the depressive symptoms abate, as they often do in primary affective disorders.
3. Some case reports have suggested that clozapine may decrease suicidality and have a mood-stabilizing effect in schizoaffective disorder. Maintenance treatment with lithium may also decrease suicidality, according to some studies. Further clinical trials are needed.

REFERENCES

1. Adler CM, Strakowki SM: Boundaries of schizophrenia. Psychiatry Clin North Am 2003;26:1–23.
2. Berrettinni WH: Are schizophrenic and bipolar disorders related? A review of family and molecular studies. Biol Psychiatry 2000;48:531–538.
3. Evans JD, Heaton RK, Paulsen JS, et al: Schizoaffective disorder: A form of schizophrenia or affective disorder? J Clin Psychiatry 1999;60:874–882.
4. Fochtmann LJ: Treatment of other psychotic disorders. In Sadock BJ, Sadock VA: Comprehensive Textbook of Psychiatry, 8th ed. Philadelphia, Lippincott, Williams & Wilkins, 2004 [in press].
5. Janicak PG, Keck PE Jr, Davis JM, et al: A double-blind, randomized, prospective evaluation of the efficacy and safety of risperidone versus haloperidol in the treatment of schizoaffective disorder. J Clin Psychopharmacol 2001;21:360–368.
6. Levinson DF, Umapathy C, Musthaq M: Treatment of schizoaffective disorder and schizophrenia with mood symptoms. Am J Psychiatry 1999;156:1138–1148.
7. Neu P, Kiesslinger U, Schlattmann P, Reischies FM: Time-related cognitive deficiency in four different types of depression. Psychiatry Res 2001;103:237–247.

PATIENT 39

A 42-year-old woman with bizarre behavior

History of Present Illness: A 42-year-old woman was brought to the psychiatric emergency department by emergency medical services because she was noticed to be acting "bizarre" when she was arrested for having struck a woman on the subway. The patient reports that "the voices told me to hit her." She states that she has been hearing voices for many years, but over the past two days they have become louder and she cannot ignore them anymore. She also reports feeling angry because people "read my mind and tease me about having epilepsy." The patient denies being depressed and reports normal sleep and appetite. She takes multiple medications under the supervision of her boyfriend. The boyfriend confirms her account and also reports that she has epilepsy and had "a typical seizure" four days ago. He describes the seizure as characterized by sudden speech arrest, turning of her head to the right, and rigidity of her right upper extremity, followed by shaking of her whole body. He also states that she would often "talk to herself." At presentation the patient is taking molindone, 10 mg twice daily; sertraline, 100 mg daily; valproic acid, 500 mg twice daily; and phenytoin, 100 mg 3 times/day. According to the patient, she has had epilepsy since the age of 12. Because of the recent seizure, the neurology service was asked to see the patient.

Diagnostic Testing: EEG (see figure, top of p. 144): bilateral slowing, bilateral spike and wave discharges, and mostly left temporal dominant spikes in the awake and drowsy states. MRI study of the brain (see figure, bottom of p. 144): generalized cerebral atrophy with enlarged ventricles and sulci; cystic encephalomalacia in the left anterior temporal lobe.

Laboratory Examination: Valproic acid level, 55 μg/ml (50–100); phenytoin level, 18 μg/ml (10–20). Routine blood work was within normal range, and urine toxicology was negative.

Past Psychiatric History: The patient had five previous admissions for episodic psychosis. Her first psychiatric admission was at age 29 when she presented with agitation, auditory hallucinations, and paranoia. Her most recent admission was 1 year ago for major depression with a suicide attempt when she overdosed on her anticonvulsant medication. She has been treated with sertraline successfully for her depression. She has been on various antipsychotic medication in the past, including trifluoperazine, thiothixene, and haloperidol. The patient has no history of drug or alcohol abuse, no history of mania, no history of violence, and no history of mental illness in the family.

Past Medical History: The patient had her first seizure in her mid-teens and has been treated in various hospitals. She also has a history of head trauma at age 9, but the correlation with her epilepsy is not clear. Her typical seizures have been complex partial seizures with occasional secondary generalization. The current anticonvulsant regimen has had significant success in seizure control; the patient reports only 1–2 complex partial seizures/month, whereas in the past she had 3–4 seizures each week, some with secondary generalization.

Mental Status Examination: The patient looks her stated age. She is disheveled, with poor eye contact, and poorly related. Speech is nonspontaneous and monotonous, mood is mildly irritable, and affect is mood-congruent yet constricted in range. Thought process shows mild disorganization with circumstantiality. Thought content is impoverished with the persistent delusion that "people can read my mind and know I have epilepsy." She has command auditory hallucinations of "voices telling me to hit the woman." She denies any suicidal or homicidal ideation. On cognitive testing, the patient is awake and alert, and oriented to self, place, and year but unable to state the month and day. Her attention is impaired, as demonstrated by an inability to perform serial sevens. She counts the months forward but has significant difficulty in counting them backward. She is able to register 3 items after multiple trials; her recall is impaired at 5 minutes because she can recite only 2 of 3 items. She has moderate impairment in all higher-level cognitive functions (abstraction, calculation). Insight and judgment are impaired. She lacks understanding of her illness and how it affects her behavior. Impulse control at the time was poor.

Questions: What is the diagnosis? What common psychiatric illnesses are seen in patients with epilepsy?

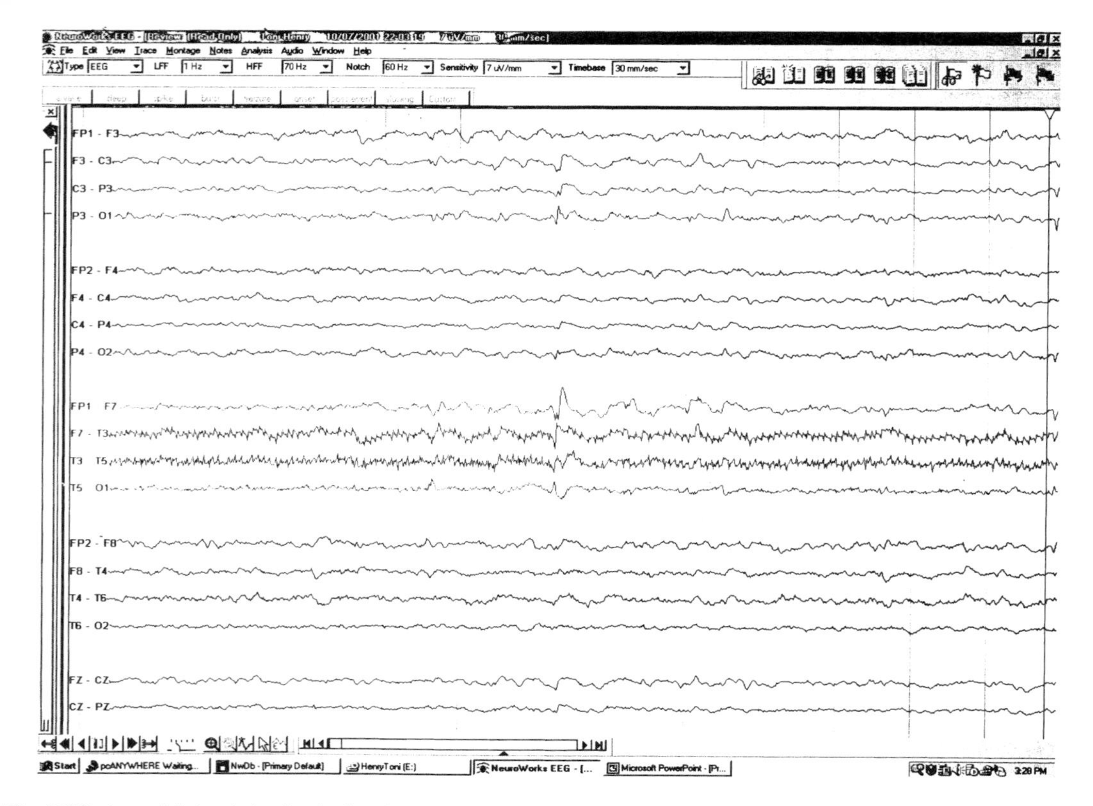

The EEG shows bilateral slowing in the sleep state, with 3–5 Hz wave and bilateral spike and wave discharges, most prominent in F7–T3 and T3–T5, which represent the left temporal lobe.

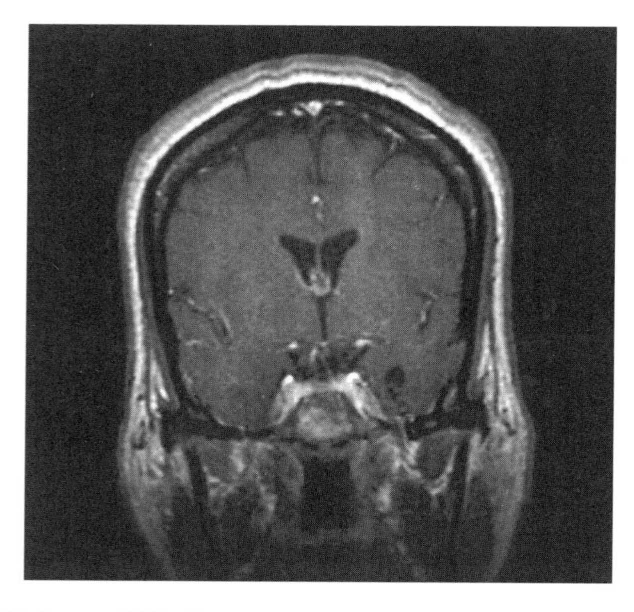

T1-weighted coronal MRI with gadolinum enhancement shows the temporal lesion.

Diagnosis: Psychosis due to a general medical condition: postictal exacerbation of interictal psychosis.

Discussion: Psychiatrists frequently are faced with having to care for patients with epilepsy. About 10% of patients admitted to an acute psychiatric inpatient unit and up to 15% of patients in psychiatric institutions for the chronically ill may have epilepsy. Psychosis associated with epilepsy is a major concern to neurologists and psychiatrists. The differential diagnosis of episodic psychosis in patients with epilepsy includes ictal psychosis, postictal psychosis, alternating psychosis with improved seizure control (forced normalization), interictal psychosis, and iatrogenic psychosis resulting from antiepileptic drugs (AEDs). In general, psychosis in patients with epilepsy is most often classified according to the time that the psychotic episode occurs in relation to the seizure.

In ictal psychosis, symptoms may be a result of concurrent epileptic charges of the brain. Except in some patients with simple partial status, scalp EEG abnormalities are present. The majority of patients have a focus in the temporal lobe, but the focus is extratemporal in 30% of patients. The psychosis resolves with anticonvulsant medication.

Postictal psychosis accounts for 25% of all psychosis associated with epilepsy. The prevalence of postictal psychiatric disorders in the general population of patients with epilepsy is between 6% and 10%. As seen in the present patient, there is commonly a delay between the onset of psychosis and the time of the last seizure. In patients with postictal psychosis, there is often an increase in the frequency of secondary generalization of seizures. There may also be a history of depression that responds to low dose antipsychotic medication. The majority of patients with postictal psychosis have epilepsy for more than 10 years before the onset of psychosis, and most suffer from partial complex seizures that are secondarily generalized. As seen in the EEG of this patient, the electrical abnormalities persist during the psychosis. The treatment is administration of low-dose neuroleptic medication until the psychosis resolves.

Alternative psychosis was a phenomenon first described by Landolt based on observations of an inverse relationship between seizure control and occurrence of psychiatric symptoms. He described "normalization" of EEG recordings with the appearance of psychiatric symptoms (psychosis and depression) and called it "forced normalization." The pathogenic mechanisms mediating this phenomenon are yet to be established. Alternative psychotic episodes should be treated by reducing and/or discontinuing AEDs until overt seizure recurrence causes a remission of psychotic symptoms. Following seizure recurrence and remission of psychotic symptoms, AEDs should be reintroduced slowly.

Interictal psychosis is seen in 0.5–9% of chronic epilepsy patients. The psychosis observed in these patients has a "schizophrenia-like" quality. It is a behavioral phenocopy with a similar course that is largely uninfluenced by concurrent seizure activity, and it responds to antipsychotics. This patient also presents with interictal psychosis with chronic auditory hallucinations and delusions. Both patients with interictal psychosis and patients with schizophrenia often show enlarged ventricles and cerebral volume loss, as seen in the MRI of the present patient. The risk factors involved in developing interictal psychosis include the presence of a left temporal seizure focus, female gender, secondary generalization of the focal seizure, high-frequency seizure activity, young age at onset, and diffuse or bilateral EEG abnormalities. The present patient has all of these features. Treatment includes optimal seizure control, since episodic psychotic exacerbations can accompany clusters of seizures. Neuroleptic medications are also used for interictal psychosis and may be required for a protracted period. The proconvulsant properties of neuroleptic drugs should be taken into consideration but should never preclude treating a patient with psychosis.

Psychotic symptoms in epilepsy may also be associated with severe depressive episodes as depressive disorders represent the most common psychiatric comorbidity in epilepsy. The prevalence of depression in patients with epilepsy is in the range of 9% to 22%, and increases to 39% in patients with medically refractory complex partial seizures with onset in the temporal lobe. This patient also had a major depressive episode (1 year before the current presentation) that resulted in a suicide attempt. Therefore, recurrent depressive symptoms need to be carefully assessed.

Depressive episodes are mostly interictal but may be seen as ictal phenomena or in the immediate postictal period. Acute dysphoria in the context of a seizure is typically followed by alterations of consciousness. It is important to note that some AEDs may have mood-stabilizing or antidepressant activity (e.g., valproic acid, lamotrigine), and their discontinuation may unmask a previously treated depression. On the other hand, some AEDs, such as phenobarbital, may precipitate depressive episodes. The cause of comorbid depression in patients with epilepsy is often multifactorial and may depend on the specific features of the seizure disorder (e.g., seizure frequency, severity, localization, type of seizure) and psychosocial factors (e.g., quality of life, stressors, unemployment). Many reports indicate a higher risk of depression in patients with temporal lobe epilepsy, particularly left-sided. Selective serotonin reuptake inhibitors are considered the first-line therapy for depressive disorders in patients with epilepsy.

Patients with epilepsy are at significantly increased risk for suicide. According to eight reports, death by suicide occurs in 5% of patients with epilepsy. Suicide is often preceded by depressive or psychotic episodes that are frequently overlooked. Suicide is a striking problem among patients with chronic epilepsy who suffer from depressive and psychotic disorders, and timely intervention to treat these symptoms is crucial.

The current patient was admitted to the psychiatric unit for further evaluation and treatment of the acute exacerbation of chronic psychosis. She was switched from molindone to olanzapine, and her psychosis responded quickly to this intervention. In addition, valproic acid was increased to 500 mg 3 times/day, and she was discharged on this dosage, along with phenytoin, 100 mg 3 times/day; olanzapine, 10 mg at bedtime; and sertraline, 100 mg/day. Follow-up in the neurology and psychiatry clinics was arranged.

Pearls

1. MRI studies have shown cerebral volume loss and amygdala enlargement in patients with schizophrenia-like psychosis of epilepsy. Amygdala enlargement has also been reported in different patient groups with epilepsy and affective disorders. Further research should be directed at whether cerebral morphometry may predict the development of affective or psychotic syndromes.
2. Depressive episodes are the most common psychiatric comorbidity in patients with epilepsy and are frequently underrecognized and undertreated.
3. The association between temporal lobe epilepsy and psychosis and depression may help us understand the underlying pathogenesis of these disorders.
4. Patients with epilepsy have a 5-fold greater incidence of suicide than the general population and therefore need to be carefully assessed for the presence of psychiatric symptoms.

REFERENCES

1. Blumer D, Montouris G, Davies K, et al: Suicide in epilepsy: Psychopathology, pathogenesis, and prevention. Epilepsy Behav 2002;3:232–241.
2. Harden CL: The comorbidity of depression and epilepsy, epidemiology, etiology and treatment. Neurology 2002;59:S48–S55.
3. Kanner AM: Psychosis of epilepsy: A neurologist's perspective. Epilepsy Behav 2000;1(4):219–227.
4. Sachdev P: Schizophrenia-like psychosis and epilepsy: The status of association. Am J Psychiatry 1998;155:325–336.
5. Tebartz van Elst L, Baeumer D, Lemieux L, et al: Amygdala pathology in psychosis of epilepsy: A magnetic resonance imaging study in patients with temporal lobe epilepsy. Brain 2002;125:140–149.

Tara Lynn Brass, MD

PATIENT 40

A 16-year-old girl with dizziness

History of Present Illness: A 16-year-old girl is brought to the emergency department by her soccer coach and a few teammates. Her coach told the doctor that during a routine practice that afternoon, the girl suddenly collapsed on the field. Her friends mentioned that following previous practices, she had also complained of "feeling sort of dizzy" but never mentioned "passing out" or losing consciousness. Her friends explain that she has been spending less time with them lately; often going straight home after practice instead of out for a snack with teammates, as she used to do. The girl says that she "had a weird pain in my chest, felt dizzy, and then just passed out." She describes several episodes of chest pain lately and apparently has been feeling more dizzy than usual. She said that these feelings occur throughout the day and are not confined to soccer practice or other periods of strenuous activity. She denied taking any medications or abusing any illicit substances. She also denied any previous medical or psychiatric illnesses or any family history of either.

When the girl's mother arrived in the emergency department, she was visibly frantic. "What happened? I told you that you were practicing too much! It's no wonder you passed out. You play soccer for more than 4 hours every day!" The patient's mother corroborates the absence of any significant past medical or psychiatric history but states that the girl "has not been herself lately. She is spending most of the weekend lying in bed instead of going out with her friends. I know she is not sleeping well—just last night I found her looking through the fridge at 3 AM!"

Physical Examination: The patient is a slim girl who is 65 inches tall, weighs 135 pounds, and has a resting pulse of 48 beats/minute in a regular rhythm. Her blood pressure is 115/60 mmHg seated and 120/67 mmHg standing. She is afebrile. She appears well nourished and hydrated but is clearly anxious and states that she feels "nervous" about being in the hospital. The head-ear-eye-nose-throat (HEENT) exam is significant for enlarged parotid glands bilaterally. The remainder of the physical exam is unremarkable.

Laboratory Testing: Serum sodium, 138 mmol/L; potassium, 2.7 mmol/L; chloride, 82 mmol/L; bicarbonate, 35 mmol/L. Venous blood gas analysis revealed a pH of 7.5. All other laboratory tests were within normal limits with the exception of hypomagnesemia (Mg level = 1.0 mmol/L). The electrocardiogram showed prominent U-waves and a prolonged QT interval.

Mental Status Examination: The patient is a slim girl who appears her stated age. Her eye contact is limited; she mostly looks down at her lap. She is cooperative throughout the interview. She appears restless, picking at her fingernails and pulling at the bottom of her shirt. Her speech is spontaneous but with soft volume. She states that her mood is "fine, I guess," and her affect is anxious and dysphoric. She denies any suicidal or homicidal ideation. She denies any auditory, visual, olfactory, or gustatory hallucinations. Her thought process is linear and goal-directed. She is oriented to person, place, and time. She is able to spell WORLD correctly both backward and forward. She performs serial sevens accurately to 65. Her insight and judgment are poor.

Questions: What is the diagnosis? How does the medical work-up confirm it?

Diagnosis: Bulimia nervosa (BN).

Discussion: The girl suffers from BN, a disorder originally described in 1979 that affects as many as 5% of adolescents and young adults. According to the DSM-IV-TR, bulimia is defined by the presence of recurrent binge eating (at least 2 times/week for 3 months); recurrent purging, excessive exercise, or fasting to prevent weight gain (at least 2 times/week for 3 months), and an excessive concern about body weight or shape. In addition, the patient cannot meet criteria for anorexia nervosa. A binge is typically characterized by the consumption of an unusually large quantity of food during a discrete period of time (e.g., 72 hours), with a perceived lack of control over eating.

Of patients that present with BN, more than 90% are Caucasian and more than 95% are female. More than 75% of patients first present during adolescence. Although patients can be of any gender, race, age, or socioeconomic class, most are from the middle- to upper-middle class. The prognosis for BN is variable, but the general consensus is that approximately 45% have good outcomes (cessation of purging) and approximately 18% have intermediate outcomes (the number of binge-and-purge episodes decreases but does not completely remit). Approximately 21% have poor outcomes. Variables shown to predict favorable outcomes include early age at diagnosis, short interval before treatment begins, good parent-child relationship, and other supportive relationships with friends and therapists.

Eating disorders are frequently accompanied by mood, anxiety, and personality disorders. In particular, bulimia has been shown to be associated with substance abuse. In the assessment of a patient with bulimia, the goals should be to establish the diagnosis, identify comorbid psychiatric illnesses, and evaluate the risk for suicide. It is also important to explore the psychosocial context of the development of the disorder, which can be quite helpful in further psychotherapeutic treatment. In the present case, a mood disorder should be included in the differential diagnosis. Note that the girl has been withdrawing from her friends and seems not to enjoy the activities that used to give her pleasure. Her mother reports an increase in isolation and notes a sleep disturbance. Her mental status exam also revealed signs of anxiety, and an anxiety disorder should also be in the differential. Of course, because the patient presented with syncope, many medical conditions should also be appropriately included, including a vasovagal episode, orthostatic hypotension, cardiac arrythmias, and seizures.

The cause of BN is a question under active research, but it is clear that biologic, psychological, and social factors are involved. Family studies have shown an increased rate of eating disorders in relatives of people with BN compared with relatives of controls. Twin studies also suggest a genetic component because monozygotic twins have higher concordance rates of BN than dizygotic twins. Current research also focuses on determining other predisposing and perpetuating factors in BN.

There are two types of bulimia nervosa: purging type and nonpurging type. In the purging type, the patient regularly engages in self-induced vomiting and/or the misuse of laxatives, diuretics, or enemas. In the nonpurging type, the patient uses other inappropriate compensatory mechanisms, such as fasting or excessive exercise, but has not engaged in purging behaviors. Some patients, like the present girl, manifest purging and nonpurging types of behaviors.

Many people tend to think of vomiting as the key feature of bulimia; however, it is actually the act of binge eating. People with bulimia are aware that their eating patterns are abnormal and, as a result, have depressive and self-deprecating thoughts. To relieve the stress associated with such thoughts, patients seek methods that will rid their bodies of the calories consumed. Such purging methods include not only self-induced vomiting but also laxative, diuretic, and enema abuse. Patients with bulimia, nonpurging type, use other inappropriate mechanisms to compensate for their consumption, including excessive exercise or fasting. The present patient clearly had elements of both purging (self-induced vomiting) and nonpurging types (excessive exercise).

It is important to recognize and treat bulimia because of potentially severe and life-threatening medical consequences. In the present patient, lab values indicate a hypokalemic, hypochloremic metabolic acidosis, which is a direct result of recurrent vomiting. The girl was brought to the emergency department after a syncopal episode. Her EKG showed U-waves and a long QT interval, which were the result of severe hypokalemia and hypomagnesemia.. The prolonged QT interval can also lead to torsade de pointes, an arrhythmia that can cause dizziness and syncope and even lead to sudden cardiac death. With the correction of the electrolyte abnormalities, the EKG changes are usually reversible. In addition to cardiac abnormalities, patients who engage in recurrent vomiting can develop esophagitis (resulting in chest pain, as in this patient) or more serious complications, such as an esophageal tear. Physical manifestations of self-induced vomiting also include swelling of the parotid glands, abnormal dentition, and abrasions on the dorsum of the hand.

Treatment for bulimia can usually be accomplished in the outpatient setting; however, patients have to be admitted to the hospital to stabilize serious medical complications. The present patient was immediately given intravenous fluids supplemented with potassium chloride. A bolus of magnesium was also given, and she was admitted to the hospital for observation.

Randomized studies have shown that cognitive-behavioral therapy (CBT) is the best-established approach to the treatment of bulimia. CBT focuses on the relationship among thoughts, affect, and behavior. For example, what thoughts and feelings make the patient choose to induce vomiting? In CBT, specific interventions are designed to reduce the maladaptive behavior. The specific focus is the value that patients attach to an idealized weight and shape, because this value leads them to restrict food intake in severe ways that leave them susceptible to episodes in which they lose control over eating (binge episode). Consequently, the patient purges as an attempt to compensate for the binge. CBT intensely aims to alter the significance of body weight and shape, which are overvalued in patients with BN. It also focuses on replacing rigid dietary restraint with more normal and regular eating patterns. Another established method of treatment is interpersonal therapy (IT), a time-limited type of therapy that addresses the interpersonal stressors thought to lead the patient toward a disordered eating pattern. Studies have shown that CBT and IT are equally effective in treating bulimia and can even be used together to achieve symptom reduction, although in some randomized control studies CBT had a more rapid treatment effect than IT.

Psychopharmacology also plays a role in the treatment of bulimia. The most studied medication in randomized, controlled trials is fluoxetine, which has demonstrated efficacy in the treatment of bulimia both in conjunction with CBT and in patients who did not respond adequately to psychotherapy. Another randomized, controlled trial showed that patients who responded to fluoxetine during the acute phase of their illness had improved outcome and decreased likelihood of relapse if they continued the medication.

The present patient was referred to the outpatient psychiatry department and diagnosed with BN after a thorough evaluation. She began therapy using a multidisciplinary team approach that included meeting with a nutritionist, a psychiatrist, and a trained cognitive-behavioral therapist. She was started on fluoxetine, and the dose was gradually titrated upward to 60 mg/day. She engaged in CBT for 12 weeks. At 6month follow-up the patient reported a total cessation in binge-purge episodes and was gradually tapered off fluoxetine. She continues to meet with her psychotherapist on a biweekly basis.

Pearls

1. Genetic linkage studies have identified several markers that may prove to be susceptibility loci for BN; in particular, chromosome 10p and 14q are now under investigation.
2. Compared with controls, patients with BN have been found to release less cholecystokinin (CCK) after a test meal, particularly after a large load. Once the patient is treated for the BN, CCK release improves. As CCK release has been found to be directly related to the feeling of satiety, this finding suggests that as patients have a reduction in the frequency of binge-eating episodes, their ability to feel satiety after a meal may improve.
3. One prospective study has shown a significantly higher risk of developing BN among patients who have the habit of eating alone and/or have parents who are divorced, separated, or widowed. This finding must be further explored, but if replicated, it may be useful for early detection or prevention of BN.

REFERENCES

1. Bacaltchuk J: Antidepressants versus placebo for people with bulimia nervosa. Cochrane Database Syst Rev 2001:(4):CD003391.
2. Becker AE, Grinspoon SK, Klibanski A, Herzog, DB: Eating disorders. N Engl J Med 1999;340:1092–1098.
3. Bulik CM: Significant linkage on chromosome 10p in families with bulimia nervosa. Am J Hum Genet 2003;72:200–207.
4. Klump KL: The evolving genetic foundations of eating disorders. Psychiatr Clin North Am 2001;24:215–225.
5. Martinez-Gonzalez MA: Parental factors, mass media influence, and the onset of eating disorders in a prospective population-based cohort. Pediatrics 2003;111:315–320.
6. Romano SJ: A placebo-controlled study of fluoxetine in continued treatment of bulimia nervosa after successful acute fluoxetine treatment. Am J Psychiatry 2002;159:96–102.

Alex Kolevzon, MD

PATIENT 41

A 28-year-old man with agitated behavior

History of Present Illness: A 28-year-old man is brought in to the psychiatric emergency department by emergency medical services (EMS) after neighbors called the police because he was yelling out the window. On the evening before presentation, the patient had an argument with his mother because he wanted to order Chinese food for dinner and his mother insisted on hamburgers. The patient became angry and started kicking his bedroom door, spit at his mother, and then hit her on the shoulder and began yelling out the window incoherently. Police were called by neighbors in an adjacent building, and staff at his group home called EMS because they feared for their safety.

The patient lives in a group home. Staff members describe him as withdrawn and isolative but prone to behavioral outbursts when specific rituals are disrupted. He has several behavioral rituals that involve walking, drinking water, and turning the light on and off. If rituals are disrupted by noise of any kind, the patient must stop and retrace his steps, take another drink of water, or turn the light on and off again. The disruptive noises may be sirens, horns, or people yelling. There have also been several recent incidents of agitated behavior on public transportation, the latest of which prompted a call to the police. Behavioral outbursts are noted to occur several times a day, but until 1 week before presentation they were self-limited and responded to verbal redirection.

Past Psychiatric History: At 3 years of age the patient had delayed language development and would have frequent tantrums when unable to communicate. Other developmental milestones were reached at the appropriate ages. His verbal abilities remain impaired to date, and he reads with difficulty. As a child he was noted to be socially isolated and apathetic and tended to follow other children rather than actually play with them. At 7 years of age he began to exhibit occasional self-injurious behavior. Rituals and repetitive behavior patterns were also common. He had to touch objects as he walked by, would turn lights on and off repeatedly, and was preoccupied with his hands, constantly staring at them and making bizarre movements. Compulsive eating eventually required him to be transferred from his parent's home to a more supervised setting.

Past Medical History: The patient has no significant medical problems. He has never experienced head trauma or had a seizure and does not use alcohol or other drugs.

Medications: Risperidone, 2 mg at night, and citalopram, 40 mg/day.

Mental Status Examination: The patient is an obese man who appears younger than his stated age. His eye contact is limited, and at times he seems distracted, possibly responding to internal stimuli. He is cooperative and eager to please the examiner. His behavior is restless, and he frequently stares at his hands and makes wringing movements. Speech is incoherent at times, with increased volume and peculiar rhythms, such as mumbling and frequent clicking sounds alternating with deep breathing. The patient describes his mood as "fine," but his affect is labile with rapid changes from apathy to irritability. Thought process is disturbed by echolalia and perseveration; he asks repeatedly when he can return home. He denies any thought content or perceptual disturbance. He also denies suicidal or homicidal ideation and, despite occasional self-injurious behavior when he is frustrated, he has no history of suicide attempts or violence. He is alert and oriented, but his cognitive abilities are impaired by concrete thought and increased distractibility. Impulse control is impaired, as evidenced by temper tantrums and self-injurious behavior. The patient's insight and judgment are limited because he lacks understanding of his illness and how his behavior affects others.

Diagnostic Testing: EEG showed cortical slowing, no signs of a seizure focus; Weschler Adult Intelligence Scale: IQ = 80.

Questions: What is the diagnosis? How might this patient be treated?

Diagnosis: Autistic disorder.

Discussion: Autistic disorder is categorized as a pervasive developmental disorder in the DSM-IV-TR. It is estimated to affect 1 out of 1000 children and is more common in boys. The precise etiology is unknown but genetic factors with an unclear mode of transmission contribute to its development. Parents and siblings of children with autism may also show milder phenotypes of the disorder with varying degrees of deficits in language, behavior, and social interaction. Current genetic linkage studies are attempting to identify genes that increase the susceptibility to autism while various neuroimaging techniques are examining associated anatomical changes.

Autistic disorder is characterized by impaired language development, impaired social interaction, and repetitive, stereotyped behavioral patterns. Parents may first suspect autism when children do not begin to speak at the appropriate age or when they do not respond when their name is called. Audiometry may be the first diagnostic test performed because affected children are often disinterested in their surroundings and may appear deaf. Reciprocal play is limited. Autistic children are usually found engaging in repetitive, solitary play with minimal imagination or creativity. It is very difficult for autistic children to remain focused, and they may not respond to attempts to engage them in activities with parents or siblings. Children may develop preoccupations with inanimate objects such as metal or buttons and become angry easily if such attachments are discouraged. Patterns of behavior are typically ritualistic and may involve rocking, hand-flapping, or jumping up and down repeatedly. As in this case, patients with autistic disorder often require specific routines and predictable expectations, such as Chinese food on Friday nights. Interruptions of routines can lead to temper tantrums, aggression, and possibly self-injurious behavior such as biting or head banging. Mood lability is also a common feature, and patients may alternate rapidly between crying and anger without apparent triggers. As patients grow older, they may become increasingly aggressive with low frustration tolerance and worsening impulsivity. If language develops, as it did in this case, it may be peculiar and disturbed by echolalia and perseveration about specific ideas or desires. The present patient asked every minute when he was going home and occasionally made clicking sounds or imitated the noise of a car engine. Meaningful language develops in only half of all children with autism. It is also estimated that up to 75% of children with autism have IQ scores consistent with mental retardation, and seizure disorders with EEG abnormalities are frequent comorbid findings. The presence of mental retardation or a seizure disorder adversely affects the prognosis.

The present patient was diagnosed with autism based on the developmental history and the presence of classic features such as social isolation and repetitive behavior patterns. Other diagnoses that were considered included mental retardation, a primary psychotic disorder, and obsessive-compulsive disorder. Records showed that the patient was not mentally retarded, and although his speech was peculiar, there was no underlying psychotic process. Although obsessive-compulsive disorder may have been present as a comorbid condition and his ritualistic behavior certainly falls within the obsessive-compulsive spectrum, the overall clinical picture is more consistent with autism. In terms of treatment, behavioral therapy is probably the most common psychosocial therapy and was used in this patient to reduce stereotyped behavior and improve social interaction. Antipsychotic medication, such as risperidone, is used frequently for aggressive behavior and in this patient showed good effect. Controlled trials with risperidone have demonstrated its efficacy in reducing aggressive and repetitive behavior, hyperactivity, and affective lability. Selective serotonin reuptake inhibitors may also be effective for aggressive, impulsive, and self-injurious behavior. Although some patients demonstrate improvements in social interaction and communication, repetitive play and ritualistic behavior tend not to improve. The majority of patients with autistic disorder, including the present patient, eventually require long-term supervised housing and residential treatment.

The present patient was hospitalized on an inpatient psychiatric unit because of his agitated behavior. His medication regimen was continued, but the doses of both risperidone and citalopram were increased. After approximately 2 weeks, he did not demonstrate any behavioral outbursts. A family meeting with the patient's mother and staff from the group home was also held to discuss behavioral techniques to reduce and manage the patient's outbursts. Soon afterward he returned to the group home where he lived and was followed by the permanent staff and a psychiatrist who was available on a weekly basis.

Pearls

1. Genetic factors play a clear role in autism, as evidenced by twin studies. Concordance rates in monozygotic twins vary from 36% to 91%, depending on the study; in dizygotic twins concordance rates vary from 0% to 10%.

2. Genetic linkage studies have identified several markers that in the future may provide evidence for an autism susceptibility gene. Chromosomes 2 and 7 have shown particular promise in recent studies.

3. MRI studies have revealed excessive cerebral growth and increased brain volume in early childhood, followed by abnormally slowed growth beginning in middle childhood and continuing thereafter. Postmortem data also indicate significant cerebellar pathology, with loss of Purkinje neurons.

4. A recent open trial has shown that divalproex sodium (Depakote) may be useful in patients with autism for associated symptoms of mood lability, impulsivity, and aggression, particularly in patients with seizure disorders or EEG abnormalities.

REFERENCES

1. Bailey A, Le Couteur A, Gottesman I, et al: Autism as a strongly genetic disorder: Evidence from a British twin study. Psychol Med 1995;25:63–77.
2. Courchesne E, Karns CM, Davis HR, et al: Unusual brain growth patterns in early life in patients with autistic disorder. Neurology 2001;57:245–254.
3. Hollander E, Dolgoff-Kaspar R, Cartwright C, et al: An open trial of divalproex sodium in autism spectrum disorders. J Clin Psychiatry 2001;62 :530–534.
4. Liu J, Nyholt DR, Magnussen P, et al for the Autism Genetic Resource Exchange Consortium; Ott J, Gilliam C: A genomewide screen for autism susceptibility loci. Am J Hum Genet 2001;69:327–340
5. McDougle CJ, Holmes JP, Carlson DC, et al: A double-blind, placebo-controlled study of risperidone in adults with autistic disorder and other pervasive developmental disorders. Arch Gen Psychiatry 1998;55:633–641.
6. Tanguay PE: Pervasive developmental disorders: A 10-year review. J Am Acad Child Adolesc Psychiatry 2000;39:1079–1095.

Thomas Stewart, B.A.
Daniel Stewart, M.D.

PATIENT 42

A 20-year-old man with grandiosity

History of Present Illness: A 20-year-old man is brought to the emergency department (ED) in handcuffs by the police. When you go to meet the stretcher bringing him into the hospital, the police sergeant takes you aside and relays the following:

> We had responded to a call that there was a man standing in the road directing traffic, but when we got there, we found him standing in the middle of the road naked, screaming at the cars to slow down. My officers tried to get him to come out of the road, but when he refused, they went out to get him. He saw them coming and climbed a tree, threatening to defecate on the officers if they tried to follow him up. Needless to say, my guys weren't happy about following him, but they did manage to get him down. We had to cuff him because he was squirming and trying to lash out the whole time, saying that we were the ones who should be chained up for interfering with his plans for a new world. My guys all think that he's on something, PCP or something, but I'm not so sure. There's something else weird about him. Anyway, Doc, he's all yours.

You thank the officer for his help, and turn back to the patient, who remains handcuffed to the stretcher, surrounding by several police. When you introduce yourself, he says, "Shall I say, I am Lazarus, come back from the dead, come to tell you all, I shall tell you all?"

You begin a discussion with him about removing the handcuffs. He states, "I am not bound by your physical laws. I am only in handcuffs because I allow myself to be, for your sake." Further attempts to elicit a history are met with similar replies. He refuses to allow lab work and to give urine for a toxicology screen. You decide to give him an antipsychotic and a benzodiazepine, but when you offer them to him, he refuses, stating, "I am the one who comes from many, the many that comes from one. You shall not give me your poisons. I will smite you down for this act of cowardice." He agrees to a physical examination, which you perform with security standing nearby.

After his physical examination, he agrees to lab tests and gives urine, stating that he will do anything to "help me get out of here more quickly." He is able to tell you how to contact his family and gives you permission to speak with them. He answers most other questions by saying, "In time, it will be my will that will be done."

Corroborative Data: The patient's mother expresses shock to hear that her son is in the ED under these conditions. She states that he has never had any similar episode before and expresses concern that one of his friends "slipped him something to make him this way." She reports that he had always been a decent student, getting Bs and Cs throughout high school. "When he left for college this year, he was fine," she states. "But when he came home around Christmas, he seemed different." She relates that at the Christmas dinner he had seemed more energized than usual, talking incessantly. He appeared to have boundless energy, staying up very late at night (often the entire night). He was quite happy with himself and had reassured her that he had "never felt better." She worried that he was using drugs at college and that the drugs were responsible for the changes. When his grades arrived, they were Bs and Cs. This report relieved her because she had decided that if he were doing drugs, he would not have been able to keep up his grades. His friends are unreachable for corroboration, but drug-induced psychosis or a manic episode is high on your differential diagnosis.

Laboratory and Diagnostic Testing: Urine toxicology screen is negative. Physical examination shows no signs of infection or head trauma, and laboratory work and head CT scan are unremarkable.

Course of Presentation: When re-interviewed over the course of the night, he remains grandiose and psychotic and is given the tentative diagnosis of bipolar disorder, type I, manic episode. He is admitted to the inpatient service and started on an antipsychotic and a mood stabilizer. Over the next two weeks on the inpatient service, his manic symptoms appear to resolve, but he remains psychotic. He no longer has his inexhaustible energy, and his mood seems less labile. His speech becomes less pressured, and he is able to hold conversations with the inpatient doctors and nurses. However, his delusions persist. He also reveals that he knows that he is special because he has heard the voice of god in his head for many months now, since shortly after starting college. The voice has told him that he is chosen for a special purpose that will be revealed to him in time, but it has also rebuked him violently for any sexual encounters that he has had over the past few months. He states that he would not normally reveal this information, but he does so to convince you that he is "not crazy."

Mental Status Examination (on the inpatient unit): The patient is a cooperative and attentive young man, dressed in a hospital gown and robe, who demonstrates no abnormal involuntary movements, psychomotor retardation, or psychomotor agitation. His speech is normal in rate, rhythm, and volume. His mood is generally euthymic, but his affect seems inappropriate at times, although no longer labile. On the dimension of thought process, he remains somewhat disorganized but is generally coherent. He does appear, however, overly vague and somewhat overly inclusive. His thought content is remarkable for ongoing grandiose delusions and auditory hallucinations of god's voice. His insight and judgment are poor.

Questions: Why should you reconsider the diagnosis of bipolar disorder, type I, manic episode? What is the more probable diagnosis?

Diagnosis: Schizoaffective disorder, bipolar type.

Discussion: Schizoaffective disorder is categorized in the DSM-IV-TR as a psychotic disorder because the psychotic process is believed to be the primary pathology. The diagnostic criteria for schizoaffective disorder combine the diagnostic criteria for schizophrenia with the diagnostic criteria for a mood disorder (either major depression or bipolar disorder). Essentially, the patient must meet criteria A for schizophrenia, which includes the presence of delusions, hallucinations, disorganized speech or behavior, catatonia, or negative symptoms (e.g., flat affect, alogia, avolition). In addition, the patient must meet the diagnostic criteria for either a major depressive episode or a manic episode. Importantly, the patient's psychotic symptoms must be present for at least two weeks in the absence of prominent mood symptoms (establishing it as a primary psychotic disorder). However, the mood symptoms sufficient for diagnosis must be present for a substantial portion of the total duration of both the active and residual phases of the illness. There are two subtypes of schizoaffective disorder-bipolar type and depressive type. Depressive type is covered in case 38. The remainder of this discussion focuses on the bipolar type.

Psychosis has an exhaustive differential diagnosis that is covered elsewhere in this book. Obviously, as this case demonstrates, one must always be on the look out for organic causes, such as infection, cerebral hemorrhage, tumors, and drug use (including PCP, cocaine). When a patient presents in a manic episode, the major psychiatric differential is between bipolar mood disorder and schizoaffective disorder. In bipolar disorder, which is primarily a mood disorder, the patient very well may be psychotic. However, the psychosis should not exist outside the context of the mania itself. In other words, the psychosis should not predate the appearance of mood symptoms, and the psychosis should not persist after the resolution of mood symptoms. In this case, the patient was diagnosed with bipolar disorder on presentation largely because there was no clear indication that overt psychotic symptoms were present before the onset of his mood symptoms. For example, when he came home for Christmas, it appeared that he had mood symptoms without obvious psychotic elements. Based on this information, it is logical to suspect bipolar disorder. However, when, after the resolution of his mania, his psychotic symptoms persisted, serious doubt is cast on the diagnosis of bipolar mood disorder, because, by definition, the psychotic symptoms resolve with or even before the successful treatment of the mood symptoms. Schizoaffective disorder, on the other hand, is defined by the persistence of psychotic symptoms outside the context of the mood symptoms and so becomes a more likely diagnosis.

Differentiating schizoaffective disorder from schizophrenia can be equally difficult. Although the presence of mood symptoms seems to be an easy way of telling the two apart, some of the manifestations of schizophrenia can look like the symptoms of a mood disorder. For example, when a patient with schizophrenia presents with pronounced negative symptoms, he can appear quite depressed. He often sits idly in his chair; he may not engage the interviewer or even answer questions; he may have an increased latency in his responses (the time it takes for him to answer after a question is asked). These symptoms can often lead a physician to make the diagnosis of schizoaffective disorder, depressed type. Similarly, patients with schizophrenia can present with disorganized, rambling, and even pressured speech, which can lead to the mistaken diagnosis of schizoaffective disorder, bipolar type. In either case, the diagnosis is made prematurely without exploring the full history of symptoms. It is not enough to have some symptoms that suggest a mood disorder; the patient must meet the full diagnostic criteria for the mood disorder in question, which involve more than amotivation or pressured speech. Failing to attend to this important element has led to what many consider a rampant overdiagnosis of schizoaffective disorder in both community and inpatient populations.

There is an ongoing debate about whether schizoaffective disorder exists as a distinct diagnostic entity. Some have argued that these patients represent the most severe cases of bipolar disorder, because mood-stabilizing medications have such a profoundly beneficial effect. Others argue that these patients should be categorized as schizophrenic, because the primary disorder is psychotic in nature. Mood symptoms in this case are considered either accessory or comorbid, but they do not constitute the need for a separate diagnosis. For example, a patient with hypertension and high cholesterol does not qualify for a new, third diagnosis that accounts for the presence of both symptoms. Similarly, a patient with schizophrenia and major depression should be described using both diagnoses rather than a third.

Advocates of a relevant and separate diagnostic entity in schizoaffective disorder tend to cite literature that demonstrates neuropathologic findings, psychological functioning, premorbid functioning, and prognostic factors as somewhere between those of schizophrenia and mood disorders. In any event, schizoaffective disorder remains poorly delineated in the DSM-IV-TR, especially given the importance of longitudinal factors in distinguishing schizophrenia, schizoaffective disorder, and bipolar disorder. For example, patients who present initially with manic symptoms are more likely to have their diagnosis changed over the long term than patients who present with symptoms of schizophrenia or depression, at least in European samples. In another longitudinal study of a first-admission sample of patients who presented with psychosis, schizoaffective disorder was among the least stable diagnoses, and patients were most likely to shift to a diagnosis of schizophrenia at 2-year follow-up.

The general use of mood stabilizers and antipsychotics are covered in other cases, but an additional and important treatment decision comes from the distinction between schizoaffective disorder, bipolar type and bipolar mood disorder that presents with psychosis. Both tend to be treated in the acute phase with a mood stabilizer and antipsychotic medication; however, the maintenance phases tend to be handled differently. In both cases, the mood stabilizer is often continued prophylactically. But in the case of bipolar disorder, it is typically suggested that the antipsychotic be withdrawn after the resolution of the psychotic episode to reduce a patient's exposure to neuroleptics, which can have serious adverse consequences, especially with prolonged use. In schizoaffective disorder, on the other hand, ongoing antipsychotic use during the maintenance phase is often indicated to prevent the recurrence of psychotic symptoms with accompanying decompensation.

Despite the lack of clear and convincing evidence about the treatment of schizoaffective disorder, several meaningful general concepts can be applied to the use of psychotropic medications. There appears to be some benefit to subtyping patients and treating accordingly. For example, in patients who have a primarily "schizobipolar" presentation with pronounced affective symptoms, lithium, carbamazepine, and valproate have been found to be effective to varying degrees. On the other hand, if these "schizobipolar" patients present with more pronounced schizophrenic-like symptoms, antipsychotics are often considered as first-line treatment. In this case, clozapine has the most support for efficacy; however, concerns about agranulocytosis prevent its use as a first-line treatment. Instead, clinicians tend to use other atypical antipsychotics in this case, although the decision for long-term use must be weighed carefully, given the risks of tardive dyskinesia, new-onset hyperglycemia or diabetes, progression of coronary disease, and possibly an increased risk of stroke.

The present patient was maintained on both valproic acid and risperidone. His mood symptoms and psychosis were well controlled by the time of his discharge, but he was too impaired after his psychotic break to return to college. Instead, he entered a vocational training program and moved back home with his family.

Pearls

1. Ongoing debate continues about the validity of schizoaffective disorder as a diagnosis; however, increasing amounts of evidence seem to suggest that it is at least distinctive from either schizophrenia or bipolar disorder/major depression in neuroanatomic findings and neuropsychological performance.
2. Regardless of the validity of the diagnosis, treating psychosis early and aggressively is an agreed-upon practice. Psychotic episodes appear to contribute to functional decline, regardless of diagnosis; as such, they are often thought of as "the fever of the brain."
3. Close monitoring of schizoaffective disorder patients is necessary due to the instability of their presentation. Monotherapy may be insufficient, and combinations of mood stabilizers and antipsychotics are often necessary.

REFERENCES

1. Baethge C: Long-term treatment of schizoaffective disorder: Review and recommendations. Pharmacopsychiatry 2003; 36:45–56.
2. Eliot TS: Prufrock and Other Observations. London, The Egoist, Ltd., 1917.
3. Kaplan H, Sadock B (eds): Comprehensive Textbook of Psychiatry, vol. 1, 6th ed. Baltimore, Williams & Wilkins, 1995.
4. Marneros A: Schizoaffective disorders: Clinical aspects, differential diagnosis, and treatment. Curr Psychiatry Rep 2003;5:202–205.
5. Marners A, Deister A, Rhode A: Stability of diagnoses in affective, schizoaffective and schizophrenic disorders: Cross-sectional versus longitudinal diagnosis. Eur Arch Psychiatry Clin Neurosci 1991;241(3):187–192.
6. Schwartz JE, Fennig S, Tanenberg-Karant M, et al: Congruence of diagnoses 2 years after a first-admission diagnosis of psychosis. Arch Gen Psychiatry 2000;57:593–600.

Sander Markx
Daniel Stewart, MD

PATIENT 43

A 38-year-old medical doctor with marital problems

History of Present Illness: A 38-year-old medical doctor walks into the office and says that he is seeking psychotherapy because his wife insists that he needs psychological help. The patient says that his wife is considering a divorce, stating that she can no longer tolerate his constant need to control everything, his coldness toward her, and his long work hours. The client starts the session by stating that he is here only because his wife demands it. He does not see any problems at all; he says that the marriage is going just fine.

When asked about his job, the patient looks quite worried. He reports that he is one of the hardest-working gastroenterologists in a prestigious hospital and has to have a certain number of publications in reputable journals every year. He says that if he fails to accomplish this goal, he might not become a professor within the next ten years. He never lets the opportunity pass to write another article, and he describes himself as a perfectionist because he is never satisfied with the end result. Furthermore, the patient is constantly correcting the work of his coauthors because he thinks their writing does not meet the criteria for what he considers a high-quality article. He becomes highly irritated with what he considers their lack of discipline. Because the patient is constantly correcting other people's work, he falls behind on his busy schedule, which stresses him even more. As unfinished work piles up, the patient becomes paralyzed, not knowing where to start. He is having a hard time making decisions and has been making schedules for when to finish what. Most of the time the patient does not succeed in finishing tasks on time, which leads to 14-hour working days. His colleagues are complaining that because of his rigid fixation on details and because of his inability to let other people be responsible for the end result of the articles, his efficiency is diminishing.

The patient has two children: a 9-year-old son and a 7-year-old daughter. When he talks about them, it appears as if he sees them as another reason to worry since taking care of them makes him lose valuable time that he could use to finish his work. However, when explicitly asked about his feelings toward them, he displays clearly visible affection. When asked about his wife, he describes her as "a great friend," a person to whom he is really close, someone whom he can trust and build upon. The patient does not understand why she is not satisfied with their marriage. He denies any symptoms of depression, including neurovegetative symptoms, as well as symptoms of anxiety, mania, and psychosis.

Past Psychiatric History: The patient is the oldest son with one younger brother. His father was an accountant and an exceptionally hard worker, and his mother was a housewife. While growing up, the patient always felt that he had to prove himself with great achievements and that the time to do so was always running out. He has always been considered a "high achiever," someone who wanted to be the best. He spent most of his time studying and felt that he had no time to become involved with girls seriously since there was too much work to do. Consequently, the patient was 29 years old when he had his first serious relationship with a woman. During vacations, the patient always had a hard time relaxing, constantly thinking about things he had to do. When people would say something about this preoccupation, he would usually become irritated and would start shouting and slamming doors. He has never been hospitalized in a psychiatric hospital, suffered from any psychiatric condition, or even seen a psychiatrist before.

Mental Status Examination: The patient is a thin man, dressed very neatly with his hair meticulously combed. During the interview, he sits in a stiff, upright position and rarely moves his arms or legs. He makes good eye contact, looks very serious, and rarely smiles during the interview. He is cooperative, although rigid and stubborn when discussing his point of view. The patient describes his mood as "fine," but he comes across as highly serious and anxious with constricted affect. When asked a specific question, he frequently gives an unusually detailed answer. When confronted with his problems at work and with his wife, the patient uses rationalization and intellectualization as defense mechanisms. He denies any perceptual disturbances. As to disturbances in the content of his thought, the patient reports his preoccupation with his work and his obsession with becoming the best gastroenterologist that he can be. The patient denies suicidal or homicidal ideation at this time. He is alert and oriented, and no disturbances in memory functions are evident. Concentration, attention, and impulse control seem nonimpaired. The patient's insight and judgment are limited as evidenced by his lack of understanding how his behaviour affects others and his explanations for his trouble at work and in his marriage.

Questions: What is the diagnosis? How might this patient be treated?

Diagnosis: Obsessive-compulsive personality disorder (OCPD).

Discussion: OCPD is categorized as a Cluster C—Anxious Cluster—personality disorder in the DSM-IV-TR. The exact prevalence of OCPD is unknown, but it is thought to be more prevalent in men than in women. The disorder is more often diagnosed in the oldest child in a family, and it is also more frequently diagnosed in people who come from families with strong discipline. People who have experienced childhood abuse or neglect are also considerably more likely to develop personality disorders, including OCPD. Furthermore, OCPD is more often diagnosed in first-degree biologic relatives of patients with the disorder than in the general population. It is now widely accepted that personality disorders have a genetic basis. The exact etiology of OCPD and the nature of its relationship to obsessive-compulsive disorder (OCD) and "obsessive-compulsive spectrum disorders" are still unknown, but increasing data are being published on specific genetic, neurochemical, neuroanatomic, neurodevelopmental, and environmental factors that may be involved.

A personality disorder is a pervasive and persistent pattern of behavior that usually begins by late adolescence or early adulthood and is consistent across a number of contexts. OCPD is characterized by a preoccupation with order, perfectionism, and control in both mental and interpersonal arenas. These qualities are present at the cost of flexibility and efficiency. Patients with OCPD must have four or more of the following: (1) a preoccupation with rules, order, organization, neatness, schedules, and details; (2) a devotion to work and productivity that excludes leisure and friendships; (3) an overconscientiousness and inflexibility about ethical or moral issues; (4) an inability to discard worthless items; (5) reluctance to delegate tasks unless in total control of the situation; (6) miserliness; and (7) rigidity and stubbornness. The typical patient with OCPD—like the 38-year old physician described above—presents in a formal and serious manner and often lacks a sense of humor. Patients are often unable to tolerate what they perceive to be interference with their rules or schedules. Accordingly, they lack spontaneity and flexibility and can be quite intolerant. Patients with OCPD can be capable of prolonged work, but only if they feel that they are in control. Their extreme devotion to work and productivity can lead to high achievement in professions where attention to detail is essential. However, as with the patient described above, a successful career sometimes comes at a high price since their significant others frequently find them difficult to live with. Although many of these patients are high achievers, some of them find that their character style interferes with task completion. Since these patients are striving for perfection, they may ruminate endlessly about small details and thereby lose track of the main purpose of a particular task.

Intimate relationships pose a significant problem to patients with obsessive-compulsive personality disorder, since they have a potential of becoming "out of control." They are unable to compromise and frequently insist that others submit to their needs. For patients with OCPD, anything that threatens their routines or perceived stability can precipitate a great deal of anxiety that is otherwise bound up in rituals, schedules, and organizational schemes. Because of this trait and the sometimes excessive devotion to work, patients have a hard time investing in more intimate relationships. Although a stable marriage is not uncommon, patients with OCPD have few friends.

Many patients with psychiatric disorders may present with obsessive-compulsive traits. Crucial for establishing the diagnosis of OCPD is the assessment of whether the obsessive-compulsive traits significantly impair occupational or social life. When recurrent obsessions or compulsions are present, the patient most likely has obsessive-compulsive disorder (OCD). In patients with OCD, the symptoms are seen as problematic, and the patient typically wants to get rid of them. In OCPD, the traits are lifelong patterns of behavior, and some patients (as the patient described above) may even regard them as highly adaptive. It should also be noted that some patients with personality disorders, including OCPD, may also present with delusional disorder.

The course and prognosis of OCPD are not predictable. During the patient's life, obsessions or compulsions may reoccur from time to time. In some patients, the symptoms persist or even tend to increase over the years. Patients with OCPD may do well in professions involving detailed work; however, they remain vulnerable to unexpected changes. The symptoms of this patient have been relatively stable, but his functioning at work and his relationship with his wife are becoming increasingly problematic. OCPD is associated with an elevated risk for suicidal ideation and behavior during adolescence as well as with an elevated risk for depressive disorders, especially those of late onset. The patient described above denied suicidal ideation or behavior and other symptoms of depressive disorders.

Patients with OCPD may benefit from individual, group, and behavior therapy. In contrast with other personality disorders, patients with OCPD often have some insight into the impact of their behavior on their lives. Unlike the patient described above, who clearly displays a lack of insight, patients with OCPD may seek treatment on their own. Pharmacotherapeutic options typically include medications used to treat OCD, such as clonazepam, fluoxetine, or clomipramine. Although these medications may be of use when obsessive-compulsive symptoms are evident or severe, there is currently no consensus on their role in the treatment of patients with OCPD. For the 38-year-old gastroenterologist, a course of psychotherapy was initiated with consequent improvement in his home and work functioning; as a result, pharmacotherapy was not indicated.

Pearls

1. Increasing data are being published on the neurobiologic basis of personality disorders and specific personality disorder features, such as obsessive-compulsive traits. It is still unknown how OCPD, OCD, and other "obsessive-compulsive spectrum disorders" are related in terms of etiology and pathophysiology.
2. Several lines of neurochemical evidence (e.g., data from pharmacologic, functional imaging, and postmortem studies) suggest a crucial role for dopaminergic, glutamatergic, and serotonergic neurotransmitter systems, all of which are functionally intertwined.
3. Neuroanatomically, frontal-striatal-thalamic circuits are thought to be particularly important. Dysfunction in these neural circuits may be associated with obsessive-compulsive symptoms. Neuroimaging studies show abnormalities in prefrontal, striatal, and thalamic anatomy and activity in patients with obsessive-compulsive traits.
4. The genetic component of personality disorders such as OCPD is polygenic and highly complex. Researchers have begun to identify specific genes (e.g., COMT, MAOA and DRD4) that seem to be involved in the development of psychiatric disorders with obsessive-compulsive symptoms.

REFERENCES

1. Kaplan HI, Sadock BJ: Concise Textbook of Clinical Psychiatry. Baltimore, Williams & Wilkins, 1996.
2. Rosenberg DR, Hanna GL: Genetic and imaging strategies in obsessive-compulsive disorder: Potential implications for treatment development. Biol Psychiatry 2000;48:1210–1222.
3. Stein DJ: Neurobiology of the obsessive-compulsive spectrum disorders. Biol Psychiatry 2000;47:296–304.
4. Nestadt G, Addington A, Samuels J, et al: The Identification of OCD-related subgroups based on comorbidity. Biol Psychiatry 2003;53:914–920.
5. Reif A, Lesch K-P: Toward a molecular architecture of personality. Behav Brain Res 2003;139:1–20.

Lori Pellegrino, MD

PATIENT 44

A 38-year-old man with suicidal ideation

History of Present Illness: A 38-year-old man is sent to the psychiatric emergency department directly from his internist's office. That morning the patient and his wife presented to the doctor's office without an appointment, and the patient expressed feelings of being overwhelmingly depressed. He had developed a plan to commit suicide, which included taking a bottle of Tylenol and drinking "as much vodka as it takes." The doctor performed a thorough evaluation, drew lab tests and called 911 to have the patient brought to the emergency department.

When you encounter the patient, he is visibly upset and clinging to his wife. The couple explains that they separated a month ago, because the patient "just couldn't be a husband anymore." Over the past 6 weeks, he had become isolated, complained of decreased energy, concentration, appetite, and sleep. He had lost his job as a house painter 6 months earlier. The patient no longer enjoyed the caretaking of the couple's two children, ages 4 and 6—a drastic change from the role he had previously enjoyed as a father.

You ask the patient when he first began feeling down. He states clearly, "When my mother died, one and a half years ago." He said that he has been feeling guilty over the circumstances of her death and wishing that he had been closer to her in the years preceding her death. The wife notes with concern, "That was just about when you started drinking so heavily, as well." As you question further, you determine that the patient has been drinking daily since the death of his mother. He estimates that he is drinking 6 beers a day. He admits that his drinking is a problem, and he actually tried to stop drinking 2 weeks before the visit to the emergency department. The patient said, "My wife had kicked me out of the house, I missed my kids, I didn't have a job.... I knew something was wrong." He noted that in the days after stopping drinking, he experienced some shakiness and symptoms "like there were bugs under my skin." He added that having a beer made these symptoms subside. Last night he had become very upset after calling his wife to check on the children and finding that they were not home. He sat in his hotel room and thought, "I can't go on living like this." He called his wife at 6 the next morning and said that he thought he might kill himself. She immediately brought him to the doctor's office.

Past Psychiatric History: The patient has never been hospitalized psychiatrically, nor has he seen a psychiatrist before. He recalls having been depressed only once earlier in his life, during his 20s, but he did not seek treatment at that time. Although the patient is currently suicidal, he denies any past suicidal thinking and has not made previous suicide attempts.

Past Medical History: Hypertension, hypercholesterolemia.

Medications: Metoprolol, 50 mg 2 times/day orally.

Family History: The patient's father has a history of alcohol dependence, and his mother had hypertension and coronary artery disease before dying of a myocardial infarction. The patient denies any history of psychiatric illness in the family.

Substance Abuse History: The patient has been drinking 6 beers/day for the past year and a half; before that, he was not drinking on a daily basis. He has a remote history of similar drinking in his 20s during his first divorce, but he was able to quit "cold turkey" and has never been to any detoxification facilities. He experienced symptoms of withdrawal when he quit but has no history of withdrawal seizures. He denies use of marijuana, heroin, cocaine, or other recreational substances. He smokes one-half pack per day of cigarettes.

Social History: The patient describes a chaotic childhood, since his father was "unpredictable" because of his drinking. He was able to finish high school and then went to vocational school. He became a house painter and has worked sporadically. He was married in his early 20s and has a 17-year-old daughter who is being raised by her mother. He married his current wife 8 years ago; the marriage was functioning well until the recent drinking became a problem.

Mental Status Examination: The patient is a white male who appears exhausted and mildly disheveled in a sweatshirt, baseball cap, and jeans. He frequently becomes teary throughout the evaluation and has poor eye contact, although he is cooperative with the interview. His stature is slumped, even seated in the chair, and he often leans forward and hides his face in his hands. His speech is notable for increased latency and paucity of words. His affect is dysphoric, congruent with the context of the discussion, and does not brighten throughout the interview. His thought process is linear and logical, and thought content is notable for preoccupation with his mother's death. The patient has no overt delusions; he denies ideas of reference and paranoid ideation. He also denies experiencing auditory, visual, olfactory, or gustatory hallucinations. He is expressing suicidal ideation with intent and plan but denies homicidal ideation. His insight and judgment are fair at this moment in that he knows he needs treatment. Cognitive exam is grossly intact.

Laboratory Examination: Alcohol level: 130; aspartate aminotransferase (AST): 68 IU/L; alanine aminotransferese (ALT): 45 IU/ L; gamma-glutamyl transferase (GGT), 35 U/L; other liver function tests are within normal limits. Hemoglobin: 13.4, hemotocrit: 41, MCV: 95 μm^3, triglycerides: 200 mg/dl.

Questions: What is the diagnosis? What are the important differential diagnoses to consider in this patient?

Diagnosis: Substance-induced mood disorder-specifically, alcohol-induced mood disorder with depressive features, with onset during intoxication.

Discussion: Chronic use and abuse of substances can cause mood disorders and psychotic disorders. The diagnosis substance-induced mood disorder was so termed for the DSM-IV; previously substance-induced disorders were classified under the heading "organic mood disorders." However, the term *organic* is ambiguous and has since been replaced because current research consistently validates a biologic basis for most psychiatric disorders. In the current patient, alcohol has caused a major depressive episode. Any substance of abuse or dependence can cause a mood disorder, including prescription, illicit, or over-the-counter agents. Medications, according to some sources, may be more frequent causes of substance-induced mood disorders. Antihypertensives (particularly reserpine and methyldopa), steroids, stimulants, and antineoplastics are among the long list of medications that cause depression. Some of these same medications, such as steroids, can also cause mania. In making the diagnosis of a substance-induced mood disorder, it is important to specify the type of substance causing the mood disorder and the type of mood disorder experienced (i.e., depressive type, manic type, or mixed).

For a mood disorder to be substance-induced, it logically follows that the symptoms of the mood disorder were not present before use of the substance(s). According to the DSM-IV-TR, substance-induced mood symptoms may develop at any time within 1 month of ceasing to use the substance. The current patient had not experienced symptoms of depression or mania outside his present drinking history and the episode of drinking in his 20s. This fact is important to tease out with patients, because a patient with a primary mood disorder may become dependent on substances; one theory holds that such patients are self-medicating their psychiatric symptoms with the substance of abuse. Substances can obscure uncomfortable feelings of depression, mania, anxiety, and psychosis. For example, a patient with depression might find that using cocaine gives energy and the sensation of being able to concentrate. Alcohol is also an effective anxiolytic, and patients frequently use it to treat panic attacks and other anxiety symptoms. Although there is no consensus in the epidemiologic data, some researchers have postulated that substance abuse is more likely to occur after the onset of bipolar disorder and before the onset of depression.

In the current patient, mood symptoms developed during the protracted daily use of a substance. However, mood symptoms may develop during withdrawal from a substance as well. It is not uncommon for patients to experience severe depression when withdrawing from cocaine, and they often feel suicidal during this uncomfortable (but not lethal) withdrawal. Anxiety is also a common symptom during withdrawal from both alcohol and opiates. It is important to note that not every patient who has depressive symptoms while intoxicated or withdrawing from substances meets criteria for a substance-induced mood disorder because the symptoms experienced must be in excess of those usually experienced with intoxication or withdrawal.

The comorbidity between substance abuse and mood disorders is quite strong. Eighty percent of alcoholic persons report histories of intense depressions, but only 5-10% of these patients actually meet DSM-IV-TR criteria for major depressive disorder when they are not drinking heavily. Epidemiologic data show that the lifetime prevalence of any affective disorder in patients with alcohol dependence is 13.4%. The symptoms of a substance-induced mood disorder are likely to improve rapidly with abstinence. In a recent study of 200 men with alcohol dependence, 40% had symptoms of major depression after 1 week of abstinence, but after 4 weeks of abstinence, only 5% had these symptoms. The key point in the history taking is to delineate which came first, the patient's mood symptoms or the substance abuse. Approximately one-third of cases of depression in people with alcohol dependence represents a primary depressive illness. It is also important to note that recovering patients are at a higher risk of relapse if they develop a mood disorder during times of abstinence.

The treatment of substance-induced mood disorders is controversial. As previously mentioned, many studies indicate that the patient's mood symptoms may abate through sobriety alone. Therefore, antidepressant or mood-stabilizer therapy (if the patient has bipolar symptoms) is often not necessary. However, studies also indicate that antidepressant therapy may reduce the likelihood of relapse in people with alcoholism who experience comorbid depression and may also improve depressive symptoms even in substance-induced depression. Thus, although pharmacotherapy is not uniformly practiced, evidence supports pharmacologic treatment of substance-induced mood disorders. However, antidepressant treatment has not been shown to prevent relapse in alcoholic persons who do not experience depressive symptoms. In addition, psychosocial support for both depression and sobriety, such as day programs, 12 Step Programs, and individual counseling, are beneficial to patients with both mood and substance disorders.

The differential diagnosis for the current patient includes major depressive disorder, adjustment disorder, and bereavement. The patient experienced a similar depressive episode earlier in his 20s. Clarifying the temporal relationship between this patient's depressive symptoms and his drinking allows us to delineate between primary depression (MDD) and depression secondary to substance abuse. When the patient's mother died, he began drinking daily. If, on the other hand, the patient had stated that he began to feel depressed after his mother had died but began drinking 1 year after her death, we would be more suspicious of major depression.

Because the death of the patient's mother is clearly an event that marks the onset of his psychiatric symptoms, adjustment disorder with depressed mood is also on the differential. Adjustment disorder criteria require the onset of depressive symptoms within 3 months of the stressor (his mother's death). The patient and his wife are able to clearly delineate the timeline of his symptoms: his mother's death and onset of drinking took place one and a half years ago, with the development of depressive symptoms 6 weeks ago. Therefore, the onset of the patient's depressive symptoms was not closely related to the death of his mother.

One might also consider bereavement as a potential explanation for both the patient's mood and substance dependence. Normal bereavement, by DSM definition, may last different lengths of time in varying cultural groups, but the average duration is set at 2 months. Major depressive disorder may be distinguished from bereavement by five key symptoms, which include suicidality, excessive guilt, significant psychosocial difficulties, hallucinations, and psychomotor retardation. The facts that the current patient experienced suicidality and that the majority of his symptoms did not begin until more than 1 year after his mother's death make bereavement unlikely.

The patient had a 10-day admission on the locked psychiatric unit in the hospital. During the first 5 days he was on a benzodiazepine taper to prevent withdrawal symptoms from alcohol dependence. He was also started on a selective serotonin reuptake inhibitor (SSRI) with the hope that it would facilitate remission of his depressive symptoms and help support his sobriety. By day 9 of his admission, the patient was notably brighter in affect and was no longer expressing suicidal ideation. He was discharged from the psychiatric unit with the aftercare plan of seeing a psychiatrist and psychotherapist and attending evening groups at the hospital's Addiction Recovery Program. He also was given the lists of Alcoholics Anonymous meetings in his neighborhood. His wife was supportive of the patient's recovery and eager to begin couples' counseling. She also began attending Al Anon meetings while the patient was still in the hospital. On discharge the patient went home with his wife. A phone message from the patient 1 month later reported that he was still sober and that he and his wife were getting along well.

Pearls

1. Laboratory analysis of patients with alcoholism may show elevated ALT, AST, GGT, and mean corpuscular volume (MCV). These levels may return to normal with abstinence and, for MCV, with proper dietary intake.

2. For all patients suspected of substance abuse, a toxicology screen (both serum and urine) should be done on initial evaluation, and, if indicated, random toxicology screens may be instituted.

3. Medical attention should also be given according to the specific drug of abuse. For example, if the patient had been abusing cocaine, a cardiac history and EKG should be done. Or, if the patient had been abusing intravenous drugs, serologic tests for HIV and hepatitis C should be performed.

REFERENCES

1. Hasin D, Liu X, Nunes E, et al: Effects of major depression on remission and relapse of substance dependence. Arch Gen Psychiatry 2002;59:375–380.
2. Hales R, Yudolsky S, Tabot J: APA Textbook of Psychiatry, 3rd ed. Washington DC, APA Press, 1999, pp 363–373.
3. Kaplan HI, Saddock BJ: Comprehensive Textbook of Psychiatry, 7th ed. Baltimore, Williams &Wilkins, 2000, pp 924–960.
4. McGrath J Nunes E, Quitkin FM: Current concepts in the treatment of depression in alcohol-dependent patients. Psychiatr Clin North Am 2002;23:695–711.

F. Tuna Burgut, MD

PATIENT 45

A 36-year-old woman with depressive symptoms

History of Present Illness: A 36-year-old Caucasian woman presents to the psychiatric emergency department with her mother because of suicidal thoughts. The patient reports that she came at the insistence of her mother and does not believe that "anyone can help her." She states that she feels sad all of the time and that she does not enjoy anything. She also feels that she is worthless and has become a burden to her family. The patient reports wishing that "I was dead." She denies any current suicidal plans as well as past attempts but has ongoing passive death wishes. She also reports a 10-pound weight loss and insomnia over the past 4 weeks. The mother describes the patient as becoming more isolative and not taking caring of herself. She is apparently not eating well and not bathing; she spends most of the night awake and crying. The mother reports that she has also been only intermittently compliant with her medications from her neurologist, which include interferon beta 1a (33 μg intramuscular injection weekly) and baclofen (10 mg twice daily).

The patient denies any past episodes of depression but describes feeling very sad for almost a week when she was first diagnosed with multiple sclerosis 5 years ago. She did not have any previous depressive episodes, manic episodes, or any other past psychiatric symptoms. The patient denied any drug or alcohol abuse. This is the patient's first psychiatric evaluation.

Past Neurologic History: The patient was diagnosed with multiple sclerosis 5 years ago when she presented with sudden visual loss in her right eye. Diagnostic work-up at the time included cerbrospinal fluid studies and a brain MRI, which revealed multiple periventricular demyelinating lesions. Three years later she presented with left-sided hemiparesis, which was treated in the hospital with high-dose intravenous steroid treatment. Her last relapse was 1 year ago when she presented with sudden paraparesis and incontinence and was diagnosed with transverse myelitis. At that time she was started on interferon beta 1a to reduce the relapse rate and disease progression.

Family History: The patient's grandmother suffered from a depressive episode and was treated with electroconvulsive therapy in 1966.

Social History: The patient is divorced from her husband and blames their divorce on her illness. She has worked in the past as an accountant but has been on disability for 2 years. She has been living with her parents since her divorce 1 year ago.

Mental Status Examination: The patient looks older than her stated age; she is disheveled with unkempt hair and stained clothes and makes poor eye contact. Speech is nonspontaneous, with low volume, and monotonous, Mood is described as depressed, and her affect is mood-congruent but constricted in range. Thought process is linear and well organized. Her thought content is impoverished, without signs of paranoid delusions, but preoccupied with guilt and perceived feelings of worthlessness and being a burden to her family. She denies experiencing any auditory, visual, or olfactory hallucinations. She expresses passive suicidal ideations but denies any plans. She denies homicidal ideation. On cognitive exam she is oriented to year and month but did not know the day. She has difficulty with tasks that measure attention, as demonstrated by her limitations with serial sevens (which would have been an otherwise easy task, considering her occupation as an accountant). She also had mild difficulty in working memory tasks, as demonstrated by a reduced digit span: she was able to recite only 4 numbers forward and 2 backward, whereas normal capacity would have been 7 forward and 4 backward. She is able to register 3 items after multiple trials, and her recall is impaired at 5 minutes because she can only recite 2 of 3 items. Insight and judgment are limited because she lacks understanding of the severity of her illness and had not wanted to come to the hospital. Impulse control at the time of the interview was intact.

Diagnostic Testing: An MRI of the brain with and without gadolinium enhancement revealed multiple foci of increased signal in the periventricular white matter on T2-weighted images.The findings ar suggestive of diffuse demyelination (see figure).

Laboratory Examination: TSH level and routine blood work are within normal range. Urine toxicology screen is negative.

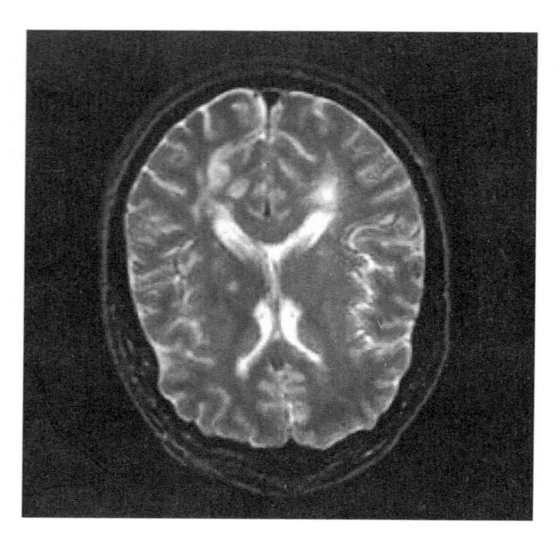 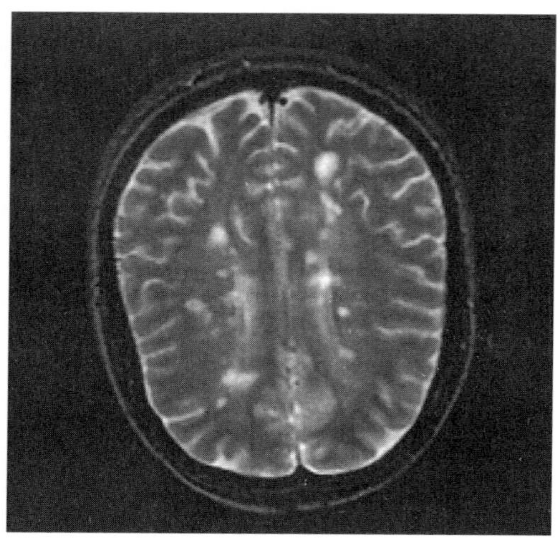

T2-weighted axial images show multiple foci of increased signal in the periventricular white matter suggestive of diffuse demyelination (figure on the right is a higher cut).

Questions: What is the diagnosis? What are the psychiatric illnesses commonly seen in patients with multiple sclerosis?

Diagnosis: Mood disorder due to multiple sclerosis with major depressive-like episode.

Discussion: Multiple sclerosis (MS) is an inflammatory disorder affecting the central nervous system and believed to be triggered by an unknown etiologic agent, perhaps viral, in a genetically susceptible host. MS occurs in 0.1% of the population of the United States and has a similar prevalence rate in Europe. It is the most common cause of neurologic disability in young adults and affects women nearly as twice as often as men. The diagnosis of MS requires the occurrence of at least two neurologic events consistent with demyelination in the central nervous system and separated temporally and anatomically. Early onset and long duration of illness result in tremendous individual, family, and societal costs as well as reductions in quality of life and work productivity.

From the earliest descriptions of MS to the present, psychiatric manifestations of the disease have been considered paramount. Affective disturbances in MS include depression, bipolar disorder, and pathologic laughter and weeping. Of great concern is the elevated risk of suicide, reported to be 7.5 times that of the general population, with a cumulative risk of 2%.

Depression is among the most commonly identified affective disorders in MS. Lifetime incidence studies examining depression in MS populations indicate that approximately 50% of patients develop depression. There are many risk factors associated with depression, and psychosocial risk factors in particular are thought to contribute to the etiology of depression in MS. The unpredictability of the disease, patients' perceived lack of control, and the frequently encountered losses, such as divorce and unemployment, are examples of common stressors encountered by young patients with MS. The present patient also expressed lack of control over her life and had experienced cognitive loss that led to loss of her job. Cognitive dysfunction is associated with depression and social stress, and may be the source of depression in many patients with MS. Cognitive dysfunction can occur early in the course of the illness, and the most common deficits associated with MS relate to memory, attention, speed of information processing, and executive dysfunction.

Affective disorders can also appear as a symptom of MS relapse. For example, the destructive lesions found in the temporal, parietal, and frontal lobes as well as in the limbic cortex and left arcuate fasciculus have been implicated in the development of depression. Such patients probably should be treated with combination therapy of high-dose steroids and antidepressants. There has also been some concern about the use of interferon therapy for long-term immunomodulation of MS. Even though debate exists in the literature, clinical depression has been observed to be a side effect of interferon treatment, particularly in the first 6 months. However, the present patient had been on interferon therapy for over a year without any initial side effects. The reduction of relapse rate with interferon therapy is key in the long-term treatment of patients with MS; therefore, interferon therapy is often temporarily stopped during the initial treatment of depression but reinstituted once depressive symptoms are treated.

There are few published controlled studies of treatment for depression in MS. One double-blind, placebo-controlled clinical trial showed that desipramine was effective, although side effects developed in one-half of the treated group. Despite the lack of controlled studies, a variety of antidepressants, including selective serotonin reuptake inhibitors and tricyclic antidepressants, are often successfully used to treat depression in patients with MS. In addition to pharmacotherapy, individual psychotherapy and cognitive behavior therapy are also clearly effective for depression. Electroconvulsive therapy has also been shown to be effective for patients with MS and more severe or intractable depression.

Bipolar disorder appears to be much less common than depression in the MS population. However, one study proposed a possible association between MS and bipolar disorder because 10 patients from Monroe County in New York had both conditions concurrently, despite the fact that epidemiologic data would indicate the expected number to be 5.4. Although patients rarely complain of classic mood cycling, rapid mood swings and cyclothymia are common in the MS population. The treatment of bipolar disorder in patients with MS should follow the APA practice guidelines, which dictate the use of lithium, anticonvulsants, and atypical antipsychotics. Pharmacotherapy for disabling mood swings and irritability in the absence of formal psychiatric diagnoses such as major depression or bipolar disorder may also improve the quality of life for many patients with MS and should be carefully considered.

Pathologic laughing and crying (PLC) may also occur in MS. PLC is characterized by an inability to control outbursts of laughter and crying that may not be associated with subjective feelings of mirth or sadness, respectively. The patient with PLC does not necessarily experience the emotion that is displayed. PLC often responds quickly and completely to low doses of tricyclic antidepressants.

The current patient was admitted to the psychiatric unit for treatment of her major depressive symptoms. She was placed on close observation due to the risk of suicide and self-neglect. Bipolar disorder was also considered in the differential diagnosis due to the higher risk present in patients with MS and the family history of an unspecified affective disorder in the patient's grandmother. The patient had no prior history of mania; sertraline was therefore started at 50 mg and titrated to 100 mg with close monitoring of mood. Adjustment disorder was ruled out due to the acute presentation of depressive symptoms in the presence of a chronic stressor. An MRI of the brain was done to look for possible new MS lesions. Although there was no evidence of prominent new lesions, periventricular demyelinization was seen. The patient's mood stabilized after several weeks, and she was scheduled to follow up in the neurology and psychiatry clinics.

Pearls

1. Proposed reasons for the association between MS and depression include the psychosocial effects of disability and direct effect of brain lesions. The complex interplay between these two factors needs further investigation.
2. Depressive episodes are the most common psychiatric comorbidity in patients with MS and are frequently underrecognized and undertreated. Symptoms of irritability, sadness, tearfulness, and affective instability are also common in the MS population and should be effectively treated even in the absence of a formal psychiatric diagnosis.
3. Patients with MS have greater than a 7-fold increase in the incidence of suicide compared with the general population and therefore need to be carefully assessed for precipitating psychiatric symptoms.
4. High-dose steroid therapies used to alleviate the neurologic symptoms in MS relapses may cause mania and psychosis. If these symptoms emerge, they are typically managed with anticonvulsant therapy or low doses of antipsychotic medication, which are given throughout the course of steroid treatment.

REFERENCES

1. Chwastiak L, Ehde DM, Gibbons LE, et al: Depressive symptoms and severity of illness in MS: Epidemiologic study of a large community sample. Am J Psychiatry 2002;159:1862–1868.
2. Feinstein A, Feinstein K: Depression associated with multiple sclerosis: Looking beyond diagnosis to symptom expression. J Affect Disord 2001;66:193–198.
3. Krupp LB, Rizvi SA: Symptomatic therapy for underrecognized manifestations of multiple sclerosis. Neurology 2002;58: S32–S39.
4. Schiffer RB, Wineman NM, Weitkamp LR: Association between bipolar affective disorder and MS. Am J Psychiatry 1986; 143:94–95.
5. Scott TF, Carol Cheiffe C, Burgut T: Affective disorders in patients with multiple sclerosis: Pathophysiology and approaches to management. CNS Drugs 1999;12:431–436.

PATIENT 46

A 32-year-old man with threatening, aggressive behavior

History of Present Illness: A 32-year-old man is admitted to an inpatient psychiatric unit for suicidal ideation. After two days of admission, he begins to argue with another patient. The resident on call is summoned to the unit, and by now the argument has progressed to loud yelling. According to the patient, he was eating breakfast and asked another patient if he could have his toast, and the other patient replied "yes." However, the other patient maintains that his toast was actually stolen, and both men began yelling at each other. The nursing staff overheard the 32-year-old man threaten the other patient, and he was quickly placed in locked seclusion. After an hour, the resident again interviewed the patient, who said that he felt "calmer," was no longer angry, and agreed that the argument was "silly." He denied any feelings of wanting to hurt the other patient and agreed to "stay out of his way." The patient was anxiously awaiting his discharge the next day and appeared concerned about potentially affecting his discharge date. He reported being in the hospital only because "my girlfriend kicked me out because I was drinking too much." Furthermore, he disclosed that he had lied to the admitting doctor about feeling suicidal "just so I could get admitted."

During the second interview, the patient denied any active suicidal or homicidal ideation, and the resident discontinued the seclusion order. After being let out of seclusion, he calmly approaches the other patient and cuts him across the neck with a razor blade taped to his body. He states that the other patient "got what he deserved" and did not appear to feel any remorse for his actions, despite the obvious pain and disfigurement that he caused.

Past Psychiatric History: The patient has a history of multiple psychiatric hospitalizations, dating back to childhood. His first psychiatric contact was at age 10, when he killed the family dog with a B.B. gun. A review of old charts notes that his mother reported frequent episodes of theft and truancy. He was frequently suspended from school for fighting, and his mother described him as the "school bully." He was able to finish high school and obtain an associates degree, but he was unable to hold a job for long because of alcohol and sporadic cocaine abuse. He made several attempts at detoxification and rehabilitation for his substance abuse but was often discharged because of fighting and surreptitious drug use.

The patient also has a history of self-injurious behavior and describes superficially cutting his wrist in the past "because I was bored." He has been arrested several times for domestic violence, and his current girlfriend has an order of protection against him. His past psychiatric diagnoses in childhood include conduct disorder and attention deficit/hyperactivity disorder. In adulthood, he has been diagnosed with alcohol dependence, alcohol-induced mood disorder, major depressive disorder, and even bipolar disorder during one hospitalization.

Mental Status Examination: The patient is well kempt in hospital pajamas. He appears his stated age and has good eye contact. He is cooperative with the interview and displays no psychomotor agitation or retardation. The patient is actually quite pleasant, almost charming. His speech is of normal rate and volume and well articulated. He describes his mood as "fine," and his affect is congruent and euthymic. He does not appear to be responding to internal stimuli. Thought process is logical and goal-directed. He denies any suicidal or homicidal ideation, stating that he "only wanted to nick him a little bit." He does not want to hurt anybody else but states that he "doesn't know what I'll do if someone gets on my case." He denies any auditory or visual hallucinations. He is alert and oriented, and his concentration, recall, and retention are not impaired. The patient's insight and judgment are intact because he is aware of what he is doing and understands the results of his actions. His impulse control, however, is clearly impaired, as evidenced by recent behavior.

Diagnostic Testing: Urine toxicology screen: negative. Blood alcohol level: negative

Question: Which diagnosis can explain the patient's history and present illness?

Diagnosis: Antisocial personality disorder (ASPD).

Discussion: According to the DSM-IV-TR, ASPD is defined by a pervasive disregard for, and violation of, the rights of others from the age of 15 (with evidence of conduct disorder before the age of 15). It is important to note that the definition and diagnosis of what is now called ASPD has undergone several changes since its first description. In 1835, James Pritchard first described symptoms of "moral insanity," which later was termed "sociopathy." In Psychopathic Personalities (1958), Kurt Schneider describes 10 discrete, socially deviant personality types, which led to the use of the term "psychopath." In the 1940s through the 1950s, Cleckley, McCord and McCord, and Karpman described a personality type that lacked features of guilt, anxiety, and loyalty. In 1968, this personality type became antisocial personality disorder in the DSM-II.

The prevalence of ASPD in the general population is approximately 3% for males and 1% for females. In clinical settings, the prevalence can be as high as 30%, with even higher rates in forensic and substance-abusing populations. In prison populations, a review of the literature reveals a wide range of the prevalence of ASPD: from 11% to 78% in males and from 12% to 65% in females. It has also been noted that ASPD may be underdiagnosed in females due to the many aggressive items required to meet the diagnosis of conduct disorder.

The etiology of ASPD involves both genetic and environmental factors. It is more frequent among first-degree relatives of probands with ASPD. Of interest, it has been found that biologic relatives of women with ASPD have a higher risk for developing ASPD than biologic relatives of men with ASPD. Adoption studies also support the presence of both genetic and environmental factors because adopted and biologic children of parents with ASPD have a higher risk of developing the disorder. In addition, the presence of conduct disorder before the age of 10 and comorbid attention-deficit/hyperactivity disorder increase the risk of developing ASPD in adult life. ASPD is also more likely to develop from conduct disorder when parenting is erratic, inconsistent, or neglectful.

Among the differential diagnoses, it is important to distinguish the impulsive and high-risk behavior characteristic of ASPD from acute mania. In bipolar I disorder, mania occurs in an episodic fashion and is associated with euphoric mood. The current patient's mood was euthymic, with stable, appropriate affect, and he did not display thought process disturbance or grandiosity typical of a manic episode. In addition, ASPD can be distinguished from other personality disorders, such as narcissistic and histrionic personality disorder, by the presence of significant criminality and aggression.

Patients with borderline personality disorder may become violent, but they also typically display pronounced affective instability and the need for nurturing. The current patient also had an alcohol-related disorder, and the increased prevalence of substance abuse (alcohol in particular) has been well documented in ASPD. The diagnosis of ASPD is sometimes complicated by the presence of irritability, low frustration tolerance, and depressed mood, and clinicians may mistake the presentation for major depressive disorder. In general, patients with ASPD are also at increased risk for comorbid impulse control disorders, major depression, and somatization disorder.

As difficult as the diagnosis of ASPD may be to confirm, treatment is often even more elusive. Most people with personality disorders see their lifestyles as normal and seldom refer themselves for treatment. They seek help only when maladaptive behaviors culminate in intolerable marital, family, or career distress with associated anxiety, depression, or substance abuse. This pattern was seen clearly in the above patient, who entered the hospital only after his alcohol abuse led to discord with his girlfriend.

Many psychotherapeutic techniques have been tried to treat ASPD. Because so many have failed, it has been said that patients with ASPD are resistant to existing psychotherapeutic treatments. However, it is possible to treat coexisting axis I disorders, such as substance abuse or major depression. If the patient with ASPD wants to enter treatment, he or she should identify specific and concrete goals for treatment at the outset (e.g., to drink less). With regard to psychopharmacology, medications may be used in two ways: to correct the neurobiologic dispositions underlying the patient's deviant traits (called causal treatment) or to treat specific behaviors and symptoms of ASPD (called symptomatic treatment).

In causal treatment, the doctor attempts to promote harm avoidance, decrease novelty seeking, and reward dependence, which are proposed underlying themes of symptoms seen in ASPD and are postulated to reflect differences in serotonergic, dopaminergic, and noradrenergic neurotransmitter systems. This treatment strategy is still experimental and not widely practiced.

In symptomatic treatment, the physician targets aggression, mood dysregulation, anxiety, or possible psychotic symptoms and treats them accordingly. For example, a patient with predatory aggression, as seen in the above case, may benefit from an antipsychotic or mood stabilizer. Several randomized, controlled trials have shown that lithium reduces affective display and aggression in both normal and impulsive people. However, lithium has not been found to reduce nonaggressive antisocial behavior, such as lying or stealing.

In treating a patient with ASPD, the therapist must use firm and frequent limit-setting techniques and be aware that patients can often manipulate even the best therapists. It is important to note that people with ASPD often do not tell the truth and cannot typically be trusted to adhere to any standard of morality. In this case, because there was no evidence of any comorbid axis I diagnosis besides alcohol dependence and because the patient did not cut the other patient in response to internal stimuli (i.e., psychosis), the unit chief called the police, who charged the current patient with attempted murder and removed him from the unit.

Pearls

1. One aid in diagnosing a patient with ASPD is the Minnesota Multiphasic Personality Inventory (MMPI), which contains a special scale, called the psychopathic deviate (Pd) scale. This scale was designed to assess specific aspects of antisocial personality disorder (e.g., lack of empathy, callous disregard for others, glibness, failure to accept responsibility for one's actions). The Pd2 subscale has emerged in recent literature as a marker of ASPD because its items refer explicitly to illegal actions and callousness.
2. Despite their often ridiculous explanations for their behavior, people with ASPD have been noted to have a heightened sense of reality and frequently impress clinicians with their good verbal intelligence.
3. The high prevalence of ASPD in forensic populations may be secondary to misdiagnosis of an axis I disorder. For example, patients may have psychiatric symptoms (such as paranoid delusions and auditory hallucinations) that they deny. Instead they act out violently in response to these symptoms, thus receiving the label of ASPD. In addition, some authors see antisocial behavior in prison as a "game" that inmates and officers "play." As a result of this game, inmates are diagnosed incorrectly with ASPD.

REFERENCES

1. Kaplan H, Sadock B: Comprehensive Textbook of Psychiatry, 7th ed. Philadelphia, Lippincott Williams & Wilkins, 2000, pp 1723–1764.
2. Lilienfeld SO: The relation of the MMPI-2 Pd Harris Lingoes subscales to psychopathy, psychopathy facets, and antisocial behavior. J Clin Psychol 1999;55:241–255.
3. Rotter M: Personality disorders in prison: Aren't they all antisocial? Psychiatr Q 2002;73:337–349.
4. Rutherford MJ, Cacciola JS, Alterman AI: Antisocial personality disorder and psychopathy in cocaine-dependent women. Am J Psychiatry 1999;156:849–856.

Corbett Schimming, MD

PATIENT 47

A 42-year-old man with hallucinations and agitation

History of Present Illness: As a resident on the psychiatry consult-liaison team, you are called to evaluate a 42-year-old man on the orthopaedic surgery service who has acutely developed "hallucinations and agitation." The patient was admitted to the hospital approximately 48 hours ago and underwent an uncomplicated shoulder surgery with minimal blood loss. However, over the past several hours, the orthopaedics resident noted the patient to be agitated, anxious, and combative, yelling at the nurses to "get the hell out of my room," constantly trying to crawl out of bed to "leave this prison," and accusing various staff of trying to hurt him. The patient also appeared terrified of some holes in the ceiling tiles, saying, "Don't you see all those ants crawling up there?" In addition, the patient has been commenting excitedly on the "little weasels that keep crawling under my bed."

When you see the patient, he is tremulous and mumbling to himself while trying to remove the blood pressure cuff from his arm. He quickly says, "Oh great, the psychiatrist! I just came in here to get my shoulder fixed....now they've got me imprisoned in here so they can kill me. By the way, I don't know what kind of hospital lets animals run around in the rooms!" During the interview the patient complains of nausea, excessive sweating, insomnia, seeing bugs crawling all over the ceiling, and seeing various small animals running around his room and under his bed. Furthermore, the patient loudly accuses the doctors and nurses of "having it in for him." When questioned about alcohol and drug use, the patient vehemently denies either, screaming: "I don't do any of that stuff! Damn it, I'm not talking to you anymore! Interview over."

Past Psychiatric History: Luckily, the patient's wife arrives at this time to provide additional history. She is shocked to see him in this state and reports that he has no history of hallucinations or paranoid ideation. Of note, she says, "He does drink alcohol pretty often." When asked to approximate how much the patient drinks, she replies: "I don't know, I guess he just drinks socially." She denies any knowledge of illegal drug use but adds, "I've seen him take a little white pill once in a while...when he gets really upset." The patient has no formal psychiatric history, and his wife denies previous psychiatric hospitalizations or outpatient visits. She says that "sometimes he seems to get kind of depressed after he's been under too much stress at work." However, she denies suicide attempts or knowledge of any suicidal ideation. Finally, she reports: "his father was a pretty heavy drinker....one time, when he went for surgery, he had a seizure in the hospital. The doctors didn't seem to know what was going on."

Mental Status Examination: The patient is a diaphoretic, obese man who appears older than his stated age. A coarse tremor is grossly obvious in both hands. He makes adequate eye contact but is occasionally distracted by other stimuli. The patient is uncooperative with the interview, answering only some of the questions. His speech alternates between loud and soft mumbling. He demonstrates significant psychomotor agitation, pulling on his hospital gown, looking around the room, and trying to get out of bed. When asked about his mood, he replies: "Pissed off at this hospital!" The patient's affect is agitated and labile, quickly ranging between anger and apprehension. His thought process fluctuates between logical and somewhat disorganized, and his thought content is disturbed by hallucinations (animals in room), illusions (bugs on ceiling), and paranoid ideation (staff trying to hurt him). The patient denies suicidal or homicidal ideation. Surprisingly, he is alert and oriented to person, place, and time, but he becomes highly agitated when asked these questions. Both insight and judgment are significantly impaired.

Vital Signs: Temperature, 37.1°C; heart rate, 110 beats/min; blood pressure, 152/90 mmHg; respiratory rate, 20 breaths/min.

Questions: What is the cause of the patient's agitation and psychotic symptoms? How should he be treated?

Diagnosis: Alcohol withdrawal with perceptual disturbances.

Discussion: Alcohol withdrawal is a syndrome that occurs in the context of cessation or reduction in alcohol use that has been heavy and prolonged. This syndrome consists of at least two of the following symptoms: autonomic hyperactivity; hand tremor; insomnia; nausea or vomiting; transient visual, tactile, or auditory hallucinations or illusions; psychomotor agitation; anxiety; and grand mal seizures. As with many drugs of abuse, after the brain has chronically been exposed to high levels, a decrease in blood levels of the substance can lead to symptoms of withdrawal. The symptoms are generally the opposite of the physiologic changes caused by the substance. In the case of alcohol, a central nervous system depressant, the above symptoms can be understood as the inverse of symptoms of alcohol intoxication. For example, the low blood pressure sometimes seen in alcohol intoxication is replaced by autonomic hyperactivity, and sedation is replaced by anxiety and psychomotor agitation.

The alcohol withdrawal syndrome generally follows a time course that corresponds to declining levels of alcohol in the blood. The onset of symptoms is usually heralded by tremors and increased heart rate about 4–12 hours after cessation of alcohol, and most withdrawal symptoms generally peak in intensity after approximately 48 hours. Symptoms then diminish and usually improve on the fourth or fifth day of abstinence. Of course, these numbers are highly variable, with symptoms sometimes taking days to appear and peaking significantly later, with a range of 5–10 days. Very few people who undergo alcohol withdrawal develop more severe complications. For example, alcohol withdrawal seizures ("rum fits") occur in fewer than 3% of patients.

An even more dreaded complication is alcohol withdrawal delirium (also known as delirium tremens or "DTs"), in which the patient develops a fluctuation in level of consciousness or a change in cognition, generally along with the "three Ts" (tremor, increased temperature, and marked tachycardia). As with other forms of delirium, the patient becomes unable to focus or sustain attention and becomes confused, with transient disorientation or loss of memory. Alcohol withdrawal delirium is quite rare, occurring in approximately 1% of any single withdrawal, but its incidence is increased in people who have also had seizures. This feared complication of alcohol withdrawal is extremely dangerous. Left untreated, it is associated with a mortality rate of 20%. Alcohol withdrawal delirium is most likely to develop in patients with concomitant medical problems, such as liver failure, pulmonary infections, gastrointestinal bleeds, or electrolyte disturbances.

The current patient shows clear signs of alcohol withdrawal, corresponding to cessation of alcohol intake at the time of hospital admission (48 hours). Patients commonly present with withdrawal in the postoperative context, and the clinician should be on guard for this syndrome, especially in patients who suddenly appear psychotic without a past psychiatric history. This patient manifests many classic signs and symptoms of withdrawal, including tremors, tachycardia, diaphoresis, agitation, anxiety, hallucinations, and illusions. Although the patient's wife gives a vague history of his alcohol use, it should be assumed that, given his clinical presentation, he drinks more than just "socially."

Other diagnoses that might be considered are alcohol withdrawal delirium (DTs), benzodiazepine withdrawal, a primary psychotic disorder, or substance-induced psychosis. Alcohol withdrawal delirium can be ruled out based on the patient's lack of disorientation or memory loss and the absence of fever or marked tachycardia (heart rate > 125 beats/min). However, the patient should be carefully monitored for the development of this complication over the next several days, as the incidence of DTs peaks approximately 4 days after the last drink. Benzodiazepine withdrawal may also present in a similar fashion, and because of the wife's statement that he takes pills "once in a while," this diagnosis must be kept in the differential. However, alcohol withdrawal is a more common phenomenon, and the patient has both a presentation and a family history more suggestive of alcohol withdrawal. Although urine toxicology studies might help sort this out, treatment for both withdrawal syndromes is the same.

A primary psychotic disorder (e.g., schizophrenia) is not particularly likely, as this middle-aged patient has no previous psychiatric history and developed psychotic symptoms with an acuity uncharacteristic of primary psychotic disorders. Finally, alcohol-induced psychotic disorder can be ruled out because, although the patient demonstrates prominent hallucinations within a month of alcohol intoxication/withdrawal, the symptoms are not in excess of those typically associated with the alcohol withdrawal syndrome.

The etiology of alcohol withdrawal stems largely from the effects of chronic alcohol exposure on the brain. This exposure is postulated to lead to an upregulation of N-methyl-D-aspartate (NMDA) receptors and downregulation of gamma-aminobutyric acid (GABA) receptors. Increased NMDA receptor density may result in the neuronal hyperactivity seen in alcohol withdrawal, since drugs that act as antagonists at NMDA receptors are helpful in reducing the symptoms of withdrawal. In addition, downregulation of GABA receptors probably contributes to the signs and symptoms seen in alcohol withdrawal, since both benzodiazepines and barbiturates activate GABA receptors and are used to eliminate the signs and symptoms of withdrawal.

Treatment of the current patient should begin with benzodiazepines. A tapered course of either lorazepam (Ativan) or chlordiazepoxide (Librium) is the current treatment of choice because both agents safely provide sedation, increase the seizure threshold, and relieve withdrawal symptoms. Although both are acceptable choices, lorazepam has the advantage of more predictable clearance and renal metabolism, whereas chlordiazepoxide undergoes hepatic metabolism to four different active metabolites-with half-lives greater than the parent drug. This difference may be of particular importance in patients experiencing alcohol withdrawal. In addition, adequate hydration should be ensured, and nutritional supplementation should be given, including thiamine (to prevent Wernicke-Korsakoff syndrome), folic acid, and vitamin B complex. The clinician should always administer thiamine before giving the patient glucose, because thiamine is required for glucose metabolism. If glucose is given without thiamine, the rapid metabolism of already depleted thiamine stores can cause or worsen encephalopathy. Other components of treatment include frequent neurologic exams and seizure precautions. Finally, long-term treatment options for alcohol cessation should be discussed when the patient is stable.

The current patient is started on a tapered course of lorazepam, with additional doses given as needed for breakthrough withdrawal symptoms. Over the next 24 hours, the nursing staff notes that the patient is no longer tremulous, is sleeping peacefully in bed, and has normal heart rate and blood pressure. By the time you see him again, he is a bit sleepy but no longer agitated or having hallucinations. He says, "Sorry for the way I spoke to you, doc....I guess I've been drinking too much." You continue to follow the patient while he is in the hospital, discussing various options for long-term treatment while monitoring mental status and vital signs. The patient remains stable and is tapered off benzodiazepines. When he expresses a desire to stop drinking, you arrange close follow-up in the outpatient psychiatry clinic and make plans for him to attend local meetings of Alcoholics Anonymous.

Pearls

1. The alcohol withdrawal syndrome tends to follow a typical time course. Withdrawal symptoms usually begin within 4 to 12 hours and peak in intensity at approximately 48 hours. Alcohol withdrawal seizures typically occur within 6 to 48 hours, and alcohol withdrawal delirium usually begins 48 to 96 hours after the cessation of alcohol.
2. A recent randomized, controlled trial demonstrated that symptom-triggered (as-needed) treatment of alcohol withdrawal with benzodiazepines can shorten the time course of detoxification and decrease the quantity of medication used compared with a fixed-dose schedule of benzodiazepine administration. Importantly, symptom-triggered therapy was found to be just as safe and comfortable for the patient.
3. Several lines of evidence point to an upregulation of brain NMDA receptors and a downregulation of brain GABA receptors after chronic alcohol consumption as a molecular mechanism contributing to the symptoms of alcohol withdrawal.
4. Oral topiramate, an antiseizure medication, has been shown in a randomized, controlled trial to reduce the number of drinks per day and the craving for alcohol in patients with alcohol dependence. Topiramate is postulated to decrease mesocorticolimbic dopamine activity after alcohol intake and to antagonize chronic changes caused by alcohol at glutamate receptors.
5. Acamprosate, a drug not yet approved in the United States, shows promise as an agent for treating many aspects of alcohol dependence. This medication works by suppressing NMDA receptor activity, thereby reducing alcohol withdrawal and preventing relapse. Acamprosate was shown to begin working at 30 to 90 days of treatment and to help maintain abstinence for up to one year of treatment.

REFERENCES

1. Chang PH, Steinberg MB: Alcohol withdrawal. Med Clin North Am 2001;85:1191–1212.
2. Daeppen J-B, Gache P, et al: Symptom-triggered vs fixed-schedule doses of benzodiazepine for alcohol withdrawal. Arch Intern Med 2002;162:1117–1121.
3. Edwards G, Gross MM: Alcohol dependence: Clinical description of a provisional syndrome. Br Med J 1976;1(6017): 1058–1061.
4. Gulya K, Grant KA, et al : Brain regional specificity and time course of changes in the NMDA receptor-ionophore complex during ethanol withdrawal. Brain Res 1991;547:129–134.
5. Johnson BA, Ait-Daoud N, et al: Oral topiramate for treatment of alcohol dependence: A randomised controlled trial. Lancet 2003;361:1677–1685.
6. Mason BJ: Treatment of alcohol-dependent outpatients with acamprosate: A clinical review. J Clin Psychiatry 2001;62(Suppl 20):42–48.
7. Mayo-Smith MF: Pharmacologic management of alcohol withdrawal: A meta-analysis and evidence-based practice guideline. JAMA 1997;278:144–151.
8. Rossetti ZL, Carboni S : Ethanol withdrawal is associated with increased extracellular glutamate in the rat striatum. Eur J Pharmacol 1995;283:177–183.

Sander Markx
Daniel Stewart, MD

PATIENT 48

A 29-year-old woman with feelings of being too dependent on friends

History of Present Illness: A 29-year-old, well-dressed woman walks into the office and sits down, sighing heavily. The patient is here because of anorgasmia, frequent headaches, and feelings of being unwanted and too dependent on family and friends. The patient has been working as a research assistant in the department of internal medicine at a hospital in the city. During the interview, she is eager to give detailed answers to all questions. She talks about the intensity of her job and how she is always busy and working late. When asked what her daily responsibilities are, the patient gives an excessively superficial description without concrete examples and does not directly answer the question.

The patient talks at length about her colleagues and how close she is with all of them. She says that she became best friends with two female colleagues with whom she goes shopping "at least once every month!" She has had numerous relationships, all with "very attractive men," but each has lasted less than a year. When asked about these relationships, the patient becomes flirtatious and asks seductively "Well, what do you want to know specifically?"

The patient states that she enjoys the feeling of being attractive. She says that she loves it when men are talking about her at work during the lunch break. After having said this, the patient repeatedly asks whether it is wrong to feel attractive as a woman. Then, all of a sudden, she starts to cry and says that she sometimes thinks that nobody really loves her. After a few minutes, the patient stops crying and continues to talk about work.

Throughout the interview, the patient appears highly emotional. At many points she becomes overtly enthusiastic, and at the next moment she seems angry or sad. When asked whether she acknowledges these feelings, the patient reacts with surprise and says that she is not that emotional about such matters. She denies depressed mood; states that her sleep, appetite, and energy are fine; and denies all symptoms of psychosis, mania, and anxiety.

Past Psychiatric History: The patient is the oldest child in the family with a sister who is younger by 2 years. She describes her youth as happy and uneventful. She talks fondly of her father and says that she has always been "daddy's little girl." The patient says that she is also very close with her mother, with whom she would always go shopping and visit beauty salons while talking about her boyfriends and asking her mother for advice. She says that when she was 17, her father became an alcoholic, which has had an enormous effect on her well-being. She says she was quite depressed around that time and starts to cry again. After a minute or two, she cleans herself with her handkerchief and continues to talk about how happy she was during the years that she lived with her family. The patient does not talk about her sister other than mentioning that she owns a clothing store and that the two of them are also quite close.

Mental Status Examination: The patient is an attractive woman, dressed in a flamboyant purple suit and wearing heavy make-up. During the course of the interview, she frequently makes dramatic gestures when giving answers. She is cooperative, attention-seeking, and overtly seductive during the interview. The patient describes her mood as "great," but her affect is labile with rapid changes from sadness with tears to anger with temper tantrums. When asked specifically, the patient denies being emotional at these moments. She also denies suicidal ideation or behavior. The patient is alert and oriented, and no disturbances in memory functions are evident. Concentration, attention, and impulse control appear to be within normal limits. The patient denies any thought or perceptual disturbances. Her insight and judgment are limited, as evidenced by her lack of awareness of her own true feelings and how her behavior affects others.

Questions: What is the diagnosis? How can we understand the patient's presentation?

Diagnosis: Histrionic personality disorder (HPD).

Discussion: A personality disorder is a pervasive and persistent pattern of behavior that usually begins by late adolescence or early adulthood and is consistent across a number of contexts. HPD is categorized as a Cluster B personality disorder—the Dramatic Cluster—in the DSM-IV-TR. The prevalence of HPD is estimated at approximately 2–3% in the general population and at about 10–15% in mental health settings. HPD is diagnosed more frequently in women than in men. People who have experienced childhood abuse or neglect are also considerably more likely to develop personality disorders, including HPD. It is now widely accepted that personality disorders have a genetic basis. However, the etiology of HPD is still unknown. In contrast to other personality disorders (e.g., antisocial, borderline, schizotypal) very little research has been done on HPD. To date, no neurobiologic, neuroimaging, or genetic studies have been conducted.

As with the 29-year old woman described above, the behavior of patients with HPD is characterized as dramatic, extroverted, and emotional. The diagnosis is made by observing at least five particular characteristics. One of the main features is that patients are uncomfortable in situations in which they are not the center of attention. In their attention-seeking behavior, patients tend to exaggerate, dramatize, and display flirtatious, seductive behavior. Patients often have rapidly shifting and shallow emotional expression; however, this expression tends to be overly dramatic and exaggerated. They consistently use their physical appearance to draw attention to themselves, and they tend to consider relationships to be more intimate than they actually are. Their speech is often lacking in detail. Finally, they are suggestible and easily influenced by others.

When patients with HPD do not receive enough praise, attention, or approval, they may become extremely angry or sad, displaying temper tantrums or bursting into tears. When asked to elaborate on these expressed feelings, they may react with surprise or simply deny being emotional, as did the current patient. Patients with histrionic personality disorder have an extreme need for reassurance; they may act on their sexual impulses to reassure themselves that they are attractive to the other sex. Some female histrionic patients may be anorgasmic (as was the current patient), and male histrionic patients may be impotent. Defense mechanisms include dissociation, repression, and emotionality itself. By becoming intensely yet superficially emotional, patients may try to defend against deeper emotions. Frequently, they are unaware of their deeper feelings and tend to forget or deny previous emotional events.

As with other Cluster B disorders, associations with other psychiatric conditions have been found, including depression, anxiety (especially around separation), alcohol and other substance abuse, and somatization disorder. There is clinical overlap between patients with histrionic and borderline personality disorder, although suicide attempts and brief psychotic episodes are more likely to occur in the latter. The distinction between the two can be quite difficult, and both disorders can also be diagnosed in the same patient. In the past, a distinction was made between the diagnosis hysterical personality disorder for "healthy"/high-functioning patients, and the diagnosis histrionic personality disorder for the more "sick"/dysfunctional patients. However, others have argued that these two types of personality disorders are simply gradations along the continuum of HPD, as defined by the DSM-IV-TR.

As patients with histrionic personality disorder grow older, they tend to show fewer symptoms. In many patients, however, the attention-seeking behavior may persist, although not as clearly visible as in the years of their youth. When patients become more "fixed" in their life as an adult with a regular job, a partner, and children, their histrionic features become less overt. Of course, under significant emotional stress or other specific circumstances (e.g., alcohol or substance use), the behavioral and other personality features may be easily triggered. Psychoanalytically oriented psychotherapy is probably the treatment of choice. Psychotherapy often focuses on helping patients become more aware of their emotions. Pharmacotherapy, such as antidepressants or anxiolytics, can be used adjunctively in patients with psychiatric comorbidity, but large-scale trials for any treatment modality in HPD are lacking.

Pearls

1. Genetic factors play a role in the pathogenesis of HPD, as evidenced by twin studies. The genetic component of personality disorders like HPD is most likely polygenic and highly complex. However, the specific etiology remains unknown.
2. Histrionic personality disorder is more frequently diagnosed in women, and patients may have experienced childhood neglect or abuse. Furthermore, epidemiologic studies have suggested that HPD is more prevalent in some cultures than in others.
3. Some psychiatrists and psychologists make a distinction between hysterical personality disorder for the "healthy"/high-functioning patients, and histrionic personality disorder for the more "sick"/dysfunctional patients. Whether these PD clusters represent different etiologic entities or are simply gradations along a continuum remains controversial.

REFERENCES

1. Kaplan HI, Sadock BJ: Concise Textbook of Clinical Psychiatry. Baltimore, Williams & Wilkins, 1996.
2. Gabbard GO: Psychodynamic Psychiatry in Clinical Practice. The DSM-IV Edition. Washington, DC, American Psychaitric Press, 1994.
3. Johnson JG, Cohen P, Skodol AE, et al: Personality disorders in adolescence and risk of major mental disorders and suicidality during adulthood. Arch Gen Psychiatry 1999;56:805–611.
4. Lenzenweger MF: Stability and change in personality disorder features. Arch Gen Psychiatry 1999;56:1009–1015.
5. Johnson JG, Cohen P, Brown J, et al: Childhood maltreatment increases risk for personality disorders during early adulthood. Arch Gen Psychiatry 1999;56:600–606.
6. Reif A, Lesch K-P: Toward a molecular architecture of personality. Behav Brain Res 2003;139:1–20

PATIENT 49

A 6-year-old boy with nightmares

History of Present Illness: A 6-year-old boy, usually in good health, is brought to the pediatrician by his parents in the context of several recent episodes in which the child suddenly began screaming in his sleep. The episodes occurred approximately 90 minutes after the child had gone to bed and lasted anywhere from 1 minute to 7 minutes. The parents attempted to soothe the child but to no avail. The child was inconsolable, and they had great difficulty comforting him. When the child finally calmed down, he looked around the room, asked where he was, and went back to sleep. The parents thought that he had simply suffered from a severe nightmare and were thus quite surprised in the morning when they discovered that he did not remember anything of the previous night's events and claimed that he did not dream. The next four nights were uneventful and the child slept well. However, similar episodes on the fifth and sixth nights, with a single enuretic episode on the sixth night, prompted the current evaluation. The pediatrician deemed the child physically healthy and subsequently referred him to a child psychiatrist.

The boy lives with his parents and 2-year-old brother. The family moved from the Midwest to the East Coast 3 months ago. The boy recently started first grade in public school and has been doing well academically but reportedly has difficulty making friends and is frequently picked on by some of his peers.

Past History: The parents described the boy as a colicky baby for the first 6 months of life, with subsequent frequent nighttime awakenings. From the age of 6 months until recently, however, he slept well. The child met all developmental milestones on time. He has been toilet-trained since the age of 3 with occasional and infrequent nocturnal enuresis. He was noted to have had several sleep-walking episodes at 4 years of age, at the time his younger brother was born. He is nevertheless described as a happy child and appears to have a relatively well-functioning family with supportive, married parents.

Mental Status Examination: The patient is well groomed and clean, with normal size and weight for age. He is shy but attentive and cooperative and fairly well related with good eye contact. Behavior is appropriate without psychomotor retardation or agitation. Speech is of normal volume, rate, and rhythm. The patient describes his mood as "okay," but his affect appears mildly dysphoric. Thought processes are logical and goal-oriented. He denies any suicidal or homicidal ideation. He also denies auditory or visual hallucinations, and there is no evidence of paranoid ideation. His concentration and memory are normal. The patient's insight is fair, and his judgment is good.

Diagnostic Testing: The parents used a camcorder to document the episodes for the pediatrician to see. Nighttime polysomnography was not indicated at this time. EEG was not currently indicated.

Question: What is the most likely diagnosis?

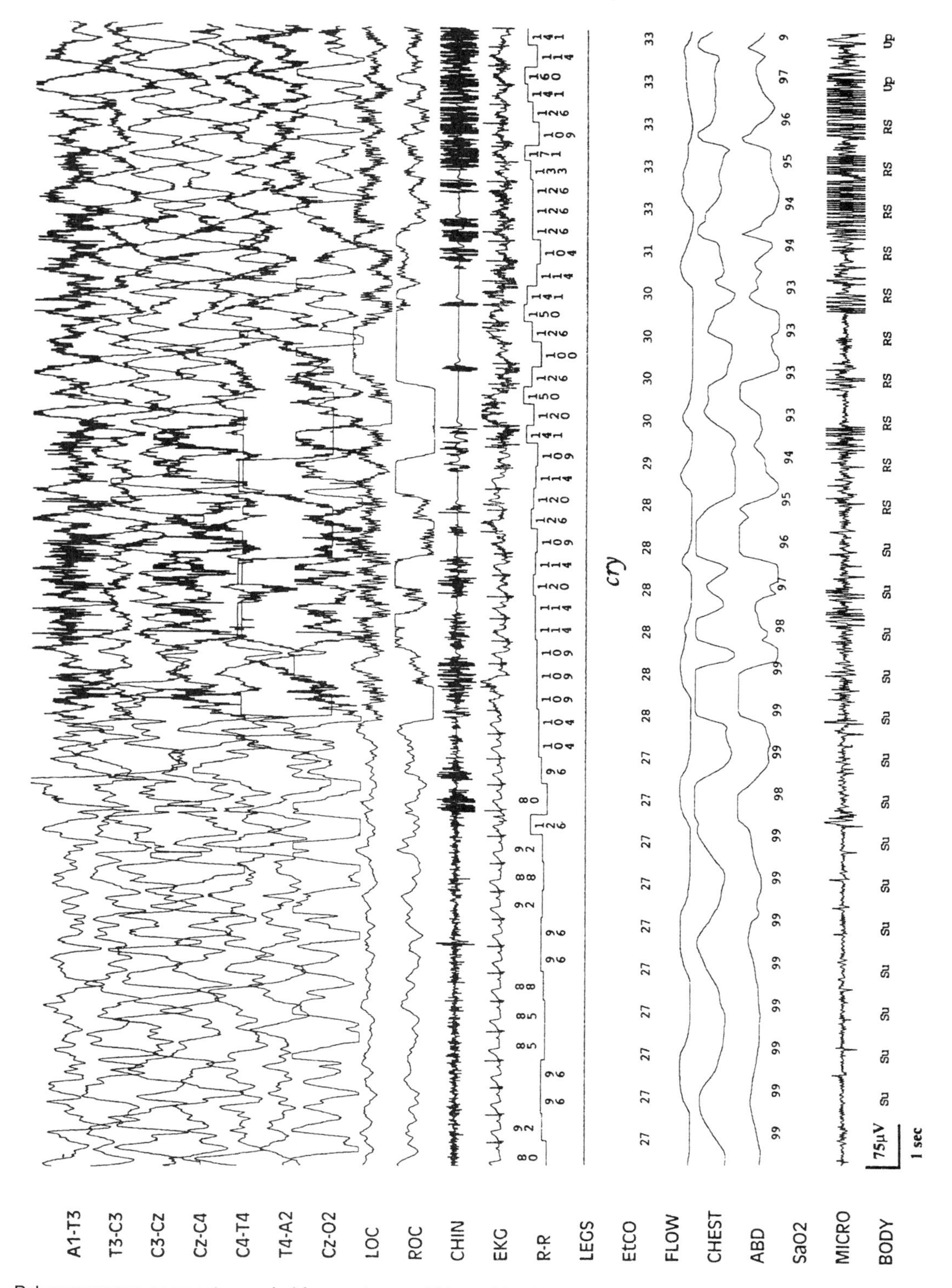

Polysomnogram segment recorded from a 4-year-old boy with a history of abrupt onset of screaming during sleep. The recording demonstrates slow-wave sleep. Note the abrupt and sudden arousal with movement and muscle artifact in the chin lead. Slow, 0.1-Hz EEG background activity is present. Increases in respiratory and heart rate are also associated with this episode. (From Sheldon SH, Riter S, Detrojan M: Atlas of Sleep Medicine in Infants and Children. Armonk, NY, Futura Publishing Company, 1999, with permission.)

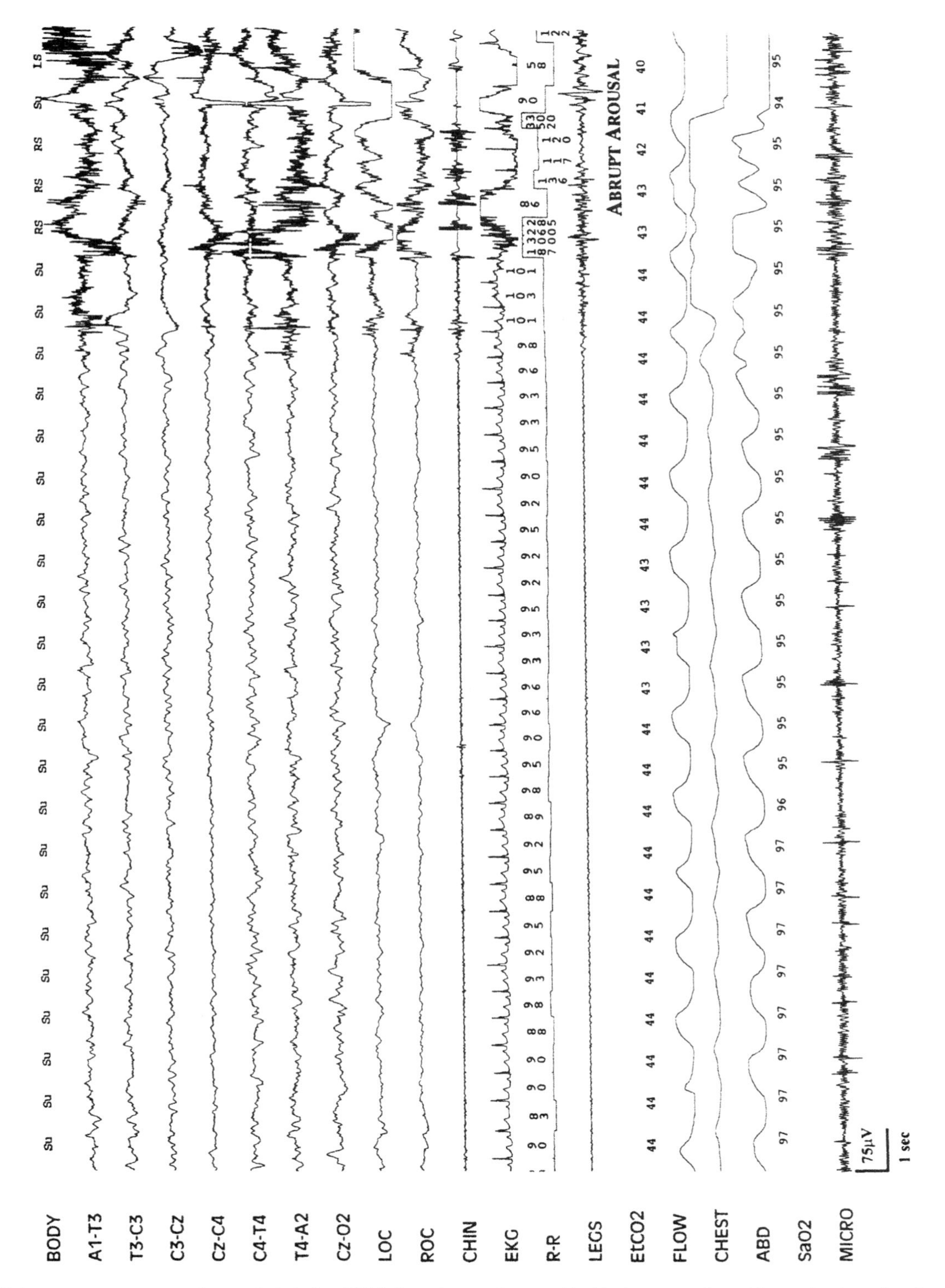

Polysomnogram segment recorded during REM sleep from a 5-year-old girl who was referred for evaluation of early morning wakenings and vivid nightmares occurring 2 to 3 times per week. Note the abrupt arousal and awakening from REM sleep. Heart rate is mildly elevated during the arousal, but no other symptoms of autonomic arousal are present. After the episode, the patient was easily comforted by her mother and returned to sleep with only minimal delay. (From Sheldon SH, Riter S, Detrojan M: Atlas of Sleep Medicine in Infants and Children. Armonk, NY, Futura Publishing Company, 1999, with permission.)

Diagnosis: Sleep terror attack.

Discussion: Sleep disorders are divided into four broad categories in the DSM-IV-TR: (1) primary sleep disorders (dyssomnias and parasomnias); (2) sleep disorder related to another mental disorder; (3) sleep disorder due to a general medical condition, and (4) substance-induced sleep disorder. This discussion focuses on the primary sleep disorders, dyssomnias and parasomnias.

The **dyssomnias** are disturbances in the amount or timing of sleep whether insufficient, inefficient, or excessive. Dyssomnias are further divided into the intrinsic, extrinsic, and circadian rhythm dyssomnias. The intrinsic dyssomnias originate from causes within the body and consist of obstructive sleep apnea syndrome and narcolepsy, which is the only dyssomnia of rapid-eye-movement (REM) sleep. The extrinsic dyssomnias are due to external factors and are termed primary insomnias in DSM-IV-TR. They are defined as disorders of initiating and maintaining sleep. The circadian rhythm dyssomnias occur because of inappropriate timing of sleep within the 24-hour day. They are due to prolonged periods of sleep deprivation or persistent irregularities in sleep hygiene, which inevitably lead to delayed sleep phase syndrome (DSPS) or a disruption of the biologic clock.

The **parasomnias** are abnormal behaviors or physiologic events that occur during sleep and intrude on ongoing sleep. The parasomnias are subdivided into (1) arousal disorders (sleep/night terror disorder, sleep-walking disorder, and confusional arousals); (2) sleep-wake transition disorders (sleep-talking, nocturnal leg cramps, rhythmic movement disorder [head-banging, sleep starts, body-rocking]); (3) REM parasomnias (nightmares and REM sleep behavior disorder); and (4) miscellaneous parasomnias (sleep bruxism, sleep enuresis).

The present patient was diagnosed with sleep terror attacks. Sleep terror attacks occur with a sudden autonomic sympathetic system discharge, such as screaming, crying out, palpitations, irregular respiration, and diaphoresis. The attacks last from 30 seconds to 10 minutes, and it is difficult to arouse patients because they are typically not reactive to external stimuli. When awakened, the patient shows mental confusion and disorientation; retrograde amnesia for the episode is characteristic. The attack occurs in the first 1 to 2 hours after sleep onset, which is the time of transition from non-REM (NREM) stage IV sleep to REM sleep. Sleep attacks are most commonly associated with partial arousals from stage III or IV NREM sleep.

Occurrences of sleep terror attacks are sporadic and thus difficult to predict. They are more frequent in children between the ages of 2 and 6 years old and have an estimated prevalence of between 3% and 7% in this population. They are more likely to occur during periods of illness, stress, or sleep deprivation, but they can also occur without any obvious associated stress. People with one form of parasomnia are also more likely to manifest symptoms of another form (e.g., somnambulism/sleep-walking), and a family history of parasomnias is common.

The main differential diagnosis for sleep terror attacks is nightmares. In comparison with sleep terror attacks, nightmares are frightening arousals from REM sleep associated with dream reports that are anxiety-laden. Nightmares predominate during the second half of the night during REM sleep. Stress, especially traumatic experiences, increases the frequency and severity of nightmares. In comparison to sleep terrors, nightmares are usually easily recalled in the morning.

The differential diagnosis also includes temporal lobe epilepsy that occurs at night, as manifested by hallucinations, incomplete arousal, fear, and automatic behavior. Suspicions of seizure activity when awake, a large degree of autonomic activation, and enuresis during the episode warrant an electroencephalogram (EEG).

Sleep terror attacks, nightmares, and primary sleep disorders in children are treated with behavioral and supportive methods. An understanding of the underlying anxiety or major life stressor and the provision of parental support, reassurance, and encouragement for the child are imperative for alleviating sleep disorders. Angry threats, ridicule, and punitive measures should be avoided. The focus of treatment is on reducing stress and fatigue (due to association of sleep deprivation with sleep terrors). Benzodiazapines and tricyclic antidepressants have also been used in the treatment of sleep terrors because they suppress stages 3 and 4 of the sleep cycle. There are no studies to confirm their efficacy, however.

The boy was evaluated by a child psychiatrist. After getting the history, interviewing the child, and viewing the tapes of the nighttime episodes, the psychiatrist concluded that the boy is suffering from sleep terror attacks. He reassured the parents that these attacks are benign, have an excellent prognosis, and are usually self-limited. The psychiatrist explained to the parents that sleep terror attacks are usually associated with major life stressors such as the families' recent move, starting a new school, and having difficulty with peer relationships. He instructed the parents to remain patient and supportive of the child. If the episodes recurred, he advised them simply to sit by the boy's side and comfort him as the episodes passed instead of trying to wake him. The psychiatrist also recommended that the child be enrolled in after-school activities and that the parents arrange play dates with children in his class to improve his social skills and increase peer interactions. The parents asked the psychiatrist whether he thought on EEG was indicated since a family friend has a child with a seizure disorder who frequently urinates in his bed during a seizure episode. The psychiatrist again reassured the parents by stating that bedwetting is also precipitated by stressful life events and that it is not uncommon for children to have an occasional enuretic accident throughout childhood. The parents were further instructed to keep a log book of the sleep terror and enuretic episodes.

One month later, the parents and child were seen in a follow-up appointment with the psychiatrist. As per recommendations, they had enrolled the child in two after-school programs. He also has weekly play dates and is now invited to some of his classmates' homes on the weekend. There were two more sleep terror attacks since the child was last seen, but this pattern represented a significant decrease in frequency. The enuretic episodes had ceased. Both the parents and psychiatrist noted the child's brightened affect and significant improvement in mood. The next follow-up was scheduled for 3 months.

Pearls

1. Sleep terror attacks occur in the first third of the sleep cycle and are partial arousals from stage III or IV NREM sleep. Nightmares occur in the last third of the sleep cycle during REM sleep.
2. Sleep terror attacks are usually not remembered the morning after the episode, but nightmares are usually well remembered.
3. Nightmares are significantly more common than sleep terror attacks: 3-7% of children 2 to 6 years of age suffer from sleep terror disorder, whereas 10-50% of children 2 to 6 years of age suffer from nightmares.
4. Sleep terrors are usually self-limited and may be related to a specific developmental conflict, a precipitating traumatic event or major life stressor, or illness.

REFERENCES

1. Andres TF, Eiben LA: Pediatric sleep disorders. J Am Acad Child Adolesc Psychiatry 1997;36(1):9–20.
2. Blum J, Carey WB: Sleep problems among infants and young children. Pediatr Rev 1996;17:87–92.
3. Chokroverty S: Diagnoses and treatment of sleep disorders caused by co-morbid disease. Neurology 2000;54(5 Suppl 1):S8–S15.
4. Coleman J: Sleep apnea. Part II: Overview of sleep disorders. Otolaryngol Clin North Am 1999;32(2):187–193.
5. Ferber R: Sleep disorders. Part I: Childhood sleep disorders. Neurol Clin 1996;14(3):493–511.
6. Laberge L, Tremblay RE, Vitaro F, Montplaisir J: Development of parasomnias from childhood to early adolescence. Pediatrics 2000;106(1 Pt 1):67–74.
7. The Merck Manual, 17th ed. Merck & Co., Inc., 1999, pp 2247–2248.
8. Sheldon SH, Riter S, Detrojan M: Atlas of Sleep Medicine in Infants and Children. Armonk, NY, Futura Publishing, 1999.

Rebecca L. West
Amir Garakani, MD

PATIENT 50

A 33-year-old man with rage and threatening behavior

History of Present Illness: A 33-year-old man is brought into the psychiatric emergency department by police after he attacks another man in a bar and threatens to "rip [your] throat out with [my] bare hands." The patient apparently returned from the restroom in the bar to find the man putting an arm around his girlfriend. The patient states that he immediately became "enraged" and began to scream obscenities. The shouting quickly escalated into a full-blown bar brawl, and the police intervened when the patient wrapped his hands around the man's throat and pinned him against the bar.

The patient admits to numerous incidents of this nature and has found himself in fights several times each year since late adolescence. Two months ago, he was arrested for smashing a car window with a baseball bat when a man "cut him off" on the highway. The patient was also fired from several jobs in his late 20s due to his "hot temper" with coworkers who were trying to "slight him." The patient believes that his actions are sometimes unreasonable, but the combination of heightened energy, racing thoughts, and anger makes his urges nearly impossible to resist.

The patient's girlfriend claims that he is a fun-loving and charming man between episodes but starts arguments with her approximately twice a week. She claims that during his verbal attacks he will often make demeaning and devaluing remarks about her. On several occasions he has broken her personal belongings during trivial arguments. The patient acknowledges that he regrets these episodes, but they usually subside within a half an hour and provide an instant sense of relief.

Past Psychiatric History: No psychiatric history or past use of psychiatric medications is reported. The patient denies symptoms of a mood disorder. He admits to 1 or 2 alcoholic drinks per week and a history of marijuana experimentation in his late teenage years.

Mental Status Examination: The patient appears well built and sharply dressed and looks his stated age. He is awake, alert, and oriented to person, place, and time. Behavior is appropriate, and eye contact is good. Speech is clear and coherent with normal rate, rhythm, and volume. Mood is euthymic, and affect is full. Thought process is logical and goal-directed. Thought content does not include delusions, ideas of reference, paranoid ideation, suicidal ideation, or homicidal ideation. Impulse control is poor, as noted by his recent violent outbursts. Insight is limited because he does not recognize the maladaptive nature of his behavior. Judgment is impaired, as evidenced by his inability to behave in socially accepted ways. Reliability is fair.

Laboratory Testing: Sodium, 141; potassium, 4.2; chloride, 106; carbon dioxide, 23; blood urea nitrogen, 9; creatinine, 0.6; glucose, 91. Blood alcohol level and urine toxicology screen are negative.

Diagnostic Testing: CT of the head shows no signs of mass, lesion, or bleeding. Electroencephalogram is unremarkable without signs of slowing or seizure foci.

Physical Examination: The man appears healthy, and the exam is within normal limits without remarkable findings.

Questions: What is the diagnosis? How should you proceed with treatment?

Diagnosis: Intermittent explosive disorder (IED).

Discussion: Intermittent explosive disorder (IED) is a controversial diagnosis in the psychiatric literature. The symptom of aggression is seen in a wide range of medical and psychiatric diagnoses, and many authorities have difficulty in viewing IED as an independent diagnostic entity. However, IED is classified as an impulse control disorder in the DSM-IV-TR, and its central feature is the failure to resist an impulse to perform an act that is harmful to self or others. The person feels an increasing sense of tension before the act and then experiences relief at the time of committing the act. Of note, people with IED have high rates of other lifetime DSM-IV-TR diagnoses. One study of patients with IED noted the following comorbidities: major depressive disorder (37%), bipolar disorder I or II (51%), substance abuse (48%), anxiety disorders (48%), and other impulse control disorders (44%). Therefore, IED is probably best understood as a distinct disorder that is highly comorbid with other psychiatric conditions.

IED is characterized by several discrete episodes of failure to resist aggressive impulses that result in serious assaultive acts or destruction of property. The degree of aggressiveness expressed during the episodes is grossly out of proportion to any precipitating psychosocial stressor. According to the DSM-IV-TR, the aggressive episodes are not better explained by another mental disorder and are not due to the direct physiologic effects of a substance or medical condition. The assaultive acts include either physical assault of another person or verbal threats to physically harm another person. The outbursts may take the form of frequent, low-intensity episodes or infrequent, high-intensity episodes. Low-intensity episodes may include verbal attacks, whereas high-intensity episodes may involve physical assault, destruction of property, "road rage," or even homicide. Research has demonstrated that approximately 70% of patients display both aggression patterns, as noted in this case.

The current patient was diagnosed with IED based on the presence of all of the above features. Other diagnoses that may have been considered include antisocial personality disorder, borderline personality disorder, mania, psychosis, conduct disorder, head trauma, or seizure disorder. Although the patient exhibited some symptoms suggestive of mania or psychosis, including heightened energy, racing thoughts, and anger, the duration of these episodes is too short to meet criteria for a manic episode. A thorough interview of the patient and his girlfriend ruled out a history of premeditated, volitional, or purposeful violent acts, as might be seen in borderline personality disorder or conduct disorder. A substance use disorder is unlikely given his negative blood alcohol level and toxicology screen as well as his history of limited alcohol intake at the present time. A CT scan, EEG, and review of his medical records failed to demonstrate a history of traumatic brain injury or seizures in the past.

IED was presumed to be rare in the past due to exclusion criteria such as antisocial or borderline personality disorder imposed by previous editions of the DSM, but it is now diagnosed with increasing frequency. A recent survey using the Structured Clinical Interview for DSM-IV Diagnoses demonstrated that 3.8% of subjects met current and 6.2% met lifetime criteria for IED. IED is seen more often in men. However, it is becoming more commonly recognized in women. Some women have also reported an increase in IED symptoms during the premenstrual period. The onset of this disorder may occur from childhood through the early twenties. The course in variable and may be chronic in some cases but episodic in others. Although familial linkage has not been established by genetic studies, family history data suggest a hereditary component. Childhood abuse is thought to be a risk factor for the development of IED.

Several etiologic theories have been proposed. One of the leading psychodynamic explanations is narcissistic vulnerability. As in this case, assaultive episodes result from a real or perceived insult to self-esteem or as a reaction to a perceived threat of rejection or abandonment. The most common presentation of IED is a large man who reacts to feelings of worthlessness or impotence with aggressive behavior.

Patients treated for IED may achieve symptom resolution; however, the treatment takes approximately 3 to 5 years and is typically a significant clinical challenge. Cognitive-behavioral therapy and anger management techniques are thought to be helpful. Anger management techniques may involve various relaxation tools, cognitive restructuring, and communication skills training. Some therapists have also tried systematic desensitization. However, pharmacology is usually needed in addition to therapy. Numerous medications have been tried in this population. One controlled study demonstrated that selective serotonin reuptake inhibitors (SSRIs) reduce overt aggression and irritability by 67% in patients with personality disorders and a history of impulsive aggression. Other controlled studies have revealed that both lithium and phenytoin reduce impulsive aggression in prison populations. Carbamazepine was shown in one controlled trial to decrease impulsive aggression in people with borderline personality disorder. Treatment of IED with antidepressants or mood stabilizers requires a trial period of 3 months, and patients are likely to return with discontinuation of the medication. Atypical antipsychotic medications and beta receptor antagonists are less well-studied but may also be useful in the treatment of IED. At this point, few controlled trials of treatments for IED have been published using DSM-IV criteria, and more investigation is needed.

As seen in this case, IED can have a tremendous impact on interpersonal and professional relationships. A clear understanding of IED is of substantial importance due to the social and clinical implications of its course on affected patients. In this case, the patient was referred to an anger management program and was started on an SSRI. At 6 months of treatment, there was clear improvement with only one episode of road rage and reduced severity of verbal attacks on his girlfriend.

Pearls

1. Some investigators have demonstrated altered serotonin metabolism in cerebrospinal fluid and platelets of patients with IED, suggesting that serotonin may play a key role in IED. PET scan studies have demonstrated that people with intermittent explosive disorder have less serotonin activity in the orbital-frontal cortex than controls.
2. In the DSM-IV criteria for IED, antisocial and borderline personality disorders are no longer exclusion criteria. Therefore, IED is diagnosed more frequently in the clinical setting.
3. Characteristics of intermittent explosive disorder that suggest a link to bipolar disorder include the presence of mood and energy changes, the substantial comorbidity with bipolar disorder, and the treatment response to mood stabilizers.
4. Neurologic soft signs, nonspecific EEG changes, and mild abnormalities on neuropsychological testing have been recorded in patients with IED. These findings are compatible with a diagnosis of IED and preempt the diagnosis only if they are indicative of a diagnosable medical condition.

REFERENCES

1. American Psychiatric Association: Diagnostic and Statistical Manual of Mental Disorders, 4th ed, Text Revised. Washington, DC, American Psychiatric Association, 2000.
2. Barratt ES, Stanford MS, Felthous AR, Kent TA: The effects of phenytoin on impulsive and premeditated aggression: A controlled study. J Clin Psychopharmacol 1997;17:341–349.
3. Coccaro EF: Intermittent explosive disorder: Taming temper tantrums in the volatile, impulsive adult. Curr Psychiatry 2003;2: 42–60.
4. Gardner DL, Cowdry RW: Positive effects of carbamazepine on behavioral dyscontrol in borderline personality disorder. Am J Psychiatry 1986;143:519–522.
5. McElroy SL: Recognition and treatment of DSM-IV intermittent explosive disorder. J Clin Psychiatry 1999;60(Suppl 15):12–16.
6. McElroy SL, Soutullo CA, Beckman DA, et al: DSM-IV intermittent explosive disorder: A report of 27 cases. J Clin Psychiatry 1998;59:203–210.
7. Sadock BJ, Sadock VA: Comprehensive Textbook of Psychiatry, 7th ed. Baltimore, Williams & Wilkins, 2000, pp 1709–1711.
8. Thompson JW, Winstead DK: Impulse control disorders. In Current Diagnosis and Treatment in Psychiatry. New York, McGraw-Hill, 2000, pp 453–454.
9. Zimmerman M, Mattia J, Younken S, et al: The prevalence of DSM-IV impulse control disorders in psychiatric outpatients (APA new research abstracts no. 265). Washington, DC, American Psychiatric Publishing, 1998.

PATIENT 51

A 35-year-old woman with anxiety

History of Present Illness: The patient is a 35-year-old divorced woman who works as a kindergarten teacher. She has no formal psychiatric history, and her medical problems include a history of childhood leukemia, hypothyroidism, and chronic migraine headaches. She presents for intake at the outpatient psychiatry clinic with the vague complaint of "anxiety." When asked to elaborate, she describes being referred by her school counselor after she started showing up late to work on a fairly regular basis about 1 month ago. She reports being too ashamed to tell her superiors that she was late because she feared getting on the subway and instead made up excuses ranging from "problems putting my contact lenses in" to broken elevators in her building. Her primary concern at present is wanting to be able to use the subway expeditiously, but she mentions that other problems have started to bother her as well—namely, going to the movies (she cannot sit in the middle of the row), having lunch with coworkers, and "just feeling anxious for no reason at all."

In describing her symptoms related to the train, she feels that people are too close to her and that there is too much talking. She feels overwhelmed, fearful of not being able to escape. Similar fears plague her at the movies. Her heart starts racing, she becomes short of breath, her lips tingle, and she feels "out of it" and has the sensation that she is going to die. These symptoms are exacerbated when, in the midst of the 10-minute episode, she realizes that there is nowhere she can go for help, no way to escape. Since she has started to have these experiences daily, she has been avoiding crowded places: "I feel best when I'm either alone or with a good friend, and especially if we have some wine—though the next day I seem to be worse." If she stays home or avoids the above-mentioned areas, she experiences no overt discomfort.

When asked in greater detail about the preceding few months of her life, she relays the story of a long and complicated divorce that was just finalized about 4 months ago. "Why, when I should be so relieved that it's finally over and I can get on with my life, does this start happening to me?" She also notes the recent stressor of an increased financial burden with the loss of the second income from her ex-husband. She denies any associated neurovegetative symptoms of sleep, appetite, or energy changes as well as depressed or elevated mood, anhedonia, guilt, suicidality/homicidality, ritualistic behavior, counting, checking, or hoarding, and delusions or hallucinations.

Past Psychiatric History: The patient has never been to a psychiatrist, psychologist, or social worker and has never received psychotropic medications. She denies any history of suicidal ideation, attempts, or other form of deliberate self-harm.

Past Medical History: As stated above, the patient had childhood leukemia (treated with chemotherapy), chronic migraine headaches, and hypothyroidism that developed after treatment for Graves' disease. She currently takes levothyroxine, 100 μg daily, but no other medications besides vitamins.

Substance Use: She drinks an average of 1–2 glasses of wine every other day. She smoked some cannabis in college. She reports no use of cocaine, heroin, hallucinogens, or inhalants. She does not smoke cigarettes and drinks 1–2 cups of coffee per day.

Family History: The patient reports that her mother was "a nervous wreck" who "would have these spells where every once in a while she just ran away to be by herself for about half an hour."

Mental Status Examination: The patient is an attractive woman of average build, wearing jeans and a sweater. Although she is calm and cooperative, she appears to be on edge but not overtly jumpy. There is no psychomotor agitation or retardation. Speech is spontaneous with a normal rate, rhythm, and volume. Mood is euthymic. Affect is mildly constricted and primarily nervous but appropriate to content and congruent with mood. No formal thought disorder is present. Thought content primarily concerns these episodes of intense and acute anxiety, as described in the history above. No delusional material was elicited. No illusions or hallucinations are present, and the patient does not appear to be preoccupied with or responding to internal stimuli. She is neither suicidal nor homicidal. Insight and judgment are generally intact, as is impulse control. Attention and concentration are intact.

Laboratory/Imaging Studies: None completed. She was referred from the counselor at her place of employment without having a medical work-up first. She states that she does not know her thyroid hormone levels, but her dosage of hormone has not changed in years.

Questions: What is the diagnosis? What etiologic theories have been proposed?

Diagnosis: Panic disorder with agoraphobia.

Discussion: The patient was diagnosed tentatively with panic disorder with agoraphobia, although formally she should have been given the diagnosis of anxiety disorder not otherwise specified. Anxiety disorder due to a general medical condition (hyperthyroidism) should be ruled out because a medical cause of her symptoms was still quite possible.

Her main presenting complaint was agoraphobia. By definition, agoraphobia is a morbid fear of open spaces or of leaving the home or other familiar setting. Different studies have reported different prevalence rates of agoraphobia, but most conclude that most cases occur in the context of comorbid panic disorder. Clinically, the agoraphobic patient enacts certain avoidant behaviors, specifically in response to a fear of developing panic symptoms. People who fear having panic attacks in public may retreat to a place of safety and comfort—a place where help is easy to find if necessary. Although the current opinion among researchers and clinicians is that agoraphobia is usually a secondary reaction to panic attacks, we do not yet know what importance comorbid agoraphobia has to a diagnosis of panic disorder other than to increase the degree of impairment. And what about treatment implications? To date, no reproducible and consistent biologic differences have been found between patients with panic disorder with agoraphobia and patients with panic disorder without agoraphobia. For a discussion of the clinical presentation and treatment options for panic disorder, see Patient 23. Although agoraphobia is not specifically mentioned, the same general principles of treatment (pharmacotherapy and cognitive behavioral therapy) apply.

The etiology of panic disorder is currently a topic of intense research, specifically on genetic, neuroanatomic, biochemical, and psychological fronts. Genetic research has found a 7- to 8-fold increased risk of panic disorder in first-degree relatives of patients with the illness. Twin and population-based studies have determined that inheritance is polygenic and multifactorial, with a genetic contribution of 30–40% to the disorder's etiology. Biologic theories surround dysregulations of the adrenergic system (misfiring of the locus coeruleus) as well as the serotonergic and the GABAergic systems (effective treatment includes serotonergic drugs and benzodiazepines). Neuroanatomic studies have focused on the interactions among the limbic (emotion and memory) system, the locus coeruleus, the raphe nuclei, and the inhibitory properties of the frontal cortex; most results point to a dysregulation in a complex feedback circuit involving all of these areas. Biochemical studies have found that inhalation of a 35% solution of carbon dioxide or infusion of sodium lactate (intravenously or orally) can precipitate panic attacks in patients with panic disorder but not in normal controls. Hypotheses of a false suffocation alarm have been well-studied with mostly positive results. During hyperventilation a drop in the carbon dioxide content of the blood causes the patient to feel dizziness, tinnitus, headache, numbness in the face and hands, and a paradoxical feeling of breathlessness, mimicking and hence increasing the fearful symptoms inherent in a panic attack. Psychologically, 60–96% of cases first manifest in the context of separation or loss, relational problems, or the development of new responsibility.

Although panic disorder is a chronic condition, reports differ as to whether the illness waxes and wanes or follows a more stable course. Scientifically based knowledge about the long-term course as well as predictors of outcome are generally lacking, although exacerbations certainly occur at times of increased stress. Of note, there is no general consensus about operationalized remission criteria for panic disorder, and different studies have used different outcome criteria. This lack of uniformity tends to confuse the issue, especially since there may be a dissociation between panic attack frequency and other outcomes. For example, patients may reduce the frequency of attacks by avoiding certain situations, and such agoraphobic avoidance may become chronic regardless of the presence or absence of panic attacks. Rates of general improvement after psychotherapeutic or medication treatment are similar on average, although different studies cite different numbers. At up to 10 years after treatment, 30% of patients are "well," 40–50% are improved but still symptomatic, and 20–30% are unchanged. Prognosis is generally good: if the patient has not experienced complete remission, he or she will most likely experience a much reduced symptom load. Most treatment failures are due to inadequate dosing of medications and inadequate length of medication trials. Indicators of poor prognosis include lower socioeconomic status, poor education, increased duration of disorder, presence of a psychiatric comorbidity (including a personality disorder), death of a parent, divorce, or other intense and acute psychosocial stressors.

The differential diagnosis of panic disorder includes all disorders that can have panic attacks in their symptom profiles, from psychotic-level syndromes to anxious states of hypochondriasis, social phobia, specific phobia, generalized anxiety disorder, and obsessive-compulsive disorder. However, in these differential diagnoses, the panic attacks are always situationally bound. Thus, although panic attacks are a common symptom, they are nonspecific, except when they are spontaneous and unprecipitated—a pattern that occurs only in panic disorder. But even in panic disorder they may become situationally related at some point, and having the patient keep a diary of symptoms can assist in making this distinction clinically apparent. The presence of anticipatory anxiety and agoraphobic avoidance also are important in distinguishing panic disorder from other possibilities. In each of the abovementioned differential diagnoses, the anxiety and avoidance are dependent on a certain stimulus or feared consequence, whereas in panic disorder the anxiety and fear are related to concerns about future panic attacks.

All of this information taken into account, there is significant comorbidity between panic disorder and other anxiety disorders: social phobia (15–30%), generalized anxiety disorder (15–30%), and obsessive-compulsive disorder (10%), to name a few. Furthermore, many patients have unexpected panic attacks during the course of a major depressive episode. Panic disorder should not be diagnosed unless at least 1 month of persistent worry about having future attacks and associated behavior changes are present. In this setting, both disorders may be diagnosed concurrently. The lifetime prevalence of comorbid major depressive disorder in panic disorder approaches 50%. One-half of these patients developed the two illnesses concurrently, whereas one-quarter developed one before the other.

The comorbidity of panic disorder is highly visible and clinically salient in the increased incidence of suicide attempts. Study results vary regarding the incidence of suicide attempts in patients with panic disorder with and without comorbidities: 1–7% in patients who are free from comorbidity (so-called uncomplicated panic disorder—present in only one-third of patients with panic disorder); up to 20% in patients with comorbid major depression; and up to 75% in patients with comorbid depression and alcohol-related disorders. Of note, as may have been evident in the current patient, approximately one-third of patients with panic disorder abuse alcohol, many in an effort to self-medicate. Forty to 50% of patients with panic disorder have a comorbid personality disorder, primarily from the anxious cluster (i.e., avoidant, obsessive-compulsive, and dependent). Medical comorbidities include irritable bowel syndrome, migraine headaches, pulmonary diseases (especially chronic obstructive pulmonary disease and asthma), and mitral valve prolapse, although the etiologic factors in these medical comorbidities are unknown. In treatment, medical and psychiatric comorbidities must be appropriately addressed and should influence the choice of therapy.

Panic disorder must be distinguished from the symptoms of a general medical condition. Hyperthyroidism, hyperparathyroidism, pheochromocytoma, vestibular dysfunctions, seizure disorders, and cardiac conditions can cause panic attacks with resulting anticipatory anxiety and phobic avoidance. However, the diagnosis in such cases would be anxiety disorder due to a general medical condition, and the symptoms would resolve with treatment of the medical condition. Likewise, panic attacks and their sequelae can be the result of either substance intoxication (e.g., cannabis or stimulants, including caffeine and nicotine), withdrawal (e.g., central nervous system depressants, such as alcohol and sedative-hypnotics), or past history of use (e.g., flashbacks of hallucinogen or inhalant "trips"). For a diagnosis of substance-induced anxiety disorder, the symptoms must have started within 1 month of the last use of the offending substance and must be etiologically related to the specific drug. When substances are involved in the presentation, the substance-related disorder must be treated first. The physician must take a careful history of the temporal components of substance use, because it may precipitate panic attacks or result from panic attacks in a patient's efforts to self-medicate. For both medical conditions and substance-related panic attacks, if the symptoms do not resolve after resolution of the primary disorder, a diagnosis of panic disorder is warranted. Usually, one should wait about 1 month after such resolution before assigning a primary diagnosis of panic disorder.

The present patient's symptoms fit quite nicely into the panic disorder concept. She manifests a typical constellation of symptoms inherent in a panic attack, although many different forms are possible. Although most of her panic attacks have occurred in the context of places from which escape might be difficult, she has had a few spontaneous, out-of-the-blue episodes, thus allowing the diagnosis of panic disorder rather than agoraphobia without panic disorder. Of note, even though her symptoms tend to abate when she remains home, the symptom of phobic avoidance is among the most troublesome in the syndrome because it is difficult to treat and causes the most psychosocial impairment. The patient is of the right age to develop such a disorder, and its onset follows a period of substantial loss in her life with the concurrent assignment of increased responsibilities; she is probably genetically loaded, as evidenced by her mother's vague panic-like symptoms. She is also like other people with panic disorder who tend to try to hide their symptoms out of a feeling of psychological weakness rather than acknowledge their presence and seek treatment.

At the conclusion of the initial intake interview, the psychiatrist recommended thyroid function testing as well as a complete chemistry and blood count panel to rule out a medical cause of the patient's symptoms. Cardiac concerns were minimized due to her age and lack of personal or familial history of cardiac disease. On return of the blood work with normal results, the patient was offered the choice of pharmacotherapy with a selective serotonin reuptake inhibitor (SSRI) or psychotherapy with cognitive-behavioral therapy (CBT). After a thorough presentation of the neurobiologic underpinnings and psychological understandings of panic disorder, as well as the expectations, mechanisms, and side effects of the treatments, she chose CBT, feeling that it would give her more control over her increasingly uncertain future. She underwent three and half months of weekly therapy, fully invested and participating in the treatment, and emerged symptom-free.

Pearls

1. The question remains as to whether the false suffocation alarm activated in times of stress has an evolutionary role. If one is genetically predisposed to develop such a misfiring during encounters with significant stress, can the same neuropathology be triggered de novo (i.e., out of the blue)?
2. Some recent controlled studies have concluded that the combination of pharmacotherapy and cognitive-behavioral therapy may not be better than either alone.
3. Directions for future research include (1) distinguishing among true comorbidity, symptom overlap within DSM-defined syndromes, and overlaps in fundamental psychopathology; (2) determining the ideal length of pharmacologic treatment; (3) the use of CBT vs. psychopharmacology in specific patients; and (4) the possibility of using "booster" CBT to prevent re-emergence of symptoms.
4. Panic attacks are quite common in schizophrenia and are often mistaken for overt hostility, aggression, or positive symptoms of psychosis.

REFERENCES

1. American Psychiatric Association: Practice Guideline for the Treatment of Patients with Panic Disorder. Washington, DC, American Psychiatric Press, 1998.
2. Ballenger JC: Panic disorder and agoraphobia. In Gelder MG, Lopez-Ibor JJ, Andreasen NC (eds): New Oxford Textbook of Psychiatry. Oxford, Oxford University Press, 2000, pp 807–822.
3. Goodwin R, Lyons JS, McNally RJ: Panic attacks in schizophrenia. Schizophrenia Res 2002;58(2-3):213–220.
4. Gorman JM, Kent JM, Sullivan GM, Coplan JD: Neuroanatomical hypothesis of panic disorder, revised. Am J Psychiatry 2000;157:493–505.
5. Lydiard RB, Otto MW, Milrod B: Panic disorder. In Gabbard GO (ed): Treatments of Psychiatric Disorders, 3rd ed, vols 1 and 2. Washington, DC, American Psychiatric Press, 2001.
6. Swoboda H, Amering M, Windhaber J, Katschnig H: The long-term course of panic disorder-an 11 year follow-up. Anxiety Disord 2001;17:223–232.

Matthew Rottnek, MFA
Arthur Fox, PhD

PATIENT 52

An 8-year-old boy with aggressiveness

History of Present Illness: An 8-year-old boy is brought into the psychiatric emergency department by his mother because of increasingly aggressive behavior toward himself and others. On the day of presentation, the patient threatened to strangle his 6-year-old sister when she would not let him play with her favorite Barbie doll. When his mother intervened and took the patient into her bedroom with her while she dressed, the patient became increasingly agitated and attempted to strangle himself with his mother's scarf while mocking her in front of the mirror.

The patient is prone to making suicidal and homicidal threats when he is upset and to biting his fingers and toes and pulling his hair when he does not "get his way." He has frequent difficulty with sleeping and is described by his mother as generally anxious, particularly around adult male family friends and relatives. He enjoys playing with dolls, especially styling their hair, and frequently expresses wishes that he were a "beautiful little girl" (e.g., when he sees his genitals while bathing). His mother reports that he talks with himself, sometimes "like he was really angry at someone." The patient denies this claim, stating that he has been secretly playing school with his stuffed animals under his bed.

Past Psychiatric History: The mother describes the patient as having been "incredibly sensitive and demanding" as an infant, but also affectionate and, once consoled, "extremely sweet—sweeter than the other kids, special." Imaginative play in preschool years was reported to be creative and focused but mostly solitary. In day care, the patient was described by workers as "a teacher's pet," affectionate and creative, but distractible, impulsive, and agitated when playing with peers. He sometimes had trouble sitting still in passive group activities. First- and second-grade teachers reported that the patient was extremely attentive to tasks in which he was interested, such as art and storytelling, but easily distracted by tasks requiring focused effort outside his areas of interest, such as arithmetic. Teachers also noted that the patient sometimes became sullen and silent during activities in which classmates were segregated by sex, such as gym. Being in a group of boys his own age "doesn't seem to make sense to him," reported one teacher.

One previous psychiatric consultation took place at age 6, following the imprisonment of the patient's father. The mother complained at the time that the patient was "so quiet most of the time, clingy, breaking all his toys, sometimes ripping his clothes while he's wearing them." She also stated that the patient's teachers had reported that his classroom behavior had deteriorated in preceding weeks, with frequent unexplained tearfulness. They further reported that his play with his peers-consistently girls-had become "less sweet and funny and more bossy and needy."

Social History: The patient lives with his two sisters and mother, who divorced the patient's biologic father two years before. The mother reports a history of depression and substance abuse that began during her own adolescence. The patient's father has been serving a prison sentence for abuse of a stepchild from a previous marriage for 2 years and does not have contact with the patient. The patient's mother describes the father as having been "a child himself—constantly needing attention...and [as having] a bad temper." She reports that although he never hit their son, he did admonish him for his doll play and " would get pretty worked up when the two of us were fighting."

Mental Status Examination: The patient is a thin, delicate-looking boy who appears younger than his biologic age. His eye contact is slightly hypervigilant; he is extremely attentive to the interviewer, studying her facial expressions and commenting on the colors she is wearing. He is variably related—at times he is eager to talk and solicitous, and at other times he is dreamy and seemingly indifferent. No psychomotor agitation or retardation is evident. His speech is of normal rate and volume. Language is spontaneous, sometimes precocious or odd; for example, he asked the interviewer the name of her lipstick shade. Mood is "sad on the inside, happy on the outside." Affect is euthymic but constricted. Thought process tends toward the tangential but is age-appropriate. Thought content is preoccupied with themes of doll hair, "angry people who shout at you," and the wish to be beautiful, admired, and, ideally, a girl. Insight and judgment are fair, with full gender constancy and reality testing. Impulse control is poor, and the patient becomes bossy or whines when attempts are made at redirection. The patient is alert and oriented.

Diagnostic Testing: Weschler Intelligence Scale for Children, third edition, revealed superior intellectual functioning. Rorschach testing revealed object representations of overpowering, malevolent figures; themes of annihilation, separation, and loss; and significant boundary disturbances. The predominant defense mechanism was a kind of splitting organized around gender; representations of women were particularly idealized and devalued. Structural clinical interviews revealed evidence of chronic depression and anxiety.

Questions: What is the diagnosis? What theories have been proposed to explain its etiology?

Diagnosis: Gender identity disorder (GID).

Discussion: According to the DSM IV-TR, two components are necessary to warrant the diagnosis of GID: (1) strong and persistent cross-gender identification (i.e., the desire to be or the insistence that one is of the other sex), without the motivation for cross-identification being due to perceived cultural advantage and distinct from a delusion that one actually belongs to the opposite sex, as can be seen in schizophrenia, and (2) persistent discomfort about one's assigned sex or a sense of inappropriateness in the gender role of that sex—with evidence of clinically significant distress or impairment in social, occupational, or other important areas of functioning. The presence of concurrent physical intersex condition disqualifies patients from this designation, in which case GID, not otherwise specified (NOS), can be used.

In the absence of any indications of congenital intersex conditions, rule-out diagnoses in this case included adjustment disorder, generalized anxiety disorder, and attention-deficit/hyperactivity disorder. GID is the more useful diagnosis because it not only describes the behavioral problems (impulsivity, anxiety, aggression toward self and others) but also the social integration issues that may need to be addressed in treatment. Moreover, unlike separation or generalized anxiety disorder, GID explains more specifically the kinds of developmental deficits suggested by the boy's troubles in his family and school life, because it points to the cross-gender identification and aversion to biologic sex as signals of severe deficits in psychic maturation.

Although the precise etiology of GID is contested, the most comprehensive developmental/psychoanalytic theory proposed thus far focuses on boys and holds that cross-gender identification results from the interaction of constitutional factors such as reactivity (the "inhibited"-type temperament) and environmental factors such as abuse, neglect, loss, or even subtle parental psychopathology during a developmental period when awareness of gender difference is present but self and object constancy are not yet fully established. Self and object constancy, usually established between months 24 and 36 of life, are the developmental achievements in which mental representations of self and caregiver become coded in memory. Successful self-constancy means that the child is able to tolerate stressors without losing the sense of who she or he is. Object constancy means that, in times of stress, the child can recall, or "invoke," the internal image of the caregiver as a source of comfort. When a traumatic loss occurs before these developments are established, a child can find her- or himself feeling lost and confused—with a sense that she or he may cease to exist. The child wishes for the sense of safety that comes from physical and emotional closeness with the mother. When this closeness is not available, a cross-gender identification can feel like the only available alternative. As one theorist states, "The child confuses having mommy with *being* mommy."

The child's experience of gender (the idea of maleness and femaleness) comes to serve as a venue for the establishment of a sort of alternate self, a self in which the mother is evoked and the sense of safety associated with her is regained, aggression feels coherent rather than disorganizing, and there is a sense of the self—albeit a constricted one—that feels, to the child, relatively organized and reliable. Once a child starts using such a construct as a refuge, it becomes highly important to him or her. This patient's "bossy and needy" play with girls at school reflects the urgency with which children can take hold of this identity construct—resulting in cross-gender play that sometimes seems driven, repetitive, and compulsive. The urgency of the cross-gender identification as a defense against annihilation also explains why children with GID sometimes have violent tantrums when forced to wear clothing that feels discordant with their internal gender sense.

GID is perhaps best thought of as a kind of attachment disorder syndrome in which cross-gender manifestations occur as symptoms—along with separation anxiety, depression, behavioral disturbances, and a drastic sense of confusion and aloneness. For this reason, some theorists consider the designation misguided, because focusing on the gender variance shifts attention away from the central breakdown in psychic structure and the psychic pain that underlie it.

No recent epidemiologic studies have reported the prevalence of GID, but the disorder is relatively rare and the use of the diagnosis appears to be declining in recent years. Boys are referred more frequently than girls, and men outnumber women by approximately 2- to 3-fold. Onset of GID is usually around ages 2 to 3 years and is typically precipitated by a traumatic experience such as separation, sexual overstimulation, or maternal stressors, and it always occurs within the context of disturbed family functioning. Children are typically referred around the time of school entry because of parental concern for sustained gender-variant behavior, increased distress due to peer ostracism, heightened sense of alienation, social immaturity, frustration intolerance, impaired school performance, school aversion, or truancy.

Although psychological testing may reveal cross-gender identification or behavior patterns, there is no diagnostic test specific for GID. Karyotyping for sex chromosomes and hormone assays serve only to rule out concurrent physical intersex condition and are not otherwise useful.

As in this case, boys diagnosed with GID are characterized by a marked preoccupation with traditionally defined feminine activities such as playing with dolls, dress-up, drawing pictures of beautiful girls and princesses, taking interest in female fantasy figures, and playing house. While playing house, the boys commonly assume the "mother role" and take on "feminine" mannerisms and speech patterns. They typically choose girls as their preferred playmates. They also tend to avoid "rough-and-tumble play" and competitive sports and show a general lack of interest in stereotypical boys' toys. Temperamentally, they often manifest a sense of bodily fragility, anxiety, and hypervigilance in the face of new situations; strong affiliative needs; extreme sensitivity to affect (e.g., becoming especially care-taking or solicitous when they experience their mothers as angry or depressed); vulnerability to separation, loss, and humiliation; remarkable ability to imitate; and sensory sensitivities to sounds, color, texture, odor, temperature, and pain. They also tend to be perfectionistic and highly over-adapted in their potential for extreme compliance. Boys diagnosed with GID may express a wish to be a girl or assert that they will grow up to be a woman. Many experience an anatomic dysphoria manifesting as an aversion toward the penis. They may insist on sitting to urinate or pretend not to have a penis by pushing it between their legs; in some cases, they may express a wish to remove it or a wish to have a vagina. Although the present patient was never known to make explicit statements about his penis, seeing his genitals in the bath caused him to wish he were a girl.

Girls diagnosed with GID typically show intense negative attitudes toward traditional female dress, wish to be called by boys' names, identify with powerful male figures, prefer boys as playmates, and share boys' interests in contact sports, "rough-and-tumble play," and traditional boyhood games. They typically show little interest in dolls or other traditional girlhood play, may insist on standing to urinate, claim to have a penis, express wishes not to grow breasts or menstruate, and assert that they will grow up to be men. (There is a general paucity of literature on the topic of GID in girls. It has been suggested that the reason is that masculine behavior in girls is less disruptive in many families.)

In adolescence and adulthood, preoccupation with appearance can lead to self-treatment with hormones, and, rarely, self-castration or penectomy. Relationship difficulties, school/work impairment, substance-related disorders, and suicide attempts are common. Adults diagnosed with GID are typically uncomfortable functioning as a member of their biologic sex; they may be preoccupied with a wish to live as the opposite sex, adopting to varying degrees the behaviors, mannerisms, and dress of the opposite sex; and they may seek hormonal or surgical manipulation of their bodies. Anxiety and depression are common comorbidities in adults, and personality disorders are more common in men.

According to the DSM-IV-TR, the diagnosis of GID is distinct and based on the extent and pervasiveness of the cross-gender wishes, interests, and activities, along with the presence of marked distress or impairment—from simple nonconformity to stereotypical sex-role behavior. This point has created a good deal of controversy about the diagnosis, because "simple nonconformity to stereotypical sex-role behavior" may itself cause a child significant distress in a social, cultural, and/or familial context adverse to difference, as evidenced by the fact that the majority of children diagnosed with GID are referred around school age when peer pressure to conform, harassment, and ostracism may become overwhelming. Furthermore, the experience of intersexed people with variant neuroendocrinologic function, homosexual children and adults, and heterosexual people who are not stereotypically male or female demonstrates a spectrum of viable, nonnormative gender possibilities that fall outside the conventional gender binary. Some theorists hold that the failure of traditional psychoanalytic and developmental theories to account for this variety of gender experience is rooted in a failure to recognize that conventional masculine and feminine behavior/identities are, at least partially, constructed categories that reflect the social, political, economic, and cultural forces in play at any given historical moment. Others maintain that gender—however expressed—follows largely from genetic constitution and biologic function—however variable.

Furthermore, for some theorists, the fact that the overwhelming majority of children brought to clinical attention for gender variant behavior/identification are boys manifesting feminine traits brings into question whether the issue is femininity itself—that is, whether the diagnosis of GID reflects a cultural bias that has been sustained in psychoanalytic and developmental theory. Alternatively, it has been suggested that the difficulties many women feel in sustaining and integrating experiences of agency and potency as gender syntonic in a society that continues to devalue female agency may be so significant as to invalidate the DSM qualification that the motivation (whether conscious or unconscious) for cross-identification should not be merely due to perceived cultural advantage.

The treatment of GID is psychodynamic psychotherapy focusing on attaining freedom from the inhibitions and ego restrictions that often mark the disorder. Once in therapy, these children typically manifest a strong need to be understood, great affiliative needs, and a capacity to express their inner experience in metaphor. Although some clinicians attempt to redirect the gender variant behavior in order to bring the child's behavior and sense of self more in line with parental wishes or social norms, it has been suggested that such redirection misses the reality of psychic pain underlying the gender performance; it is to ask children to resolve an inner dilemma by subordinating their subjectivity and conforming to social expectations. Moreover, evidence indicates that efforts to curb or replace gender-discordant traits with more traditional traits may be harmful to development, particularly to the child's emotional resilience, affective capacity, and future ability to sustain intimate relationships.

Most boys diagnosed with GID become accepting of their gender by late latency. Furthermore, two-thirds of boys diagnosed with GID develop a homosexual orientation, although they represent a very small subgroup of proto-homosexual boys. It has been suggested that homosexual childhoods, which remain insufficiently recognized and undertheorized, are at times mistaken for GID. Indeed, most, if not all, homosexual men seen in consultation or treatment report varying degrees of gender-discordant behaviors or traits during development.

The present patient was followed clinically into adolescence. The initial phase of treatment focused on issues of object permanence and individuation. At the beginning of each session, the patient would study the consultation room as if to make sure everything were still in its place, and he was preoccupied with questions of whether he could be himself if he were not like the therapist. Issues of anger or separation, such as those surrounding the end of the session, were frequently followed by fantasies of aggression, sometimes acted out with dolls, or, conversely, by brushing Barbie's hair, sometimes to the point of tearing it out. In fantasy play, he often expressed confusion about what was real and what pretend, what animate and what inanimate. Despite these confusions, he did not show evidence of a thought disorder. In the second year of treatment, the patient continued to be fixed on the theme of idealized women but in addition became preoccupied with "angry ladies."

After about two and a half years of treatment, the patient is no longer reporting thoughts of harming himself or other people. His teachers report that his peer relationships are still almost entirely with girls, but he seems more relaxed and less commandeering. Now in middle school, he does not protest sex-typed class separation or activities. In his weekly psychotherapy sessions, he no longer speaks of the wish to be a girl. His mood is generally euthymic, and although he complains of his mother's frequent depression and how "it rubs right off on me," he reports being generally happy at home. He also reports that he has a girlfriend at school but denies any sexual curiosity or experimentation with her. He is currently contemplating—"with some worries"—two weeks at a sleepaway camp after he completes the sixth grade.

Pearls

1. GID may be best thought of as a kind of attachment disorder syndrome in which cross-gender manifestations occur as symptoms—along with separation anxiety, depression, behavioral disturbances, and a drastic sense of confusion and aloneness.
2. GID is distinct from simple nonconformity to stereotypic sex-role behavior, homosexual childhood, intersex conditions, and the delusion that one is actually of the opposite sex. In GID, the level of distress accompanying the cross-gender behavior is high, and the cross-gender play is compulsive, rigid, and repetitive—reflecting its urgent role in preserving ego integration.
3. The etiology of GID is contested, but the most comprehensive theory to date is multifactorial and involves constitutional and environmental factors occurring in a developmental period when awareness of gender difference is present but self and object constancy are not yet fully established.
4. Intensive exploratory/supportive treatment is the best method of correcting the developmental deficits that are theorized to underlie GID. Successful treatment usually diminishes anxiety, improves mood and interpersonal functioning, and fosters self-coherence and acceptance. Gender-atypical interests and attraction usually remain.
5. GID is a politically controversial diagnosis. Many transgendered people and their advocates believe that the distress shown by children with GID is merely the result of familial and social nonacceptance of gender-atypical children. The appropriate treatment, in this view, is family therapy to enhance acceptance of the child. If gender dysphoria and distress persist as the child grows into young adulthood, facilitation of medical sex-reassignment is often recommended. Some theorists have suggested that GID as a diagnosis represents a displacement of cultural anxiety from sexual object choice to gender identity, since homosexuality was depathologized in 1973.

REFERENCES

1. Butler J: Doing justice to someone: Sex reassignment and allegories of transsexuality. GLQ 2001;7(4):621–636.
2. Coates S, Friedman R, Wolfe S: The etiology of boyhood gender identity disorder: A model for integrating temperament, development, and psychodynamics. Psychoanal Dial 1999;1:481–523.
3. Chused JF: Male gender identity and sexual behaviour. Int J Psychoanal 1999;80:1105–1117.
4. Corbett K: Homosexual boyhood: Notes on girlyboys. In Rottnek M (ed): Sissies and Tomboys: Gender Nonconformity and Homosexual Childhood. New York, New York University Press, 1999.
5. Fausto-Sterling A: Sexing the Body: Gender Politics and the Construction of Sexuality. New York, Basic Books, 2000.
6. Harris A: Gender as a soft assembly. Stud Gender Sexual 2000;1(3):223–250.
7. Isay RA: Gender in homosexual boys: Some developmental and clinical considerations. Psychiatry 1999;62(2):187–194.
8. Kessler S: Lessons from the Intersexed. New Brunswick, NJ, Rutgers University Press, 1998.

PATIENT 53

A 27-year-old-man with chest pain

History of Present Illness: A 27-year-old man is brought in to the emergency department by his wife complaining of chest pain at 2:00 AM Saturday morning. He is triaged to the medical emergency department, where a medical history is taken. The patient has no history of myocardial infarction, hypertension, or other cardiac risk factors. The man is irritable and hypervigilant; he repeatedly asks nurses if "you know what you are doing" and becomes increasingly guarded as the intern requests more details about his medical history, replying suspiciously, "You don't need to know that." The man's wife asks if she can speak to the doctor alone and says that her husband typically leaves his work as an investment banker on Friday night, stays out until late several nights a week, and has great difficulty getting to work on time in the morning. On the weekends, he often sleeps 12–18 hours a day. She has also noticed some weight loss over the past few months. Sometimes after a late night working or socializing with coworkers, he appears to be almost paranoid toward her, accusing her of cheating on him or talking about him behind his back. She denies his accusations and appears extremely concerned. She acknowledges that he has been under increased pressure at work to perform and stay late; several friends at work have been laid off in the past year. He denies feeling depressed and says that he is "just stressed out."

Past Psychiatric History: The patient denies any past psychiatric history; he has never been hospitalized in a psychiatric hospital or received psychiatric treatment. He admits that he "dabbled in drugs before, but I am here for chest pain."

Past Medical History: Other than seasonal allergies, the patient denies any past or current medical problems.

Mental Status Examination: The patient is alert and oriented and appears disheveled, dressed in work clothes that are unkempt. His speech has rapid rate and mildly increased volume but is not pressured. He is restless and looks around the room frequently but does not exhibit signs of psychomotor agitation. The patient describes his mood as "fine, just having chest pain," but his affect is extremely anxious, irritable, and guarded. Thought process is linear and goal-directed, but thought content shows some evidence of paranoid ideation toward his wife and emergency department staff. The patient denies auditory and visual hallucinations as well as suicidal or homicidal ideation. His cognition is intact. Insight and judgment are deemed to be limited.

Physical Examination: Vital signs: heart rate is 102 beats per minute, blood pressure is 170/90 mmHg, temperature is 98.6°F, and respiratory rate is 18 breaths per minute. The patient is breathing comfortably and is not in any apparent distress. He does appear somewhat thin, and there are traces of dried blood in the left nostril. Cardiac exam reveals no signs or murmurs, rubs, or gallops. The remainder of the physical exam is likewise unremarkable.

Neurologic Examination: Gait is normal. No abnormal movements are noted. Pupils are dilated bilaterally. Cranial nerves 2–12 are intact. A mild tremor is noted in both hands. There are no sensory or motor deficits.

Laboratory Testing: Creatine phosphokinase (CPK) is within normal limits, and other cardiac enzymes show no indication of MI. Urine toxicology: positive for cocaine.

Diagnostic Testing: EKG: normal sinus rhythm at 102 bpm; flipped T waves in several leads. Chest x-ray: normal study.

Question: Which diagnosis explains this man's presentation?

Diagnosis: Cocaine dependence.

Discussion: This patient easily meets criteria for cocaine intoxication: (1) recent use of cocaine, (2) clinically significant maladaptive behavioral or psychological changes (in this case, a change in sociability) and impaired occupational functioning that developed shortly after cocaine use, and (3) two of the following symptoms: tachycardia or bradycardia; pupillary dilation; elevated or lowered blood pressure; perspiration or chills; nausea or vomiting; evidence of weight loss; psychomotor agitation or retardation; muscular weakness, respiratory depression, chest pain, or cardiac arrhythmia; confusion, seizures, dyskinesias, dystonias, or coma. In addition, as far as we know at this point, these symptoms are not due to a general medical condition and are not better accounted for by another mental disorder.

The overall effect of cocaine is to stimulate the central nervous system. Cocaine exerts its most important action on neurotransmitters by inhibiting the reuptake of norepinephrine, serotonin, and dopamine. The reinforcing properties of cocaine are thought to be associated with enhanced dopaminergic neurotransmission in the mesolimbic pathways. Neurochemical studies have shown that large and fast increases in dopamine are associated with the reinforcing effects of drug abuse. Studies have also shown that after chronic drug abuse and during withdrawal, dopamine function is markedly decreased (known as the dopamine depletion hypothesis), and this decrease may be associated with dysfunction in the prefrontal regions involving multiple brain circuits, specifically those of reward, motivation, memory and learning, and control. Relatively new imaging technologies, such as PET and MRI, have provided new ways to investigate how biologic and environmental factors interact in drug addiction.

Results from the 2002 National Survey on Drug Use and Health estimate that in 2002, 19.5 million Americans, or 8.3% of the population aged 12 or older, were current illicit drug users. An estimated 2 million (0.9%) were cocaine users, 567,000 of whom used crack. Recent statistics show that the use of cocaine is on the rise. The percentage of young adults aged 18–25 who had ever used cocaine was below 1% in the mid-1960s but rose steadily in the 1970s and 1980s, reaching 17.9% in 1984. By 1996, rates had dropped to 10.1% but climbed in 2002 to 15.4%.

As far as this specific patient is concerned, the urine toxicology gives a big clue, but what else may point to a diagnosis of cocaine dependence or intoxication? During the "high" patients may be noted to be paranoid, with increased energy in the short term and decreased energy in the long term. They are also frequently irritable with significant mood lability. Although not noted here, some people also present with frank psychotic symptoms, such as hearing voices or experiencing tactile hallucinations of bugs crawling under the skin, also called "formication." It is possible that the patient may have started using the cocaine to increase work performance, or he may have been using in social situations related to work. As with other substance-related disorders, cocaine-related disorders are frequently accompanied by other primary psychiatric disorders. Major depressive disorder, bipolar disorder, cyclothymic disorder, anxiety disorders, and antisocial personality disorders are the most commonly associated psychiatric disorders.

A number of psychiatric conditions can also mimic cocaine use and/or dependence, including bipolar disorder (manic and depressed episodes), anxiety spectrum disorders, and primary psychotic disorders. A diagnosis of substance-induced psychotic and/or mood disorder must also be considered. Although this patient presents with a medical complaint, a full psychiatric evaluation is indicated. In the hours after a cocaine binge, a withdrawal phase is typically seen, characterized by depressed mood, a profound decrease in energy, irritability, and an increased need for sleep. This patient is sleeping 12–18 hours on the weekends and has difficulty making it to work on time. It is also not unusual to see some patients present with suicidality in the withdrawal phase, although we do not see it in this case. In general, cocaine may produce an array of neuropsychiatric states. Patients may present as delusional, paranoid, or with violent agitation. They may also exhibit compulsively repetitive behaviors or experience hypervigilence, anxiety, or hypersexuality. These states may last for several hours after ingestion, followed by a period of exhaustion and possibly obtundation.

On physical exam, the large, dilated pupils also point to the diagnosis of cocaine use. The elevated heart rate, increased blood pressure, and increased respiratory rate are typically seen in cocaine and other stimulant use. Of course, a full cardiac evaluation is a priority in this patient because his chief complaint is chest pain. Cocaine has been found to cause a number of cardiac conditions, including arrhythmia, coronary atherosclerosis, cardiomyopathy, and congestive heart failure. Treatment is often complicated by the concurrent use of sedative hypnotics, opiates, and alcohol in these patients. Cocaine intoxication can present in a number of ways. Signs and symptoms may include hyperthermia, seizures, toxic delirium, rhabdomyolysis, renal failure, coagulopathies, disseminated intravascular coagulation, shock, hepatic failure, arrhythmias, myocardial infarctions, cerebral infarctions (both ischemic and hemorrhagic), pulmonary complications, and death. Behavioral management with benzodiazapines is considered safest, because neuroleptics may worsen hyperthermia and arrhythmias and lower the seizure threshold. EKG changes in a young man with no cardiac or family history of cardiac disease are seen in this case. CPK and temperature should be monitored, along with renal function, to check for rhabdomyolysis and prevent subsequent renal failure.

Cocaine enters most countries as a hydrochloride salt made from treating coca leaves with hydrochloric acid. It is soluble in water and therefore can be injected or inhaled. Cocaine powder is the most common form and is typically inhaled. Freebase and crack are manufactured by different techniques. Freebase is made by dissolving the cocaine hydrochloride in water, then adding a base such as ammonia and a solvent such as ether. The base is dissolved by the ether, which is then evaporated. This method frequently results in burns when a flame is used to rapidly evaporate the ether. Crack cocaine is a mass-produced type of freebase that is made by dissolving cocaine hydrochloride in water, mixing it with baking soda, and heating until the mixture dries into a mass. It makes a cracking sound when smoked, and the euphoric effects last about 5–15 minutes. When cocaine is combined with alcohol, it produces a chemical called cocaethylene, which is reported to have an enhanced and prolonged euphoria but is also associated with increased toxicity and a higher risk of sudden death. Some users combine cocaine and heroin in a drug cocktail called a "speedball." The effects of inhaled cocaine occur within 15–20 minutes. Intravenous cocaine can be felt within minutes, and the effects of smoking occur within seconds. Cocaine's plasma half-life is about 90 minutes. It is important to note that the injectable form increases the risk for HIV and hepatitis infection.

To attain abstinence, patients may need referral to partial or inpatient hospitalization. Treatment relies on several modalities, combining rehabilitative, psychodynamic, and behavioral approaches with pharmacologic treatment when indicated. Long-term treatment in self-help groups is available for specific drug types, such as Cocaine Anonymous (CA) and Narcotics Anonymous (NA), and these groups promote abstinence and adherence to a 12-step program, similar to Alcoholics Anonymous (AA). Many patients with cocaine abuse/dependence also need detoxification from alcohol. Frequent urine toxicology screening is often necessary to monitor abstinence.

Pharmacologic treatment of cocaine addiction includes anticraving agents, dopamine agonists or blocking agents, and antidepressants, but all have mixed results. Chronic cocaine users may suffer from the same underlying catecholamine or serotonergic dysregulation as those with depression. The tricyclic antidepressant desipramine has been the most widely studied, but double-blind, controlled studies have demonstrated both positive and negative results. Disulfiram appears to be promising, especially for patients with comorbid alcohol abuse. Anticonvulsants such as gabapentin, lamotrigine, and phenytoin have also shown promise in small-scale studies and warrant further evaluation. Several stimulants approved for the treatment of attention deficit-hyperactivity disorder and narcolepsy have been used to test the catecholamine substitution approach, but with only limited success. The absence of any medication that meets FDA standards for efficacy and safety leaves physicians with little clear-cut guidance for pharmacologic treatment; more controlled clinical trials are clearly needed.

This patient was admitted to telemetry for observation and was seen by a psychiatrist while on the medical unit. The patient disclosed to his psychiatrist that his cocaine use over the past few months had spiraled out of control. He has been trying to "cut down" but found that his use actually increased to "get that same energy" (i.e., tolerance). He also states, "I know this is a problem. I don't want to end up with a heart attack, but I don't know what to do." Based on these statements and the presence of withdrawal, the patient was diagnosed with cocaine dependence. Symptoms of paranoia resolved once the initial episode of intoxication had passed, and the diagnosis of a primary psychotic disorder was excluded. After a family meeting with his wife, psychiatrist, and internist, a referral was made to an outpatient psychiatrist and daily CA meetings. When drug use is severe or the patient has failed outpatient treatment, inpatient treatment may be required. In many cases, patients may refuse to acknowledge the need for help and will enter treatment only under pressure from family, friends, employers, or the judicial system.

Pearls

1. The liver combines cocaine and alcohol into a compound called cocaethylene, which intensifies cocaine's effects and increases the risk for sudden death.
2. Cocaine use should be considered in the differential diagnosis of new-onset seizures.
3. Benzodiazapines may be a safer choice to control behavior in cocaine-intoxicated patients than neuroleptics, which may lower seizure threshold and potentially worsen arrhythmias and hyperthermia.
4. The reinforcing properties of cocaine (and amphetamine) are associated with their ability to increase synaptic dopamine levels.

REFERENCES

1. Gawin FH, Ellinwood EH Jr: Cocaine and other stimulants. N Engl J Med 1988;318:1173–1182.
2. Gold M: Cocaine and crack: Clinical aspects. In Lowinson JH, Ruiz P, Millman RB, Langrod JG (eds): Substance Abuse: A Comprehensive Textbook, 3rd ed. Baltimore, Williams & Wilkins, 1997, pp 181–199.
3. Gold M, Miller N: Cocaine and crack: Neurobiology. In Lowinson JH, Ruiz P, Millman RB, Langrod JG (eds): Substance Abuse: A Comprehensive Textbook, 3rd ed. Baltimore, Williams & Wilkins, 1997, pp 166–181.
4. Hoffman RS: Cocaine overdose: Clinical manifestations and treatment. J Clin Toxicol 2000;38:181–182.
5. Kaplan HI, Sadock BJ: Substance-related disorders. In Kaplan HI, Sadock BJ (eds): Kaplan and Sadock's Synopsis of Psychiatry. Substance-Related Disorders. Baltimore, Williams & Wilkins, 1988, pp 375–455.
6. Kleber HD: Pharmacologic treatments for heroin and cocaine dependence. Am J Addict 2003;12(Suppl 2):S5–S18.
7. Kosten TR, Singha AK: Stimulants. In Galanter M, Kleber HD (eds): The American Psychiatric Press Textbook of Substance Abuse Treatment, 2nd ed. Washington DC; American Psychiatric Press, pp 183–193.
8. NIDA InfoFacts: Crack and Cocaine, 1999. Available at <www.drugabuse.gov>.
9. Schrank KS: Acute cocaine intoxication: Current methods of treatment. NIDA Research Monograph Series 1992.
10. Seger DL: Cocaine: History of use, manufacture of preparations and related kinetics. J Clin Toxicol 2000;38:180–181.
11. Substance Abuse and Mental Health Services Administration 2003. Results from the 2002 National Survey on Drug use and Health: National Findings (Office of Applied Studies, NHSDA Series H-22, DHHS Publication No. SMA 03-3836). Rockville, MD. Available at <www.samhsa.gov>.
12. Volkow ND, Fowler JS, Wang GJ: The addicted human brain: Insights from imaging studies. J Clin Invest 2001;111: 1444–1451.
13. Woolf A: Cocaine poisoning. Clin Toxicol Rev 1995;18(8).

Patrick Runnels, MD

PATIENT 54

A 44-year-old woman with HIV complains of depressed mood

History of Present Illness: A 44-year-old woman is referred by her primary care physician after she tells him that "life doesn't feel like very much fun anymore." For the past few months, the patient has been uninterested in reading mystery novels and playing her violin, activities she used to do on an almost daily basis. She states, "Reading just seems so much harder than it used to be" and "I can't make the violin sound good anymore; playing it is so difficult now." When probed further, she elaborates that other activities have become difficult as well. Balancing her checkbook has been taking longer and longer (sometimes an entire day), writing notes has become difficult, she drops things all the time, and she comments specifically that brushing her teeth seems really difficult and takes "forever." When socializing, she finds herself frequently unable to keep up with more 'intellectual' topics, like politics, which she used to enjoy discussing. A number of her friends have commented that she seems to have a quick temper the past few weeks. She ends the interview saying: "I feel like a klutz. I feel stupid. I just don't feel like myself."

Past Psychiatric Illness: The patient reports a history of sexual abuse perpetrated by one of her uncles when she was 12 years old. She also saw a therapist for several years in her late 20s and early 30s and was diagnosed with depression during that time. She was prescribed fluoxetine for 2 years, but was tapered off and has not been on any psychiatric medications since. She also saw a psychiatrist for a few months because of depressive symptoms after being diagnosed with HIV. She stopped seeing him because "I felt okay." She has not seen another psychiatrist until now.

Past Medical History: At age 38 the patient was diagnosed with HIV, which she contracted through high-risk sexual activity. She was asymptomatic until age 47, when she developed *Pneumocystis carinii* pneumonia (PCP) and was hospitalized for 10 days. At that time, her CD4 count was 87. After discharge, she was started on highly active antiretroviral therapy (HAART), with which she has been poorly adherent. She is hepatitis C-negative.

Social/Family History: The patient currently lives by herself in an apartment and works at a bookstore around the corner. She has been divorced for 12 years with no children. She describes a number of close friendships with her coworkers and also keeps in touch with her two sisters, who live in the same town. There is no history of psychiatric illness in her immediate family.

Mental Status Examination: The patient appears mildly disheveled. She describes herself as depressed and appears so for most of the interview. Her body language, although expressive, is sluggish, as if she is moving through water. Her hands, in particular, appear as if they are in slow motion when she gesticulates. Although she is cooperative throughout the interview, she seems alternately bored and irritated by many of the questions, particularly those regarding smaller details about her life, which she has great difficulty in recalling. When asked to recall her current address, she initially tries to answer, then becomes irritated, and eventually responds without answering the question, "Wow! I guess I'll have to write that on a Post-It too!" In general, her memory of recent events is poor: she is unable to name any of the past three presidents, recall the significance of 9/11, or where she ate dinner a few nights earlier. She appears to be generally attentive throughout the interview but has difficulty with serial sevens. Writing a sentence takes 2 minutes. Although she is able to correctly interpret several proverbs, she spends a considerable amount of time thinking each one through and then seems uncertain about her answers. She is aware of the difficulties that she is having and nearly cries several times during the interview while struggling through some of the questions.

Physical Examination: The patient appears undernourished. She has weaker arms and legs than would be expected for her age and build, but this is not noticeable unless the muscle groups are directly challenged. She clearly has difficulty picking up a pen and writing a sentence. The handwriting appears a little shaky, and upon closer observation she has a small resting tremor, most noticeable in her hands. She has no difficulty rising to a standing position but walks tentatively and stumbles a few times for no apparent reason. Although she is able to touch her finger to her nose, then to the interviewer's nose and back, she is only able to perform this task slowly.

Diagnostic Testing: Blood count: CD4, 89; Viral load, 72,432; hemoglobin, 10.2; hematocrit, 31.3; MRI of Brain: normal.

Question: What is the diagnosis?

Diagnosis: HIV-dementia (AIDS dementia complex, HIV encephalopathy)

Discussion: Before the introduction of HAART in the early-to-mid 1990s, the lifetime risk for HIV-positive patients developing HIV dementia (HIV-D) was estimated to be between 15% and 20% and greater than 60% for patients with full-blown AIDS. Since the introduction of HAART, the incidence of HIV-D in patients with AIDS has dropped significantly, but exactly how significant a decline remains uncertain. At least one study reported a post-HAART incidence of HIV-D in patients with AIDS below 10%, and a cohort study of 2734 HIV-positive patients showed a 53% reduction in HIV-D from 1990–1992 to 1996–1998. Two cohort studies published within the past 2 years, however, reported that the cumulative incidence of dementia in patients with AIDS was around 25% at 1 year and 38% at 2 years.

Certain risk factors have been associated with increased incidence of HIV-D. One cohort study demonstrated that patients over 50 years of age are more than twice as likely to develop HIV-D as those under 50. Other risk factors include low CD4 count, high viral load, anemia, injection drug use, female sex, and low body mass index (BMI). A number of genetic risk factors have also been explored, but none have proved useful as predictive markers.

In the central nervous system (CNS), HIV resides mainly in microglia and macrophages. Infected cells are activated by the virus, causing the release of toxins that both lead to neuronal and astrocytic dysfunction and induce other microglial cells and monocytes to produce neurotoxins. Four chemokine receptors on these cells seem to be particularly important to the pathogenesis: CXCR4, CCR5, CX3CR1, and TNF receptor. The HIV peptide gp120 interacts with CD4, whereas cytokines conjointly interact with any of these four receptors. This synergistic action results in the activation of the intracellular MAP kinase p38, which in turn activates the intranuclear transcription factor MEF2C. The activation of MEF2C leads to the production of TNF-α and other neurotoxins that eventually damage CNS neurons. This activation pathway has recently emerged as a potential target of HIV-D therapy.

Astrocytes, although not infected by HIV, are found to be activated in HIV-D, and are also thought to contribute to neurotoxicity. Neurotoxins released by microglia/monocytes both induce the release of glutamate and inhibit reuptake by astrocytes. These cytokines also induce the intracellular production of nitric oxide and other free radicals eventually released by the astrocytes. In addition, the HIV protein Tat induces the release of MCP-1, a potent chemoattractant for monocytes/microglia, from astrocytes. Neuronal cell death then results from a combination of direct damage by HIV peptides, NMDA-induced apoptosis, and excessive neurotoxic insult leading to necrosis.

Pathologically, HIV-D affects both the cortex and subcortical structures. Neuronal cell loss leading to atrophy occurs in the frontal and temporal lobes with accompanying ventricular dilatation. Histologically, HIV-D is characterized by multinucleated giant cells, widespread reactive astrocytes with white matter pallor, cortical neuronal loss, and vacuolar myelopathy. Histologic findings are typically most prominent in the basal ganglia and thalamus.

Clinically, HIV-D manifests as deficits in cognition, behavior, and motor activity, which collectively constitute a subcortical dementia. Notably, insight is preserved. Initial symptoms of HIV-D are subtle and can either be overlooked or misdiagnosed as depression. Generally, the cognitive deficits of HIV-D are memory loss characterized by impaired retrieval and impaired ability to manipulate acquired knowledge. Common early cognitive complaints include memory loss, difficulty reading, and mental slowing, all of which are demonstrated by this patient. Personality changes may also occur and are characterized by apathy, inertia, irritability, and general slowing of all thought processes. Gait disturbances are a common motor manifestation, presenting early as frequent stumbling and progressing to ataxia. Other common motor symptoms include impaired rapid eye movements (manifested on clinical exam by abnormal saccadic movements), impaired fine manual dexterity (this patient had difficulty writing), hyperreflexia, and parkinsonism. Tremor and myoclonus are less common. As the dementia progresses, it becomes more global, and patients develop myopathies and sensory neuropathies as well.

HIV-D has a mean survival of less than 1 year from diagnosis in untreated patients. Survival in the HAART era has only recently been examined. A study of 254 patients with HIV-D showed an increase in survival from 11.9 months for those diagnosed in 1993–1995 to 48.2 months for those diagnosed in 1996–2000, with a striking 7-fold increase in survival for patients diagnosed with HIV-D in association with advanced immunodeficiency.

HIV-D is diagnosed by recognizing the compatible clinical picture in the setting of HIV infection, having ruled out other causes. MRI and CT are useful only for ruling out other possible causes of disease: both may reveal dilated ventricles, and MRI may show focal hyperintensities that light up on a T2-weighted image. Cerebrospinal fluid (CSF) has been rigorously investigated as a means for confirming diagnosis, but while multiple abnormalities are common, few are specific or predictive. Although patients with HIV-D generally have an overall higher viral load, high viral loads are common in asymptomatic patients also, and low viral loads are not uncommon in patients with true HIV-D. For patients on HAART, there is no correlation between absolute CSF viral load and the presence of HIV-D, but studies have demonstrated a significant correlation between viral load in the CSF and severity of symptoms. The induction of HAART also correlates well with rapid suppression of CSF HIV RNA levels.

The only current treatment for HIV-D is induction of HAART. Since the introduction of HAART, several studies have demonstrated both a decreased incidence of HIV-D and, once HIV-D develops, alleviation of symptoms. However, no placebo-controlled trials of HAART for HIV-D have been performed. Comparative trials for different antiviral regimens have not been undertaken for HIV-D.

The differential diagnosis in this patient is vast, and making the diagnosis requires ruling out several other possibilities. She is hepatitis C-negative, but patients with hepatic encephalopathy secondary to hepatic failure can present with a similar clinical picture and need to have liver function evaluated. Progressive multifocal leukoencephalopathy (PML), caused by JC virus, presents with an almost identical clinical picture. Patients have a decline in cognitive function of which they are aware as well as associated focal neurologic deficits, including visual disturbances in approximately 50% of patients. The MRI usually shows multifocal hyperintense lesions, usually in the occipital and parietal lobes, and the neurologic deficits usually correlate. JC virus can be detected in CSF, and at least one recent study cites a 92% sensitivity and specificity for CSF testing. Most notably, the course of PML is very short, with death occurring within 3-6 months in patients not well-treated with HAART. Other conditions that can present with a similar clinical picture are herpes simplex virus (HSV) encephalopathy, toxoplasma encephalopathy, cytomegalovirus (CMV) encephalopathy, and primary CNS lymphomas.

This patient was sent to an HIV specialist, who ran the box, clock, and Bender visual motor tasks to evaluate construct apraxia and the Trailmaking Test, parts A and B, to measure psychomotor slowing. Based on the results of these tests and the duration of symptoms, the patient was deemed to have HIV dementia and was encouraged to adhere more strictly to her HAART regimen. Despite encouragement, the patient failed to take her medications regularly, and both her cognitive and neurologic function declined over the next year. A year after the diagnosis, the patient was hospitalized with PCP and died during the hospitalization.

Pearls

1. Although HIV-D represents only 5% of AIDS-defining illnesses, the prevalence of HIV-D has risen as survival among HIV patients has increased. Of note, the average CD4 count of patients with HIV-D has risen from 70 to 170 since the introduction of HAART.
2. A more subtle version of HIV-D, termed minor cognitive/motor disorder (MCMD), is used to describe patients who display two of six symptoms: mental slowing, impaired attention/concentration, impaired memory, slowed movements, impaired coordination, or personality change/irritability/emotional lability. MCMD is estimated to be more prevalent than frank HIV-D, and, unlike HIV-D, its prevalence has not decreased since the introduction of HAART.
3. Inhibition of the p38 MAP kinase was shown in vitro to prevent induction of TNF-α and iNOS gene expression, and this is one potential therapeutic target for preventing HIV-D in the future. Memantine, an NMDA receptor antagonist, has been shown to be effective for the treatment of Alzheimer's and vascular dementia and is currently in a multicenter trial for HIV-D.
4. Single photon emission computed tomography (SPECT) has been shown to detect abnormalities in cerebral blood flow in HIV-1 patients with and without severe dementia. Most studies demonstrate hypoperfusion in patients with HIV-D, but the utility of SPECT in HIV-D treatment remains uncertain.

REFERENCES

1. Albright AV, Soldan SS, Gonzalez-Scarano F: Pathogenesis of human immunodeficiency virus-induced neurological disease. J Neurovirol 2003;9:222–227.
2. Clifford DB: AIDS dementia. Med Clin North Am 2002;86:537–550.
3. Dore GJ, Mcdonald A, Yueming L, et al: Marked improvement in survival following AIDS dementia complex in the era of highly active antiretroviral therapy. AIDS 2003;17:1539–1545.

Anthony J. Carino, MD
Harold W. Goforth, MD

PATIENT 55

A 66-year-old man with confusion and visual hallucinations

History of Present Illness: A 66-year-old man is brought to the emergency department by emergency medical services after the police find him confused and walking along a major highway in the middle of the night. The man is oriented to person but not to time nor place. He states that he is trying to visit his son but seems confused when asked how he came to be on the road. The family was contacted for further information. The patient's son explains that he visits his father every day after work to assist him. Today, the son had to go to a conference at night and departed his father's house a few hours earlier than usual. His father has a history of getting lost during the previous year but is usually found by his family wandering close to his home.

The family notes that his father's difficulties began when he was diagnosed with a movement disorder two years ago after developing problems with walking, multiple falls, and rigidity. These difficulties did not respond to a brief trial of levodopa. At that time, he appeared more forgetful and displayed "bad episodes" in which he would change from being attentive during conversations to seeming drowsy or appearing to "go blank." These episodes occur at random throughout the day and night and fluctuate over the course of several minutes to hours. The family notices increasing forgetfulness, wandering behavior, and an inability to cook and clean for himself.

The father frequently refers to nonexistent small animals in his house. The family is surprised by both the amount of detail he uses in his descriptions of the animals and his apparent amusement by them. These visions began soon after the diagnosis of his motor disorder but became more severe with levodopa. The family is growing increasingly frustrated because their father used to be a successful and intelligent teacher but now needs assistance in doing even rudimentary tasks of daily living.

Past Psychiatric History: The patient has had no lifetime history of a psychiatric diagnosis. The family states that he has a "risperidone allergy" because low doses of risperidone were prescribed at the onset of his visual hallucinations and the patient developed rigid limbs and a tremor, which resolved after the medicine was discontinued.

Neurologic Examination: The patient shows marked postural instability, and bradykinesia with an unsteady gait. The bilateral, upper-extremity tremor is coarse, increased at rest, and decreased with movement. Cerebellar function, sensation, reflexes, and strength are without focal deficit. Cranial nerves are intact.

Mental Status Examination: The patient is a tall, ectomorphic man who appears older than his stated age with mild temporal wasting and poor grooming. He rapidly shifts from being appropriately attentive with moderate eye contact to becoming distracted and looking around the room. He has a mild resting, bilateral, upper-extremity tremor. The patient has decreased volume and increased latency of speech. He describes his mood as "fine." The patient's affect is constricted and is of low intensity. The patient's thought process is very circumstantial with occasional fragmentation. He is without suicidal or homicidal ideation. He admits to seeing brown, mole-like animals, which follow him. He is oriented to person but not to time nor place. The patient scored 20/30 on Folstein's Mini-Mental Status Examination with marked deficits in recall, copying pentagons, performing serial sevens, and following three step commands. The patient's insight and judgment are impaired; he does not believe that he has an illness and continues to wander from home.

Laboratory Findings: A comprehensive delirium and dementia work-up, including complete blood count, electrolytes, vitamin B_{12}, folate, rapid plasma reagin test for syphilis, liver function tests, ammonia, electroencephalography, and brain magnetic resonance imaging (MRI), was performed. Results were unremarkable except for the presence of mild, generalized cortical atrophy on the MRI.

Questions: What is the probable underlying diagnosis? How should this patient be managed?

Diagnosis: Dementia with Lewy bodies (DLB).

Discussion: DLB is a progressive disorder characterized by cognitive decline associated with episodic confusion, recurrent visual hallucinations, and Parkinson-like motor features. DLB accounts for 10–25% of patients diagnosed with dementia and is about two times more prevalent in males than females. The mean age of diagnosis of DLB is 68 years, and the average time from diagnosis to death is 6 years.

The diagnosis of DLB is based on a comprehensive clinical examination. Diagnostic criteria are met if the patient has a dementia syndrome with two of the three core features: (1) progressive cognitive decline with variations in attention and alertness; (2) recurrent visual hallucinations; and (3) spontaneous motor features of parkinsonism. Other features, which are supportive of DLB but not necessarily diagnostic, include a history of repeated falls, syncope, transient loss of consciousness, sensitivity to neuroleptics, and systematized delusions and hallucinations.

The current patient has DLB based on the clinical history and mental status exam. Other diagnoses, which should be considered, include delirium, Alzheimer's dementia, and idiopathic Parkinson's disease. Fluctuating levels of attention and alertness are observed in 80–90% of patients with DLB and are also the core diagnostic feature of delirium. This patient has experienced intermittent periods of inability to pay attention and maintain alertness for more than 2 years and does not appear to have had an acute onset of the disturbance. Delirium, on the other hand, is typically characterized by an acute onset associated with medical illness and is present for days to weeks prior to resolution.

Seventy percent of patients with DLB experience persistent visual hallucinations and delusions. Hallucinations and delusions are characteristically present early in the course of DLB, as opposed to Alzheimer's dementia. Extrapyramidal motor features, although a hallmark of Parkinson's disease, are displayed by the current patient. However, 70% of patients with DLB demonstrate some form of extrapyramidal features, and in contrast to Parkinson's disease, DLB is characterized by cognitive changes early in the course of the disease. Dementia develops in one-third of cases of idiopathic Parkinson's disease but most frequently presents late in the course of the illness.

The pathogenesis of DLB has not been fully elucidated; however, a distinct neuropathology and neurochemistry have been identified. Lewy bodies are intraneuronal, spherical, eosinophilic, intracytoplasmic inclusion structures composed of ubiquitin or alpha-synuclein (see figure), and current theories connect the presence of Lewy bodies with the development of DLB symptoms. Lewy bodies have been identified in the neocortex, limbic cortex, subcortical nuclei, and brainstem, and evidence indicates that visual hallucinations may correlate with the number of Lewy bodies in the temporal lobe. In addition, DLB is associated with markedly decreased activity of cortical choline acetyltransferase (an enzyme which synthesizes acetylcholine), and this deficit is more pronounced at an early stage in DLB than in other types of dementia. Other studies suggest dopamine-2 receptor reduction, which is consistent with parkinsonian symptoms and neuroleptic sensitivity.

Treatment for this patient involves a combination of pharmacologic and behavioral interventions to optimize patient functioning. DLB appears to be preferentially responsive to cholinesterase inhibitors, which reflects the early, severe deficit in cholinergic function compared to other dementias. A recent randomized, placebo-controlled study demonstrated the efficacy of rivastigmine, an acetylcholinesterase inhibitor, in decreasing apathy, visual hallucinations, and delusions in DLB, but these benefits are lost when the medication is discontinued, indicating the need for ongoing management. In addition, patients with DLB have an increased sensitivity to neuroleptics due to the dopaminergic and cholinergic deficit, and neuroleptics should be avoided as a primary intervention in treating visual hallucinations unless necessary. Retrospective studies show that both typical and even atypical antipsychotics are associated with an

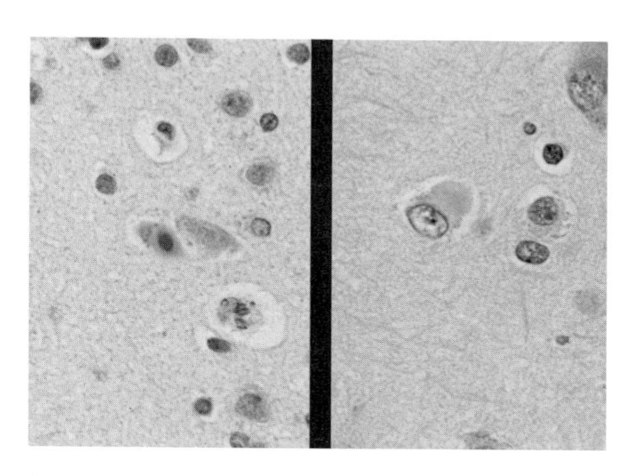

Split photo of cortical Lewy bodies. The Lewy bodies are spherical, eosinophilic, intracytoplasmic inclusion structures that have a dense core surrounded by a paler rim. The right side is stained with hemotoxylin and eosin, and the left side is alpha synuclein immunohistochemistry. (Courtesy of Daniel Perl, MD, Professor of Pathology, Mount Sinai School of Medicine.)

increased incidence of adverse events, including extrapyramidal side effects, features of neuroleptic malignant syndrome, and possibly increased mortality. Benzodiazepines should be especially avoided as a primary pharmacologic intervention, given the associated risk of confusion and falls. Other potential alternatives for control of associated agitation include low-dose mood stabilizers, buspirone, and potentially the newly approved NMDA antagonist memantine, but controlled trials are needed.

Behavioral strategies are equally important in managing a patient with dementia. Family and patient education, modification of the environment to diminish risk of falls, and provision of a supportive and highly structured atmosphere are means to decrease both patient and caregiver distress. Adult dementia day-care programs can provide additional structure for the patient as well as a needed respite for the family.

The present patient's diagnosis of DLB is supported by the presence of dementia coupled with fluctuating cognition, persistent visual hallucinations, and parkinsonian features. The diagnosis is further strengthened by the history of multiple falls and sensitivity to neuroleptics. The patient was placed on a cholinesterase inhibitor and showed substantial improvement in his fluctuating cognition and visual hallucinations. After extensive education of the patient and family, the patient began to attend adult day care, which allowed a protective atmosphere in which the patient could safely explore and receive appropriate stimulation while reducing caregiver burden.

Pearls

1. Postmortem studies indicate that DLB is grossly underdiagnosed by clinicians. It must be considered in cases of cortical dementia with extrapyramidal motor features.
2. DLB may respond preferentially to acetylcholinesterase inhibitors. One double-blind, placebo-controlled study demonstrated that rivastigmine therapy leads to a significant improvement in levels of apathy, anxiety, delusions and even hallucinations in patients with DLB.
3. Up to 57% of patients with DLB may experience the following adverse reactions to both typical and atypical antipsychotics: worsening extrapyramidal signs, sedation, immobility, fevers, or rigidity. If antipsychotics must be initiated, atypical antipsychotics with lower potency at the dopamine-2-receptor, such as quetiapine or clozapine, are preferred.
4. Cognitive changes in DLB are early, prominent, and primarily cortical. The cognitive changes of idiopathic Parkinson's disease-associated dementia, on the other hand, are more common at the end stages of the illness and are primarily subcortical in nature.

REFERENCES

1. Ballard CG, Aarsland D, O'Brien J, et al: Fluctuations in attention: PD dementia vs DLB with parkinsonsism. Neurology 2002;59:1714–1720.
2. Galvin J: Dementia with Lewy bodies. Arch Neurol 2003;60:1332–1335.
3. Khotianov N, Singh R, Singh S, et al: Lewy body dementia: Case report and discussion. J Am Board Fam Pract 2002;15:50–54.
4. McKeith I, Del Ser T, PierFranco S, et al: Efficacy of rivastigmine with Lewy bodies: A randomized, double-blind, placebo-controlled international study. Lancet 2000;356:2031–2036.
5. McKeith IG, Galasko D, Kosaka K, et al: Consensus guidelines for the clinical and pathological diagnosis of dementia with lewy bodies: Report of the consortium on DLB international workshop. Neurology 1996;47:1113–1124.
6. Serby M, Samuels SC: Diagnostic criteria for dementia with Lewy bodies reconsidered. Am J Geriatr Psychiatry 2001;9(3):212–216.
7. Verghese J, Lipton RB, Hall CB, et al: Abnormality of gait as a predictor of non-alzheimer's dementia. N Engl J Med 2002;347:1761–1768.

PATIENT 56

A 14-year-old boy with confusion and lethargy

History of Present Illness: A 14-year-old boy who was the recipient of a liver transplant due to cryptogenic cirrhosis is now in the pediatric intensive care unit (PICU) for abdominal pain and elevated liver enzymes. He was being prepared for a liver biopsy. He had recently received a pulsed dose of prednisone and was started on antibiotics, after which the abdominal pain developed. Initial labs were notable for leukopenia, which was thought to be due most probably to cyclosporine. Blood cultures were sent.

Soon after his admission, the patient began screaming unintelligibly and tearing at the sheets of his bed. Nursing staff paged the pediatrician on call and reported that the patient was agitated. When the physician arrived at the bedside, the patient was found to be sluggish and unable to cooperate with an evaluation. The pediatrician was able to ascertain that the patient was confused and not responding appropriately to staff members. He also appeared very frightened and mentioned several times that bugs were crawling on the bed and ceiling. At other times, he seemed to be responding to someone else in the room as if he were hearing voices. His ability to stay alert also seemed to vary, and he would shift between moments of lucidity and lethargy. Psychiatry was asked to see the patient to help manage the current agitation.

Past Psychiatric History: The patient had a liver transplant 7 years ago and had spent a significant portion of the current school year in the hospital. He was noted to be increasingly depressed for the last year. Child psychiatry had been consulted, and the patient was diagnosed with depression secondary to a general medical condition (chronic liver disease/transplant). The patient was started on citalopram but failed to adhere to follow-up appointments, and his mother eventually called the psychiatrist to say that he no longer seemed depressed. The mother denied that the patient has any previous history of substance abuse, psychotic symptoms, or cognitive impairment.

Past Medical History: Cryptogenic cirrhosis, on cyclosporine.

Mental Status Examination: The patient is found to be fairly groomed and well nourished, but he appears younger than his stated age. His behavior is slightly agitated, alternating with periods in which he stares at the wall and appears internally preoccupied. He utters one-word phrases addressed to the wall, but his speech at these times is indecipherable. He appears to be confused—he is oriented to person but not to place or time. When asked to describe his mood, he states "Okay," but he is anxious and angry, and his affect is clearly labile. He denies any suicidal or homicidal ideation. Thought process is perseverative: he first begins to complain about his lack of clothing in the hospital, and when the interviewer tries to redirect him, he continues to return to talking about his clothes. Poor impulse control is noted as he aggressively pushes away nursing staff when they try to assist him. On mini-mental state exam (MMSE), he is oriented to person only and is unable to recall 3 items, either immediately or after a 3-minute delay. He does not seem able to maintain concentration and quickly loses track of the task when asked to spell the word "world."

Laboratory Examinations: Complete blood count is unremarkable except for the aforementioned leukopenia (WBC = 2.3×10^6). Electrolytes and liver function tests are unchanged from admission (sodium, 140; potassium, 3.9; calcium, 8.5; alanine aminotransferase, 236; aspartate aminotransferase, 301). Urinalysis is negative, urine toxicology screen is negative, and blood alcohol level is 0. Blood cultures are pending.

Diagnostic Testing: Electroencephalogram (EEG) was performed to rule out seizure activity and showed generalized slowing but no evidence of an epileptogenic rhythm. Electrocardiogram showed a normal sinus rhythm at 96.

Question: What is the diagnosis?

Diagnosis: Substance-induced delirium.

Discussion: According to the DSM-IV-TR, delirium is categorized based on etiology and includes delirium due to a general medical condition, substance-induced delirium (including medication side effects), delirium due to multiple etiologies, or delirium not otherwise specified. In this case, the patient is probably suffering from a substance-induced delirium (secondary to prednisone administration). In general, delirium disorders share a common symptom presentation, but the DSM-IV-TR requires evidence from the history, physical examination, or laboratory findings indicating that the delirious disturbance is caused by direct consequences of the proposed etiology. In the case of substance-induced delirium, the symptoms must have developed during substance intoxication or, in the case of medications, the "medication use must be etiologically related to the disturbance."

Delirium is characterized by fluctuating levels of consciousness, difficulty in arousability, and an inability to sustain attention. Patients may not be able to focus and describe clouding or reduced clarity of awareness of the environment. Delirium typically develops over a short period; of note, its development may be preceded by several days of symptoms, such as anxiety, irritability, restlessness, fear, insomnia, drowsiness, hallucinations, and nightmares. The symptoms of delirium may last from days to weeks, and their severity fluctuates over the course of the day, ranging from severe impairment and disorganization to periods of lucidity.

The patient with delirium must suffer from either cognitive changes, such as memory impairment, disorientation, and language disturbance, or changes in mood, behavior, and perception. Patients may become very angry and agitated or describe hallucinations (particularly of the visual modality) or delusional thought. Psychomotor disturbances may manifest as either hyperactivity with increased startle response, flushing, sweating, and tachycardia, or hypoactivity, with slowed reaction time, catatonia, or depression. A disturbance of thought process is also characteristic and may include rambling, changes in the flow of speech, or incoherent speech. Patients frequently report sleep disturbance, such as insomnia, nightmares, and hypnapompic or hypnagogic hallucinations. Reversal of the sleep-wake cycle may also occur with significant daytime drowsiness.

Up to one-third of patients on surgical wards, medical wards, or intensive care units experience delirium over the course of their hospital admission. Patients with underlying dementia and the elderly in general are at the greatest risk. Other risk factors include pre-existing brain damage, a previous history of delirium, alcohol dependence, recent surgery, and malnutrition. Delirium should always be suspected in patients on medical or surgical wards with psychiatric symptoms that are new or abrupt in onset.

The most common causes of delirium are central nervous system disease, systemic disease (e.g., cardiac failure), and substance/medication intoxication or withdrawal. Postoperative delirium is also common and may be due to electrolyte imbalance, infection, fever, or blood loss. To date, the neurochemical cause of delirium is unknown, but acetylcholine has been hypothesized to be the major neurotransmitter involved.

In the present patient (as is almost always the case with delirium), a vast differential diagnosis must be considered. Psychiatric disorders, such as dementia, substance intoxication or withdrawal, depression, schizophrenia, brief psychotic disorder, mania, factitious disorder, and dissociative disorders, are possible diagnoses. Most of these can be safely ruled out in the present patient. Dementia is likely to have a more insidious, progressive onset and less likely to have impaired attention and consciousness (see Table 1) and is essentially unheard of in 14-year-olds. Major depression with psychotic features is a consideration, especially given his history of depression; however, it would not explain the acuity of his presentation or the dramatic severity of his lethargy, attentional deficit, and cognitive impairment. Mania, too, may explain some of the thought disorder, irritability, and agitation but is unlikely in this patient based on the presence of alternating periods of sleepiness and lethargy. A primary psychotic illness, such as schizophrenia, is less likely in a patient so young,

Table 1. Delirium vs. Dementia

Dementia	Delirium
Clouding of consciousness	No changes in consciousness
Significant attentional deficit	Less attentional deficit
Sudden onset (hours to days)	Gradual onset (weeks to years)
Cognitive impairments fluctuate	Gradual worsening of impairment
Duration of symptoms is transient	Duration is chronic
A precipitant is usually identifiable	An identifiable precipitant is not required

Adapted from Psychiatry Essentials: A Systematic Review. Philadelphia, Hanley & Belfus, 2001.

with no family history, and with previous normal functioning in school and social performance, but the possibility of a new-onset psychotic episode should be considered.

As far as medical differential diagnoses are concerned, many etiologies must be considered. Epilepsy, head trauma, infection, endocrine dysfunction, electrolyte imbalance, hepatic encephalopathy, and uremic encephalopathy are some of the possibilities. Toxic levels of most medications may also produce symptoms of delirium, and anticholinergics, anticonvulsants, antipsychotics, antihypertensives, sedatives, lithium, and steroids are typical offenders. Carbon dioxide toxicity, hypoxia, cardiac failure, vitamin deficiencies (e.g., thiamine, vitamin B_{12}, folate), and heavy metal poisoning must also be considered.

The present patient was under close medical observation due to his history of liver disease. He was well nourished, and his laboratory and diagnostic testing ruled out uremia, infection, pellagra, metabolic imbalance, and cardiac disease as a cause of mental status changes. An electroencephalogram (EEG) did not show the presence of a seizure disorder to explain the agitation and confusion. In fact, generalized, slow-wave patterns are typically associated with delirium. Although substance intoxication and withdrawal can often make patients appear delirious, the current patient had a negative toxicology screen. The most likely cause of the patient's delirium was thought to be the large dose of corticosteroids. Corticosteroids have been associated with confusion and aggression, and the fact that the patient was given a large dose of prednisone prior to his acute mental status change makes this a likely cause of delirium.

Agitated behavior is the most common reason for consultation in patients with delirium. Treatment requires elucidation and stabilization of the underlying etiology. Medicating the symptoms of agitation or psychosis is usually avoided, if possible, to prevent further complication of the picture. That being said, in delirium due to anticholinergic toxicity, physostigmine may be used in repeated doses. Similarly, high-potency antipsychotics, such as haloperidol, are often used to target psychotic symptoms. Patients must be carefully monitored to avoid hurting themselves intentionally or accidentally. Agitated behavior may respond to reducing sources of excessive stimulation in the environment. Disorientation can sometimes be prevented or reduced by observing daylight and nighttime switches of lighting on medical and surgical units, along with clear orienting cues (clocks and calendars).

The present patient was empirically started on a multivitamin and hydrated with intravenous fluids; corticosteroid therapy was withheld. Attempts were made to reorient him to his environment, including bringing in family members and familiar medical staff. Consideration was given to start antipsychotic medication, but this step became unnecessary because the patient's clinical course improved rapidly after tapering corticosteroid therapy. The chief complaint of abdominal pain was thought to be secondary to the corticosteroid pulse. Once blood culture results were found to be negative, the patient was transferred to the pediatric ward and eventually home.

Pearls

1. Low doses of antipsychotic drugs can control agitation, but benzodiazepines should be avoided due to possible paradoxical reactions, unless they are used specifically for alcohol or substance abuse withdrawal.
2. Visual hallucinations are more likely to occur in delirium than in a primary psychotic disorder.
3. Delirium may be divided into three subtypes: hyperactive, hypoactive, and mixed. The hyperactive subtype is characterized by agitation, disorientation, hallucinations, or delusions. Hypoactive patients are quiet, confused and apathetic. Mixed subtype patients are characterized by a combination of symptoms from both subtypes.
4. A classic sign of delirium is carphologia, in which the patient picks at bed sheets or clothes.

REFERENCES

1. Anderson SD, Hewko RA: Studying delirium. Can Med Assoc J 2003;168:755–757.
2. Gleason O: Delirium. Am FamPhysician, 2003;67(5):1027–1034.
3. Kaplan, HI, Sadock BJ: Synopsis of Psychiatry, 8th ed. Philadelphia, Lippincott Williams & Wilkins, YEAR?, pp 320–328.
4. Meagher DJ: Delirium: Optimising management. Br Med J 2001;322:144–149.

Javier A. Muniz, MD

PATIENT 57

A 31-year-old woman with fatigue and myalgia

History of Present Illness: While on the consultation liaison service, you are called to the emergency department to evaluate a 31-year-old woman who initially presented with vague physical symptoms of hoarseness, fatigue, and myalgias, but the emergency physician wants her to be evaluated for depression. The patient describes a 3-week history of worsening depressed mood, decreased energy, excessive sleeping, and crying spells. She tells you that she does not feel like doing anything anymore and that her husband is no longer attracted to her because of all the weight she has gained over the past month or so. "I don't understand why I've gained weight because I don't really feel like eating much anymore," she says as she breaks down in tears. She also describes constant worrying, especially about not being able to take care of her 8-month-old baby and being a bad mother. "It's like I can't get those thoughts out of my mind."

Past Psychiatric History: The patient denies any prior psychiatric history. The only time that she felt depressed in the past was a few days after the birth of her child 8 months ago, but her physician told her it was normal, saying that she had the "baby blues." She admits to having 1–2 drinks strictly in social situations but denies any drug use.

Past Medical History: There is no significant medical history and the patient thinks of herself as a very healthy person. She contrasts this statement by mentioning the fact that "my mother and sister have lupus."

Mental Status Examination: The patient is a slightly disheveled and overweight woman who appears her stated age. She has good eye contact and relates well to you. She is sitting on the edge of her bed with her arms to her side and barely moves during the interview. Her speech is somewhat husky, normal in rate, but low in volume, and there is a slight delay in her responses. She feels "depressed," and her affect is blunted. Her thought process is linear and goal-directed. She denies any ideas of hurting herself or others, and you are not able to elicit any delusional thought content. A quick cognitive exam shows no significant memory or obvious concentration impairment. There is some insight into the nature of her depressive symptoms, and her judgment seems adequate at this time.

Physical Examination: Vital signs: Heart rate = 64 beats/min; respirations = 18 breaths/min; blood pressure = 108/72 mmHg; temperature = 37.0°C. Physical exam reveals an obese woman in no distress. Her skin is dry and flaky. You are unable to palpate her thyroid because of her weight, but no bruits are heard on auscultation. She has no focal findings on neurologic exam, but knee reflexes are slowed at approximately 2/5 bilaterally. The remainder of her physical exam is unremarkable.

Laboratory Examination: Complete blood count shows a mild normochromic, normocytic anemia. Chemistry and liver function tests are within normal limits. Urine pregnancy and toxicology screens are negative. Thyroid function tests are pending.

Question: What underlying condition most likely explains the patient's depressive symptoms?

Diagnosis: Depressive disorder due to general medical condition: hypothyroidism.

Discussion: The patient has overt hypothyroidism. Even though thyroid function tests are pending, we can rely on her multiple physical and psychiatric symptoms to reach the diagnosis: depression, fatigue, weight gain, dry, flaky skin, anemia, and a hoarse voice. Hypothyroidism is the result of inadequate levels of thyroid hormone and can be either overt (clinical) or subclinical. In subclinical hypothyroidism, hormone levels are normal, but thyroid-stimulating hormone (TSH) is elevated or there is an exaggerated response to thyroid-releasing hormone (TRH) infusion, and the patient is by definition asymptomatic. In overt hypothyroidism thyroid hormones are low, TSH is elevated, and the patient is symptomatic. TSH is the most sensitive assay for hypothyroidism. TSH level is expected to be high in primary thyroid gland dysfunction and low in pituitary or hypothalamic pathology.

Both clinical and subclinical hypothyroidism can present with psychiatric symptoms, which may not respond to antidepressant treatment unless the underlying thyroid disorder is treated. Psychiatric manifestations are usually nonspecific but may resemble symptoms of depression, such as depressed mood, fatigue, decreased appetite, and mental slowing. Early symptoms are often attributed to aging, dementia, depression, or even Parkinson's disease. In extreme cases, "myxedema madness" syndrome has been described. This syndrome consists of hallucinations and paranoia and may result in coma or even death due to diminished cerebral blood flow. It is theorized that depressive symptoms may be a consequence of reduced central serotonin activity and a reduction in the number and function of postsynaptic beta receptors since thyroid hormone is known to affect the serotonergic and adrenergic systems.

In adults, hypothyroidism is most commonly caused by Hashimoto's thyroiditis, an autoimmune disease, but other causes include idiopathic atrophy, deficiency of dietary iodine, or hypopituitarism (from postpartum necrosis). Iatrogenic hypothyroidism is also important to consider in any patient on lithium therapy. It is estimated that the risk of developing overt hypothyroidism is approximately 20% in patients on lithium, and another 20% may develop subclinical hypothyroidism. In other words, almost half the patient population on long-term lithium maintenance therapy may have some degree of thyroid dysfunction. Some medications, such as carbamazepine, phenytoin, and barbiturates, may also lower total and free thyroid hormones by increasing their hepatic metabolism. The prevalence of clinical hypothyroidism in the general population is around 2% in women and 0.1% in men, and the prevalence of subclinical hypothyroidism is approximately 7.5% in women and 3% in men.

Medical and psychiatric symptoms of hypothyroidism usually respond well to hormone replacement, but cognitive problems may be permanent if the deficit has been prolonged. It is estimated that 10% of patients continue to have residual psychiatric symptoms after treatment with hormone replacement. There are many preparations of thyroid hormones, but levothyroxine (T_4) therapy is preferred over liothyronine (T_3) because the effects of the medication are more predictable, and it exhibits all the actions of endogenous thyroid hormone. Response should be assessed by frequent testing of thyroid function, and the return to a euthyroid state may take several weeks. Clinicians must be careful not to be too aggressive in initial treatment and thus place patients in a possible hyperthyroid state.

The present patient was diagnosed with hypothyroidism based on evidence from the thyroid function tests, which showed elevated TSH and suppressed thyroid hormone. The presence of antithyroid antibodies and histologic evidence on biopsy confirmed the etiology of Hashimoto's thyroiditis, and she was started on levothyroxine. Autoimmune diseases are more common in women and with advancing age in general. In addition, the present patient has a strong family history of lupus and was therefore at increased risk of developing an autoimmune disease herself.

After a careful discussion with the patient and her husband, you decide that she is not an imminent threat to herself or others and that her depressive symptoms can be monitored with an outpatient psychiatrist while her thyroid condition is managed by her primary care physician. Her depression and the other signs and symptoms of thyroid dysfunction improved steadily with levothyroxine treatment over the next few weeks. At her 2-month follow-up visit she reports being symptom-free, and thyroid function monitoring shows a return of TSH levels to within normal limits. The remainder of her care is transferred to the primary care physician, who recommends ongoing monitoring in addition to continued thyroid hormone replacement therapy.

Pearls

1. Both clinical and subclinical hypothyroidism can produce a variety of psychiatric symptoms.

2. Since TSH can be normal in subclinical hypothyroidism, the condition is often underrecognized and therefore not treated. Some clinicians recommend thyroid supplementation in patients who do not respond to standard antidepressant treatment even when TSH is normal.

3. There is debate in the literature about the association of hypothyroidism with treatment-refractory depression and rapid cycling bipolar disorder. Of note, both blunted and exaggerated TSH responses to TRH infusion have been found in patients with treatment-refractory depression, but the exaggerated TSH response to TRH infusion has been most associated with rapid-cycling bipolar disorder.

4. Significant controversy surrounds the bioequivalence of different oral preparations of levothyroxine products. Levothyroxine has been in use since the 1950s, and many preparations have not been reviewed by modern FDA approval processes. In 1997, the FDA committed to ensure the purity, potency, stability, safety, and efficacy of all oral levothyroxine products by August of 2003. To date, only a handful of the available products have been approved by the FDA, and some may be retired from the market.

REFERENCES

1. Altshuler LL, Bauer M, Frye MA, et al: Does thyroid supplementation accelerate tricyclic antidepressant response? A review and meta-analysis of the literature. Am J Psychiatry 2001;158:1617–1622.
2. Bauer MS, Whybrow PC, Winokur A: Rapid cycling bipolar affective disorder I: Association with grade I hypothyroidism. Arch Gen Psychiatry 1990;47:427–432.
3. Berlin I, Corruble E: Thyroid hormones and antidepressant response. Am J Psychiatry 2002;159:1441.
4. Dong BJ, Hauck WW, Gambertoglio JG, et al: Bioequivalence of generic and brand-name levothyroxine products in the treatment of hypothyroidism. JAMA 1997;277:1205–1213.
5. Geffken GR, Ward HE, Staab JP, et al: Psychiatric morbidity in endocrine disorders. Psychiatr Clin North Am 1998;1:473–489.
6. Haggerty J, Stern RA, Mason GA, et al: Subclinical hypothyroidism: A modifiable risk factor for depression? Am J Psychiatry 1993;150:508–510.
7. Hendrick VC, Garrick TR: Hypothyroidism. In Kaplan and Sadock's Comprehensive Textbook of Psychiatry. vol II, 7th ed. Philadelphia, Lippincott Williams & Wilkins, 2000, pp 1808–1812.
8. Wolkin A, Peselow ED, Smith M, et al: TRH test abnormalities in psychiatric disorders. J Affect Disord 1984;6:273–281.

PATIENT 58

An 18-year old girl with weight loss and irritability

History of Present Illness: The patient is an 18-year-old girl brought unwillingly by her parents to her pediatrician's office. The doctor asks the patient why she is there, and she responds that there is no reason for her to be there because she is fine. Her parents explain to the doctor that they went to see their daughter at college after receiving an alarming phone call from one of her friends. The friend reported that over the past few months the patient had seemed different. She seemed less happy, less social, and more irritable. She seemed "too driven" both in academics and on the long-distance track team. In addition, she seemed extremely preoccupied with her weight. Despite having lost a substantial amount of weight since the beginning of the school year, she had recently confided to her friend that she wears baggy clothing because she thinks that she is fat. When the friend tried to talk to the patient about her concerns, the patient became defensive and angry and then refused to speak with her. The patient's parents initially found it hard to believe what their daughter's friend had told them. They had noticed a few months earlier, when the patient came home for Thanksgiving dinner, that she spent a lot of time cutting her food into small pieces but then ate only a few bites. When they remarked about it, she dismissed their concern, explaining that she was "getting over a virus." After receiving the concerning phone call from her friend, the patient's parents decided to visit their daughter at college. Her face looked gaunt and tired, and her weight loss was striking. Despite the patient's extreme protests, the parents decided that she must come home with them, and they brought her immediately to her pediatrician.

The patient is the oldest of three children. Her father is a doctor, and her mother is an advertising executive. The patient is currently a freshman at a prestigious college a few hours from where she grew up. She is a premedical student and is expected to be a doctor like her father. Although the patient has received almost all As since she started college, she is extremely self-critical and does not feel that her grades are good enough. The patient is also highly competitive on the track team. In addition to the daily track team practices, she spends hours at the gym working out on her own. The patient's boyfriend of 6 months has recently broken up with her for a multitude of reasons, including her moodiness, lack of interest in social activities, and lack of interest in intimacy. The break-up is hard for the patient, and she has frequent crying spells. She also recently stopped hanging out with her friends. The patient is highly secretive, and some friends wonder if she could be using drugs especially since she only sleeps a few hours a night but never seems tired. The patient was supposed to go the track team doctor for a routine physical and drug screen; however, she keeps missing her appointments.

Past Psychiatric History: At her parents' insistence, the patient first saw a psychologist at the age of 15. Her parents were worried that she was "depressed" because she was not as outgoing as her younger siblings and was often isolative. They were also concerned because she seemed to be a perfectionist and had low self-esteem. She stopped seeing the psychologist after about 6 months, explaining to her parents that she did not need help and used her latest report card as evidence of her claim.

Mental Status Examination: The patient is a young woman wearing sweatpants and a baggy sweatshirt. Her hair is neatly pulled back in a ponytail. She is not wearing any make-up; of note is her gaunt and narrow face. She is mildly withdrawn with intermittent eye contact and uncooperative with many of the questions. Her speech is of normal rate, rhythm, and volume. She speaks articulately and with an extensive vocabulary. She reports her mood as "fine," although her affect is constricted and dysphoric at times. Her thought process is goal-directed, and she denies any thought content or perceptual disturbances. The patient denies active suicidal ideation, although she admits that at times the thought of wanting to die has "crossed my mind." She denies homicidal ideation. Her insight and judgment related to her illness are poor; she adamantly denies that there is anything wrong with her and asserts that she is not too thin.

Diagnostic Testing: CT scan of the head shows ventricular enlargement and sulci widening.

Questions: What are the characteristics of this illness? Discuss the possible treatments.

Diagnosis: Anorexia nervosa.

Discussion: Anorexia nervosa is one of three eating disorders categorized in DSM-IV-TR. Anorexia nervosa is defined as having four main characteristics, including a body weight at < 85% of that which is normal for age and height, a distorted body image, and an intense fear of gaining weight or becoming fat despite being underweight. The fourth criterion is amenorrhea—absence of at least 3 consecutive menstrual cycles—in postmenarcheal females. The DSM-IV-TR separates anorexia nervosa into two subtypes: the binge-eating/purging type and the restricting type. In the binge-eating/purging type, the person regularly engages in binge eating or purging behavior (e.g., self-induced vomiting, misuse of laxatives, diuretics or enemas), whereas in the restricting type the person does not regularly engage in any of these behaviors. People can alternate between the binge-eating/purging type and the restricting type at different periods of their illness.

The prevalence of anorexia nervosa in adolescent girls is 0.5–1%. However, it is estimated that up to 5% of all young women have symptoms of this illness but do not meet diagnostic criteria for anorexia nervosa. Although the incidence of anorexia nervosa has greatly increased in the past few decades, it is not a new illness. Well-documented case reports of anorexia nervosa can be found throughout history and date back to the Middle Ages. Of interest, throughout history it is predominately females who suffer from this illness, and at present 90% of people with anorexia nervosa are women. The most common age of onset is the midteens, and 85% have an onset between the ages of 13 and 20 years.

The precise etiology of anorexia nervosa is unknown; however, it is clear that biologic, social, and psychological factors contribute to this disorder. Evidence for a genetic contribution includes an increased incidence of mood disorders and eating disorders in first-degree relatives of patients with anorexia nervosa and studies showing a higher concordance rate of anorexia nervosa in monozygotic twins than in dizygotic twins. Although studies demonstrate a genetic contribution, the size of this contribution remains unclear. The incidence of anorexia nervosa has risen dramatically in the past few decades since Western culture has increasingly emphasized the concept that thinness is good and the equating of beauty with low body weight. These cultural elements may be a social factor contributing to the increased prevalence of anorexia nervosa. In addition, studies have demonstrated an increased prevalence of anorexia nervosa when non-Western people are exposed to Western ideals of thinness. Other social factors that increase the risk for this disorder include a troubled relationship with parents, a history of sexual abuse, and an emphasis on dieting in the family. Females active in sports that emphasize appearance, such as gymnastics, ballet, and distance running, are also at greater risk for anorexia nervosa.

Many psychological theories have been proposed to explain the development of anorexia nervosa. Cognitive behavioral theories suggest that the restriction of food intake has two main origins. The first is a need to feel in control of life. This need for control is then displaced onto controlling food intake. The second origin is an overemphasis of the effect of weight and shape on self-worth. Both of these cognitions are then reinforced by dietary restriction and weight loss. Since anorexia nervosa most often occurs during adolescence, the need to feel in control may be in part a reaction to the demands of normal adolescent pursuits, such as increased independence and increased social and sexual functioning. There are also a variety of psychodynamic explanations for the etiology of anorexia nervosa. At the root of these explanations is the belief that the patient is unable to resolve a psychological conflict, and the disorder serves as a psychological holding pattern—a way of avoiding emotional and psychological growth. In fact, anorexia nervosa does result in a halting of physical development (i.e., amenorrhea) and in the halting of psychological development because patients become preoccupied with thoughts of food and weight.

The most common differential diagnoses of anorexia nervosa include bulimia nervosa, depressive disorders, and medical illnesses that cause weight loss. Bulimia nervosa can be distinguished from anorexia nervosa because patients with bulimia nervosa do not weigh less than 85% of their expected body weight. Patients with depressive disorders can be differentiated from those with anorexia nervosa because they are not preoccupied with their weight and report decreased appetite. Although anorexia literally means "lack of appetite," people with anorexia nervosa restrict their food intake despite hunger. It is only late in the disorder that people with anorexia nervosa may have a loss of appetite. Medical conditions that can cause weight loss include Crohn's disease, hyperthyroidism, Addison's disease, and diabetes mellitus. These diagnoses can be made with a thorough history, review of systems, and medical work-up.

The present patient had all of the main characteristics of anorexia nervosa, including low body weight, fear of gaining weight, disturbance in her perception of her shape, preoccupation with her shape, and denial of the seriousness of low body weight. Like the present patient, others with the anorexia nervosa lose weight by a severe restriction of food intake and avoidance of foods that are high in fat or carbohydrates. It is also common for patients to exercise excessively and to spend many hours every day working out. In addition, people with anorexia nervosa, like the present patient, may have strange eating habits, including spitting out food, cutting food into small pieces, or rearranging food on a plate. Often patients try to hide their eating behaviors and may refuse to eat with others or in public places. Also as exhibited by this patient, people with anorexia nervosa often exhibit depressive symptoms, including social isolation, irritability, and loss of sexual appetite. Up to 50% of patient's with anorexia nervosa have comorbid major depressive disorder or dysthymic disorder. Other psychiatric symptoms often seen in anorexia nervosa include obsessive-compulsive traits or symptoms of social phobia. Low self-esteem and perfectionism are also common traits in people with anorexia nervosa.

Multiple medical problems can occur in anorexia nervosa. The most common medical problems include osteoporosis with resultant fractures, leukopenia, anemia, hypothyroidism, renal function abnormalities (including elevated levels of blood urea nitrogen), hypercholesterolemia, amenorrhea with low levels of luteinizing hormone and follicle-stimulating hormone, and hypotension. Cardiac complications include bradycardia, arrhythmias, prolonged QT interval, and sudden death. If a patient with anorexia nervosa regularly engages in purging behavior, many additional medical problems may occur, including electrolyte abnormalities (e.g., hypokalemic-hypochloremic alkalosis, hypomagnesaemia), gastrointestinal problems (e.g., esophageal and gastric erosion), dental problems, and seizures. On physical exam, the doctor may see signs suggesting anorexia nervosa such as emaciation, bradycardia, hypotension, hypothermia, pitting edema, dry skin, and lanugo (fine baby-like hair). Physical signs of purging include parotid gland hypertrophy, dental erosion, and scarring of the dorsum of the hand caused by scratching the hand during self-induced emesis.

The treatment of anorexia nervosa is difficult because the patients often do not want to be helped. People with anorexia nervosa judge their self-worth largely or even exclusively by their weight and shape and their ability to control them. The type of treatment required is determined by the severity of the illness. Possible treatment settings include outpatient therapy, a day program, or inpatient hospitalization on a medical or psychiatric unit. The decision to hospitalize is based on medical, psychiatric, and behavioral factors. Medical indications for hospitalization include very low weight (usually those weighing < 75% of that which is normal for age and height), severe electrolyte disturbances, hypoglycemia, infection, and vital sign changes (bradycardia or marked orthostatic hypotension). Other factors to consider include the potential for suicide, a history of failure using less intensive treatment, or rapid or persistent decline in oral intake. Many types of psychotherapy are used to help patients with anorexia nervosa, including cognitive behavioral therapy, psychodynamic psychotherapy, and family therapy. Medications are sometimes used as adjuncts in the treatment of anorexia nervosa. However, it is important to note that no medication has yet proved beneficial in the treatment of anorexia nervosa or in promoting long-lasting weight gain. Some preliminary evidence suggests that fluoxetine may be beneficial in preventing relapse; however, confirmatory studies are required. Medication may be indicated for patients with anorexia nervosa who have a comorbid psychiatric illness such as depressive disorders.

The course of anorexia nervosa varies greatly, and results of long-term outcome studies differ. Approximately 25% of patients recover, 25% remain chronically ill, and 50% have a partial improvement in symptoms. Poor prognostic factors include initial lower minimum weight, purging behavior, history of poor treatment response, and disturbed family relationships. It is important to remember that anorexia nervosa can be a deadly illness. Mortality usually results from cardiac arrest or suicide, and studies show a mortality rate ranging from 5% to 18%. The present patient was not admitted to the hospital, but she was referred to a treatment center that specializes in the care of eating disorders. She agreed to start psychotherapy, although she remained convinced that it would not be helpful.

Pearls

1. MRI and CT scans of patients with anorexia nervosa may show ventricular enlargement and a reduction in total gray and white matter volume. Some studies have shown that, even though white matter and ventricular volumes of cerebrospinal fluid (CSF) normalize with refeeding, gray matter deficits persist.
2. Although patients with anorexia nervosa cause themselves severe physical and psychological harm, the patient's intent is usually not consciously self-destructive.
3. Serotonin—a neurotransmitter thought to increase satiation, decrease food intake, and modulate obsessive-compulsive behaviors—may be increased in anorexia nervosa, since it has been shown that elevated CSF 5-HIAA levels (a metabolite of serotonin) are present in weight-restored anorectic patients.
4. Corticotropin-releasing factor, believed to inhibit eating behavior, has been found to be increased in people with anorexia nervosa. Of interest, this neuroendocrine product normalizes with weight restoration.

REFERENCES

1. Davis W: The anorexic adolescent. In O'Brien JD, Pilowsky D, Lewis O (eds): Psychotherapies with Children and Adolescents: Adapting the Psychodynamic Process. Northvale, NJ, Jason Aronson, Inc. 1992.
2. Fairburn CG, Cooper Z, Doll HA, Welch SL: Risk Factors for anorexia nervosa: Three integrated case control comparisons. Arch Gen Psychiatry 1999;56:468–476.
3. Fairburn CG, Harrison PJ: Eating disorders. Lancet 2003;361:407–416.
4. Halmi KA: Anorexia nervosa and bulimia nervosa. In Lewis M (ed): Child and Adolescent Psychiatry: A Comprehensive Textbook. Philadelphia, Lippincott Williams & Wilkins. 2002.
5. Halmi K: Eating disorders. In Martin A, Scahill L, Charney D, Leukman J (eds): Pediatric Psychopharmacology. New York, Oxford University Press, 2003.
6. Hendren R, DeBacker I, Pandina G: Review of neuroimaging studies of child and adolescent psychiatric disorders from the past 10 years. Am Acad Child Adolesc Psychiatry 2000;39:815–828.
7. Kaplan H, Saddock B: Kaplan and Saddocks's Synopsis of Psychiatry. Philaelphia, Lippincott Williams & Wilkins, 1998.
8. Kaye W, Nagata T, Weltzin TE, et al: Double-blind placebo-controlled administration of fluoxetine in restricting and restricting-purging-type anorexia nervosa. Biol Psychiatry 2001;49:644–652.
9. Kaye W, Strober M, Klump K: Neurobiology of eating disorders. In Martin A, Scahill L, Charney D, Leukman J (eds): Pediatric Psychopharmacology. New York, Oxford University Press, 2003.

Jacques Jospitre, Jr., MD

PATIENT 59

A 71-year-old woman with poor memory and irritability

History of Present Illness: A 71-year-old woman presents with her husband to the psychiatric outpatient department with complaints of memory impairment and increased irritability. The patient minimizes her complaints and insists that the evaluation is unnecessary. The husband is able to provide an account of what has been happening at home. He reports that she was in her usual state of good mental health until a few months ago when she started complaining about her housekeeper stealing items from the home. Later, when the same items were found, she insisted that they had been stolen and returned rather than simply misplaced. Since that time she has progressively worsened to the point that she cannot remember where her belongings are located. On several occasions, she has left the stove on or the shower running, forgetting that she turned them on. Her speech has been noted to be slower with intermittent pauses as she searches for words to express herself. Family and friends have complained to her that she is forgetting dates—birthdays and holidays. Although she worked as a shop owner and balanced the checkbook throughout their marriage, her husband took over this role about a year ago after finding several grave errors. She insisted that she had paid the bills when in fact she had not. She stopped driving at her children's insistence after she was noted to be "all over the road." Despite all of this, she still manages to enjoy her time with family and friends. She spends her free time watching television and playing bridge (although her game has suffered). Her husband insisted that she be evaluated after she got lost on her way back home from the local store.

The woman denies symptoms of mania, psychosis, neurovegetative symptoms of depression, and anxiety. She has no history of substance abuse, significant head trauma, serious infectious disease, diabetes mellitus, or hypertension. The patient is a college graduate with a long career as a successful business woman; she retired 7 years before the date of presentation. She has been taking calcium supplements and estrogen replacement since menopause at the age of 51.

Past Psychiatric History: The patient has no significant past psychiatric history. She denies any signs or symptoms consistent with a mood or psychotic disorder. Her only family history is that her mother was "very forgetful in her later years." The mother passed away from pneumonia at the age of 76.

Mental Status Examination: The patient is a healthy-looking female who appears her stated age. Her eye contact is fair. She is cooperative and engaging. She displays no psychomotor agitation or retardation. Her speech is of normal volume and tone, but she is a bit slow at times and complains of word-finding difficulty. She describes her mood as "good" and appears euthymic. Her affect is mood-congruent and stable. Thought process is linear and organized. Her thought content is focused on her belief that she is "fine," and that this psychiatric assessment is unnecessary. She denies any suicidal ideation, homicidal ideation, paranoid ideation, or perceptual disturbances. Her insight is poor, and judgment is limited, but she is in good control. She is alert and oriented to person, place, and time, and her concentration is within normal limits. Her Folstein Mini-Mental Status Exam score is 24/30; she is unable to do serial sevens and has zero recall of three words after five minutes.

Diagnostic Testing: Chemistries, liver function tests, complete blood count with platelets, and thyroid-stimulating hormone levels are within normal limits. Vitamin B_{12}, folate, and homocysteine testing are also unremarkable. Urine toxicology is negative. Head imaging shows mild atrophy that is within normal limits for stated age with no signs of cerebrovascular events or any mass.

Questions: What is the diagnosis? How should the patient be treated?

Diagnosis: Late-onset Alzheimer's disease, with behavioral disturbance.

Discussion: Alzheimer's disease (AD) is the most common cause of dementia in the geriatric population, accounting for up to two-thirds of all dementias in geriatric patients. Dementia is defined as a chronic and worsening impairment of memory and other cognitive functions, in the absence of delirium, that affects social or occupational functioning and is a clear decline from previous level of functioning. The cognitive impairment can present as worsening memory along with disturbance in language, impaired motor task activity with intact motor function, impaired object identification with intact sensory function, and a disturbance in executive functioning (i.e., planning, organizing, sequencing, and abstracting). There can also be changes in personality, mood, and/or behavior. In general, for patients to be given the diagnosis of dementia, they should have impaired memory functioning and at least one of these other cognitive deficits. The gold-standard diagnosis of AD is still made at autopsy.

When the diagnosis of dementia is being considered, other psychiatric disorders must be ruled out, such as delirium, depression, mental retardation, or amnestic disorder. Even though the present patient has cognitive impairment, which is seen in both delirium and dementia, delirium can be ruled out based on her presentation. With delirium she would have a disturbance in consciousness that rendered her unable to focus or maintain attention. Furthermore, her symptoms have evolved over months to years rather than over a short period, as is typical of delirium. Her history reveals no signs or symptoms consistent with depression, mania, or hypomania; thus a mood disorder is unlikely. The patient was a college graduate and business owner and clearly has no history of prior cognitive impairment until several years ago; hence mental retardation is unlikely. Although the patient has had memory deficits, with significant impairment to social functioning, which is consistent with an amnestic disorder, her other cognitive impairments, such as impaired executive functioning, present a picture that is better accounted for by dementia. In fact, to make the diagnosis of amnestic disorder, dementia must first be ruled out. In considering the patient's normal functioning until several years ago, with a decline in memory, getting lost, irritability, and family history of possible dementia in her mother, she is probably suffering from dementia.

The prevalence of moderate-to-severe dementia is approximately 5% in people over the age of 65 and 20–40% in people over the age of 85. Dementia can also be seen in younger adults, between the ages of 40–60, typically in patients with a strong family history and/or a known genetic mutation (e.g., Down syndrome). In people with the onset of dementia after the age of 65, AD is the most common cause (60% of cases), followed by vascular dementia (15% of cases), mixed vascular and Alzheimer's dementia (15% of cases), and other illness (10% of cases). Other illnesses that can cause dementia include frontotemporal dementia, infections (e.g., HIV or syphilis), Lewy body dementia, metabolic abnormalities (e.g., hypothyroidism), mood disorder (e.g., dementia secondary to depression), normal pressure hydrocephalus, nutritional deficiencies (e.g., folate or vitamin B_{12}), Parkinson's disease, or substance abuse. AD is a diagnosis of exclusion; patients with evidence of dementia due to another cause should undergo a careful work-up and the alternative cause should be ruled out before the diagnosis of AD is given.

The DSM-IV-TR includes six categories of dementia: dementia of the Alzheimer's type, vascular dementia, dementia due to a general medical condition, dementia due to multiple etiologies, substance-induced persisting dementia, and dementia not otherwise specified. In dementia of the Alzheimer's type, the presentation can be noted to be with or without behavioral disturbance. In the subtype with behavioral disturbance, cognitive disturbance is accompanied by behaviors such as wandering or agitation. If the patient is less than 65 years old, the dementia is with early onset; otherwise, it is with late onset.

The risk factors for dementia are age, family history, diabetes, apolipoprotein E (APOE) ε4, and hypercholesterolemia. Age is the strongest risk factor for dementia; risk increases as the patient gets older. In general, a patient with a first-degree relative with AD is at increased risk of developing AD. Seventy-two known mutations of three proteins—amyloid precursor protein, presenilin 1, and presenilin 2—are known to lead to AD. Affected patients have a strong family history of early-onset AD, which is usually autosomal dominant in transmission. The presence of the APOE ε4 genotype also appears to confer increased risk for developing AD. Some authorities argue that the presence of one APOE ε4 allele shifts the age of AD onset by about 5–10 years, whereas the presence of two alleles shifts the age of AD onset by 10–20 years in a person who is susceptible to developing AD. Recently, patients with diabetes mellitus were also found to have increased risk of developing dementia. Studies suggest that HMG-CoA reductase inhibitors (or "statins") may decrease the risk of developing AD. Other risk factors, such as extreme blood pressure, elevated homocysteine, female sex, head trauma history, low education level, impaired gait, and toxin exposure, also appear to increase the risk of developing dementia, but the data are not conclusive, and these potential risk factors remain controversial.

A clinical syndrome called mild cognitive impairment (MCI) is considered to be a prodrome of AD. Patients complain of subjective memory impairment, and examination reveals supporting evidence of their complaint. They do not have any signs of dementia except memory deficit (as opposed to dementia, in which at least one cognitive domain other than memory must be affected). Recognition of this state allows early treatment, which may result in a better overall course.

The neuritic plaques and neurofibrillary tangles that are seen in the brains of patients with AD were originally described by Louis Alzheimer in the early 1900s. The plaques and tangles are predominantly in the hippocampus, entorhinal cortex, and associated areas of the neocortex. The current understanding of the pathophysiology of AD is that the plaques are from the amyloid precursor protein (APP) that has been processed by the β-secretase on the amino terminus and the γ-secretase on the carboxy terminus. The resultant 40 and 42 amino acid β-amyloid$_{40}$ (Aβ40) and β-amyloid$_{42}$ (Aβ42) peptides later aggregate with other factors to form the extracellular plaques found in AD. The Aβ42 is less soluble and is thought to be the more amyloidogenic than the more common Aβ40.

The three secretases that process APP are known as the α-, β-, and γ-secretases. They lead to many alternative splice products of APP. The α-secretase is thought to be protective against plaque formation because it cleaves APP in such a way that the end product is p3—a small carboxy-terminal fragment of Aβ42; p3 is not plaque-forming. Normal processing of APP leads to the secretion of these different splice products. Most (about 90%) of the β-amyloid that is secreted in the cerebrospinal fluid (CSF) is the shorter Aβ40, along with small amounts of Aβ42. Studies have found a decreased amount of β-amyloid in the CSF of patients with AD.

The rare cases of autosomal dominant familial AD are associated with 10 known genetic mutations of APP (located on chromosome 21), 60 mutations of presenilin 1 (located on chromosome 14) and 2 mutations of presenilin 2 (located on chromosome 1); there are other mutations that are not yet mapped. The presenilin proteins are thought either to be the γ-secretase or to interact directly with it and/or the β-secretase. In effect, all these known mutations selectively increase the amount of Aβ42. This, in turn, leads to increased neuritic plaque formation. The neuritic plaques are thought to precipitate a cascade of inflammation, excitotoxicity, oxidative damage, and ultimately apoptosis leading to the neuronal dysfunction and eventual cell loss that is seen in AD. Of note, these plaques alone are not pathognomonic for AD; they are also found in patients with prion diseases, patients with dementia pugilistica, and patients without dementia.

The microtubule-associated protein tau (τ) is found in a hyperphosphorylated form in the neurofibrillary tangles. These paired helical filaments are the insoluble intracellular aggregates seen in AD. The overall relation between plaques and tangles is still not clear, and some researchers argue that the formation of the neurofibrillary tangles is secondary to plaque formation. Of interest, studies of the rare familial AD have found no mutations in the τ gene that are present in early-onset AD. Such mutations have been seen, however, in frontotemporal degeneration with parkinsonism. The neurofibrillary tangles are also found in other neurodegenerative disorders such as corticobasal degeneration, progressive supranuclear palsy, and dementia pugilistica as well as in patients without dementia. Studies have found an elevated amount of τ in the CSF of patients with AD.

Recent research into therapeutic interventions for AD has focused on limiting the inflammatory reactions (with NSAIDS) and the oxidative stress reactions (with vitamin E) that occur downstream of the cascade of events that follow the formation of the neuritic plaques and neurofibrillary tangles. In early-onset AD, with a strong genetic component, either excessive production of APP or excessive processing of APP by the β- and γ-secretases was found. As mentioned above, mutations of APP or the two presenilins (1 and 2), which lead to increased levels of Aβ42, have been found in these rare cases. Current research is directed at discovering potential agents that modify the activity of the β- and γ-secretases.

AD is a clinical diagnosis made by taking a careful history and by using selected laboratory tests. It is important to take a detailed history from the patient with suspected AD, especially from the family. Often the demented patient is unaware of the symptoms, or the disease itself will limit the patient's ability to recall details accurately, as was the case with the patient above. The key points to note are the onset and progression of the symptoms of memory and other cognitive deficits in the history of present illness. These symptoms are usually accompanied by a decreased capacity in the activities of daily living and increased irritability or agitation. Any history of mood disorder, psychotic symptoms, perceptual disturbances, substance abuse, or any past psychiatric history is important, as is a family history of dementia. In the review of symptoms, careful attention should be paid to symptoms suggestive of a cardiovascular illness, hypothyroidism, or head trauma. The physical exam should carefully assess the patient for any neurologic deficits, movement disorders, or other active medical problems. The mental status exam should take note of dishevelment, signs of trauma, aphasias (language disturbances), depressed mood, psychotic symptoms, and perceptual disturbances. The Folstein Mini-Mental Status Exam (MMSE) is a quick way to assess memory impairment, apraxia (impaired motor task activity despite intact motor function), and agnosia (inability to recognize objects despite intact sensory perception). Of note, MMSE scores are dependent on the patient's education level. For example, a score of 24 is normal for a patient with only a few years of education, whereas it would be highly abnormal and suggest the onset of dementia in a patient with a high school education. Having the patient draw a clock, which simultaneously evaluates multiple functional domains, including visuospatial and executive functioning, is another quick screen for dementia. Blood work should include the standard electrolytes, hepatic panel, complete blood count, and renal function tests. In addition, nutritional abnormalities (e.g., vitamin B_{12}) and endocrine abnormalities should be evaluated. A noncontrast computerized tomography (CT) or magnetic resonance (MRI) scan of the brain is helpful in assessing a past or current cerebrovascular event or neoplasm. Other diagnostic pathways should be pursued if the history supports them. Examples include testing patients for infections (e.g., urinalysis, urine micro, HIV, and syphilis), medications or drugs (urine and serum toxicology), and heavy metals.

The treatment of AD falls into three domains: safety of the environment, symptoms of the illness, and disease targets. The first issue is the safety of the environment. Patients with AD do not die from the disease itself but rather from secondary complications. They may accidentally leave the stove or gas on and be at risk for injury. They have the tendency to wander off or to have falls. They also have increased risks of motor vehicle accidents as the dementia progresses. They may not be able to handle tactivities of daily living and can decompensate as a result. These issues can be addressed by making simple changes in the patient's environment. The stove should be replaced with a microwave, or someone else should cook for the patient. Patients can wear a bracelet with identifying information in case they accidentally wander off. The furniture and overall layout of their home should be kept the same so that the patient can stay oriented. The patient should be carefully followed for any driving impairment and should stop driving at the earliest signs of worsening skills. A home health aide or nursing home placement should be instituted when necessary. Serious consideration of each of these changes is recommended for the above patient.

The overt symptoms of AD are cognitive decline and behavioral changes. Deficits in acetylcholine, found in the brains of patients with AD, correlate with changes in cognitive functioning. The acetylcholinesterase inhibitors have been found to increase acetylcholine in the synaptic cleft by inhibiting their degradation by acetylcholinesterase. Better maintenance of cognitive functioning was seen in response to these medications. It is recommended to start patients on an acetylcholinesterase inhibitor at the earliest signs of AD. Overall, these medications have been found to slow the decline in cognitive functioning and worsening behavior, but not to alter the progression of the disease. Patients treated with the acetylcholinesterase inhibitors eventually fall to the same level of deterioration as untreated patients. Ginkgo biloba has not been shown to have any efficacy in AD and is not recommended.

The most disturbing behavioral changes seen in dementia are aggressive and/or assaultive behavior. Importantly, as with all patients, behavioral changes can be the result of any number of disruptions in the body, particularly in the elderly patient. Thus, it is important to get to the root of a patient's change in behavior. For example, a change in behavior may be secondary to a urinary tract or other infection or to depression; and each has its own specific treatment. If the patient reports perceptual disturbances (e.g., auditory or visual hallucinations), Lewy body disease should be ruled out because patients with Lewy body dementia are better treated with acetylcholinesterase inhibitors (see Case 55) than antipsychotic medications. Patients who are delusional or agitated can be treated with antipsychotic medication and/or mood stabilizers. Some behaviors can also be managed with behavioral therapy.

Effective treatments to date have dealt with the environment and symptoms of AD. The future holds promise for new medications that can directly effect the progression of the disease. Several medications are directly targeted at the disease process itself. Vitamin E is an antioxidant that has been shown to confer some benefit in slowing the progression of AD. Although the evidence is controversial, the risks are minimal; thus, vitamin E is recommended for the treatment of AD. Patients placed on selegiline, a monoamine oxidase inhibitor that is effective in treating Parkinson's disease, showed no improvement; thus, selegiline is not recommended for AD. Memantine, an NMDA receptor antagonist, was found to have a minor benefit in preventing cognitive decline in moderate-to-severe

AD. Because it has limited side effects, it is recommended in the treatment of AD. Estrogen was thought to be neuroprotective, but clinical trials have shown no clear benefit in AD thus far. These studies were limited and several major trials now under way will provide a better answer in the near future. Nonsteroidal anti-inflammatory drugs (NSAIDs) are thought to help protect against AD. Unlike the other recommended medications, such as vitamin E, NSAIDs involve more risks that may outweigh the benefits; thus, they are not recommended for AD. Retrospective studies of patients on statins showed a decreased risk for developing AD, whereas patients with high cholesterol were found to be at higher risk. Studies with mice models have confirmed the theory that cholesterol contributes to the development of AD. Current research is investigating the ability of statins to prevent and treat AD.

The present patient was immediately started on an acetylcholinesterase inhibitor and vitamin E. An NMDA receptor antagonist (memantine) was later added. She tolerated the titration of the acetylcholinesterase inhibitor and the NMDA receptor antagonist without complaints of side effects. The family replaced the stove with a microwave oven. They also made a point to keep the patient's environment as consistent as possible (e.g., not rearranging the furniture). A bracelet with the patient's name and contact information was placed on her wrist. Despite these interventions, her condition continued to deteriorate gradually with worsening cognitive function reflected by a steady decline in her MMSE score. She wandered off two more times over the next 6 months. Eventually, the family had to get a 24-hour home health aide to help the patient with her activities of daily living. An atypical antipsychotic was later added for intermittent agitation. Her symptoms have been well managed with this treatment plan, and the patient has been able to continue living at home with her husband for the time being.

Pearls

1. Although the acetylcholinesterase inhibitors show better maintenance of cognitive functioning in patients with AD, they do not significantly alter the course of the underlying disease. Patients who are treated with these medications eventually decline to the same functional level as untreated patients.
2. The NMDA receptor antagonist, memantine, is the latest medication to be approved for the treatment of AD. It blocks the effects of the glutamate excitotoxicity that is thought to lead to apoptosis and eventual cell loss in AD. Although the benefits of the medication are somewhat limited, they still outweigh the risks. Memantine is recommended for moderate-to-severe AD.
3. The future treatment of AD depends on a better understanding of its pathophysiology. The β- and γ-secretases have been shown to be involved in the development of AD, and efforts to produce inhibitors to these enzymes hold promise for new therapeutic interventions that may actually slow down the progression of AD.
4. Work in immunization therapy with Aβ42 was highly effective in the mouse model, but the clinical trial had to be stopped because of a high incidence of aseptic meningo-encephilitis. Despite this major setback, immunization therapy may yield effective treatments for AD.

REFERENCES

1. Clark CM, Karlawish JHT: Alzheimer disease: Current concepts and emerging diagnostic and therapeutic strategies. Ann Intern Med 2003;138:400–410.
2. Dufouil C, Clayton D, Brayne C, et al: Population norms for the MMSE in the very old. Neurology 2000;55:1609–1613.
3. Dugué M, Neugroschl J, Sewell M, Marin D: Review of dementia. Mount Sinai J Med 2003;70:45–53.
4. Golde TE: Alzheimer disease therapy: Can the amyloid cascade be halted? J Clin Invest 2003;111:11–18.
5. Neugroschl J, Davis KL: Biological markers in Alzheimer disease. Am J Geriatr Psychiatry 200210:660–677.
6. Nussbaum RL, Ellis CE: Alzheimer's disease and Parkinson's disease. N Engl J Med 2003;348:1356–1364.
7. Reisberg B, Doody R, Stöffler A, et al: Memantine in moderate-to-severe Alzheimer's disease. N Engl J Med 2003;348:1333–1341.
8. Shulman KI: Clock-drawing: Is it the ideal cognitive screening test? Int J Geriatr Psychiatry 2000;15:548–561.
9. Younkin SG: The role of Aß42 in Alzheimer's disease. J Physiol Paris 1988;92:289–292

PATIENT 60

A 59-year-old man with memory loss

History of Present Illness: A 59-year-old man is brought to the emergency department by his sister for confusion and agitation. The sister states that he started "acting funny" after he got drunk yesterday afternoon and ate several of the marshmallow treats that she had baked for a local fundraiser. He was found stumbling aimlessly around the backyard and "totally out of it." She initially thought that he was just very intoxicated but became concerned because he did not seem any better the next day. She describes the patient as a chronic alcoholic who has lived with her family since his wife divorced him several years ago and reports that his alcohol intake has increased over the past 3-4 weeks. She also states that he subsists mostly on junk food, because he stopped eating with the family about two years ago.

In the medical emergency department he was found to be confused, apathetic, and tremulous, with elevated pulse and blood pressure. A neurologic exam revealed a slow, wide-based gait and horizontal nystagmus. Through an IV line he was given lorazepam and a "banana bag" (a solution of 100 mg thiamine, 2 gm of magnesium sulfate, and multivitamins in 1 L of normal saline, routinely given to chronic alcohol users in medical emergency departments). The patient's tremor diminished, his vital signs stabilized, and he was admitted to a medical floor for observation and a benzodiazepine taper. The following day he was more alert, and the nystagmus and gait findings improved. A psychiatric consult was called because the patient kept trying to leave his room and would cooperate with his care for only very short periods. He pulled out his IV line, stating that he did not need it, and then agreed to have it replaced after the purpose was explained to him. Five minutes later he removed it again; this cycle was repeated several times until the staff covered the IV line with strong tape that he was unable to remove. He was often agitated and belligerent towards the staff but easily redirected. The staff also reported that "he kept saying things that weren't true" and that he "couldn't remember anything." An MRI was ordered, but the patient became so anxious and agitated a few minutes after being placed in the scanner that the study could not be completed.

Past Psychiatric History: The patient has a history of multiple visits to the emergency department for intoxication and injuries secondary to falling. He has been detoxed as an inpatient several times, only to resume drinking shortly after discharge. He has never been a candidate for a rehabilitation program, having stated in the past that he likes to drink and sees no reason to quit. Although the patient's sister does not drink, she states that her father and paternal uncle were "raging alcoholics."

Mental Status Examination: The patient is a slim man who appears older than his stated age and has a red and asymmetrically thickened nose. He cooperates with questions for a minute or two and then interrupts, demanding to know why he is being interviewed. After the purpose is explained to him, he resumes cooperation for another brief period and repeats the cycle. His behavior is restless, with frequent attempts to get up and walk away, but he is easily redirected. The rate, rhythm, and volume of his speech are normal. His mood is irritable and his affect very labile. His thought process and content are marked by repeating the same questions every few minutes, although they are answered each time he asks them; he also makes up answers to questions. At one point the interviewer, who has just met the patient for the first time, asks, "Where have we met before?" The patient replies, "In the county jail." He denies any paranoid ideation, ideas of reference, suicidal ideation, or homicidal ideation. He vehemently denies hearing or seeing things that other people do not see, stating "I'm not crazy!" He has no insight into his condition, his judgment is impaired, and his impulse control is poor. He is alert and oriented to name only, and his mini-mental status exam is remarkable for the inability to recall any objects after 5 minutes as well as for making up a meaning to a nonsense proverb.

Laboratory Examination: White blood cell count, 7.6; hemoglobin, 12.3; hematocrit, 37.0; platelet count, 188; mean corpuscular volume, 109. Chemistry panel 7, within normal limits; alanine aminotransferase, 48; aspartate aminotransferase, 106.

Cerebrospinal fluid analysis: Gram stain reveals no polymorphonuclear cells or organisms; cell count reveals the following: red blood count, 6; white blood cell count, 0; protein, 46; and glucose, 52.

Diagnostic Testing: A CT of the head scan showed no signs of infarct, mass, or hemorrhage.

Question: What is the diagnosis?

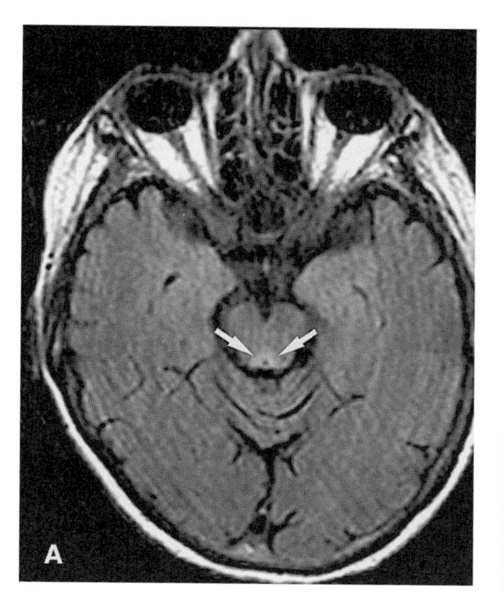

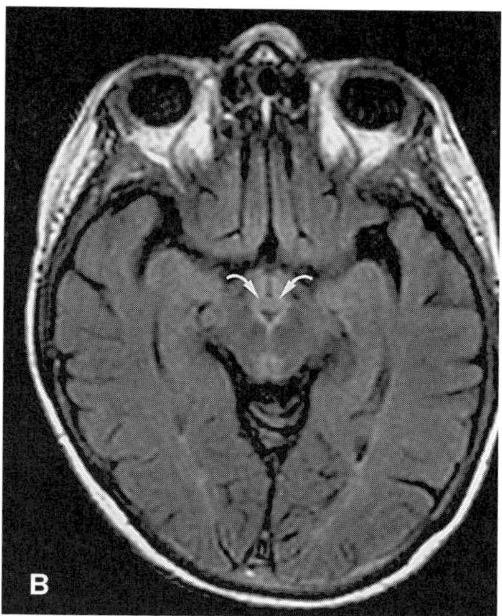

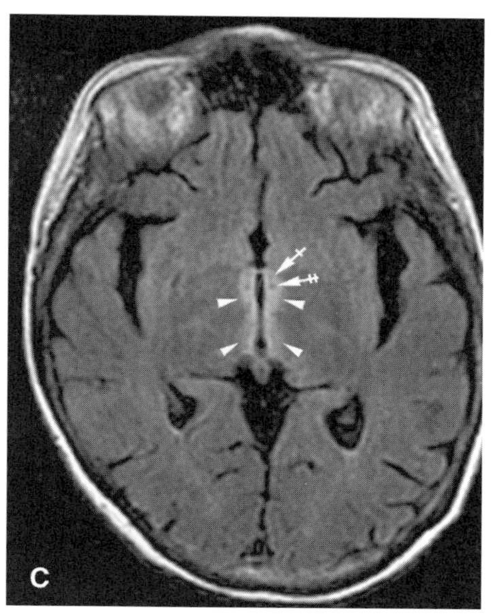

Axial FLAIR images of a patient with acute Wernicke's syndrome. *A,* At the level of midbrain there is increased periaqueductal signal (arrows), corresponding with edema. *B,* Increased signal is also seen in the mamillary bodies (curved arrows) extending anteriorly into the inferior hypothalamus. *C,* The anterior column of fornix (single-hatch arrow) and mamillothalamic fasciculus (double-hatch arrow) are seen as areas of slightly lower signal amid the diffuse hyperintensity around the third ventricle (arrowheads). (Images courtesy of Bradley N. Delman, MD, Department of Radiology, Mount Sinai School of Medicine.)

Diagnosis: Wernicke-Korsakoff syndrome (WKS).

Discussion: WKS refers to both the acute and chronic presentations of the same entity. Wernicke's encephalopathy is the acute condition, classically characterized by the triad of global confusion, oculomotor abnormalities, and gait disturbance. Approximately 80% of patients who survive Wernicke's encephalopathy have Korsakoff's syndrome, also known as Korsakoff's psychosis or Korsakoff's dementia. This chronic condition is characterized by partial retrograde amnesia, total anterograde amnesia, and confabulation. Patients are able to remember events in their lives until a certain point in time but are unable to retain new information after that point. A 70 year-old patient who has Korsakoff's syndrome might state that his age is 50, identify the year as 20 years earlier, and name the president of that time as the current president.

The diagnosis of the current patient was suggested by the history of chronic alcoholism and poor nutrition, the temporal relationship between the onset of symptoms and the consumption of the stolen marshmallow treats, and the improvement in oculomotor disturbances, ataxia, and alertness in response to the administration of thiamine. His initial presentation in the emergency department may have been consistent with severe alcohol withdrawal, but the rapid resolution of some of his symptoms (tremor, elevated vital signs) in response to lorazepam with the persistence of other symptoms (ataxia, confusion, oculomotor disturbance) suggests that the problem is more than just withdrawal. The presence of anterograde memory loss and confabulation after the ataxia, confusion, and oculomotor disturbance improved is also highly characteristic of WKS. The patient's inability to form new memories was demonstrated by the frequent need to re-orient him in order to elicit cooperation. Confabulation is defined as a false memory that the patient believes to be true and uses to fill memory gaps. They are distinguished from delusions in that delusions are fixed, false beliefs, whereas confabulations tend to be highly inconsistent. The patient's statement that he had met the interviewer before in the county jail is an example of confabulation. He did not give the same answer the second time he met that interviewer and had no memory of the first meeting.

WKS is caused by thiamine deficiency. Although the vast majority of cases occur in alcoholics as a result of poor nutritional intake, WKS can also be caused by several other conditions that result in thiamine deficiency. Examples include starvation, hyperemesis gravidarum or other causes of intractable vomiting, prolonged total parenteral nutrition, gastric bypass surgery, and long-term dialysis. Thiamine deficiency results in a disturbance of carbohydrate metabolism. The active form of thiamine, thiamine pyrophosphate (TTP), is an essential coenzyme for one enzyme (transketolase) in the pentose-phosphate pathway and two enzymes (pyruvate dehydrogenase and alpha-ketoglutarate dehydrogenase) in the tricarboxylic acid cycle. Patients with WKS show a significant increase in RBC transketolase activity after being given TTP. The exact mechanism for how thiamine deficiency causes WKS is unknown. However, one hypothesis is that a shortage of TTP causes inhibition of adenosine triphosphate synthesis, resulting in cellular injury. When patients with thiamine deficiency consume large quantities of carbohydrate, they can become acutely symptomatic, as did this patient. The precise reason why a carbohydrate challenge precipitates cellular injury in WKS is also not fully understood. However, if there is any suspicion of thiamine deficiency in a patient, it is essential to give IV thiamine before or with a carbohydrate-containing IV solution.

The characteristic neuropathologic changes in WKS are seen bilaterally in midline brain structures, including the medial thalamic nuclei, mamillary bodies, periaquductal gray area of the mesencephalon, pontine tegmentum, and superior cerebellar vermis. It is thought that the amnesia, confusion, and confabulation are related to the damage in the thalamus and mamillary bodies. CT scans have not been shown to be sufficiently sensitive in detecting any of these changes to be of diagnostic use. WKS is thought to be underdiagnosed among patients while they are alive, but autopsy studies estimate the prevalence rate to be between 0.8% and 2.8%. On MRI, an increase in T2 signal in paraventricular regions of the thalamus and periacqueductal regions of the midbrain is sometimes seen; in one study, MRI was found to have 53% sensitivity and 93% specificity in the diagnosis.

In patients presenting with the triad of oculomotor abnormalities, ataxia, and confusion, other diagnoses to consider are brainstem encephalitis, hypoxic-ischemic encephalopathy, Leigh's encephalomyelopathy, adrenoleukodystrophy, metachromatic leukodystrophy, syphilis, and AIDS. In patients who present with anterograde amnesia and confabulation, the following diagnoses should be considered: temporal lobe epilepsy, temporal lobe infarction, concussive head injury, transient global amnesia, anoxic encephalopathy, Alzheimer's disease, third ventricle tumor, and sequelae of infection with herpes simplex virus.

In any case of suspected Wernicke's encephalopathy, 100 mg of thiamine should be administered immediately, IM or IV, with additional daily doses for several days to replenish the body's reserves. Among patients who respond to thiamine, the opthalmoplegia improves first, followed by the ataxia and then the drowsiness and confusion. Patients with WKS secondary to alcoholic malnutrition, like the present patient, are generally placed on a benzodiazepine taper while in the hospital to prevent alcohol withdrawal, which can be life-threatening. The mortality rate in WKS is between 10% and 20%; once patients show evidence of Korsakoff's, approximately 80% show chronic memory problems, often requiring long-term care. Memory improvement among the 20% who recover can take up to 1 year. Agitation in these patients is managed symptomatically, generally with neuroleptics.

After the completion of his benzodiazepine taper, the present patient's anterograde amnesia persisted and he was discharged to a long-term care facility. Whether he is one of the fortunate 20% whose memory problems resolve remains to be seen.

Pearls

1. IV thiamine should always be given before IV glucose if there is any suspicion of chronic alcoholism or other possible causes of thiamine deficiency. WKS is underdiagnosed, and thiamine is harmless and potentially very helpful. When in doubt, give thiamine.
2. CT scans are of little help in establishing the diagnosis. On MRI, however, changes are sometimes seen in the paraventricular regions of the thalamus and the periacqueductal regions of the midbrain.
3. Confabulation and anterograde memory loss are prominent features of the syndrome.
4. Not all patients with severe thiamine deficiency develop WKS, leading researchers to believe that some patients may be predisposed to WKS because of variability in genes that code for thiamine-dependent enzymes.

REFERENCES

1. Antunez E, Estruch R, Cardenal C, et al: Usefulness of CT and MR imaging in the diagnosis of acute Wernicke's encephalopathy. Am J Roentgenol 1998;171:1131–1137.
2. Kinsella LJ, Riley DE: Nutritional deficiencies and syndromes associated with alcoholism. In Goetz (ed): Textbook of Clinical Neurology. Philadelphia, W.B. Saunders, 1999.
3. Munir A, Hussain SA, Sondhi D, et al: Wernicke's encephalopathy in a non-alcoholic man: Case report and brief review. Mt Sinai J Med 2001;68:216–268.
4. Reuler JB, Girard DE, Cooney TG: Current concepts: Wernicke's encephalopathy. N Engl J Med 1985;312:1035–1039.
5. Sacks O: The Lost Mariner. New York Review of Books, February 16, 1984.
6. Zubaran C, Fernandes JG, Rodnight R: Wernicke-Korsakoff syndrome. Postgrad Med J 1997;73(855):27–31.

INDEX